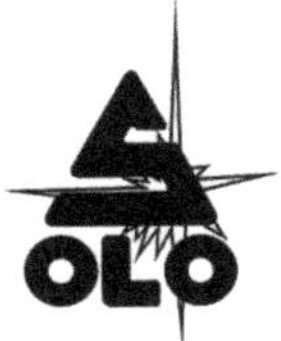

ISBN: 978-0-9996249-3-7

DISCLAIMER: Emergency medicine is an ever-changing field, and although the author and publisher have made every effort to ensure that the information in this book was correct at press time, the author and publisher do not assume and hereby disclaim any liability to any party for loss, damage, injury, or disruption caused by errors or omissions, whether such errors or omissions result from negligence, accident, or any other cause. This book has been designed as a companion resource to specific SOLO Wilderness First Responder courses, and the possession of this book in no way implies or confers upon the owner or user any level of expertise whatsoever. The author and publisher advise readers to take full responsibility for their safety and know their limits—do not take risks beyond your level of experience, aptitude, training, standard of care, licensure, and comfort level.

NOTE: SOLO students appear in some of the photographs and images in this book, and they have granted permission for this use as part of their agreement to take a SOLO course. And while we stress the use of personal BSI protection equipment (e.g., latex gloves) when working on patients, we do not always require its use during mock teaching scenarios—so some people may appear without gloves in some images.

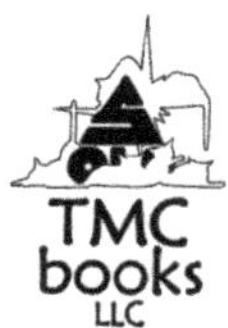

TMC books LLC

731 B Tasker Hill Rd.
Conway, New Hampshire
03818
U.S.A

SOLO WILDERNESS FIRST RESPONDER

Frank Hubbell, DO

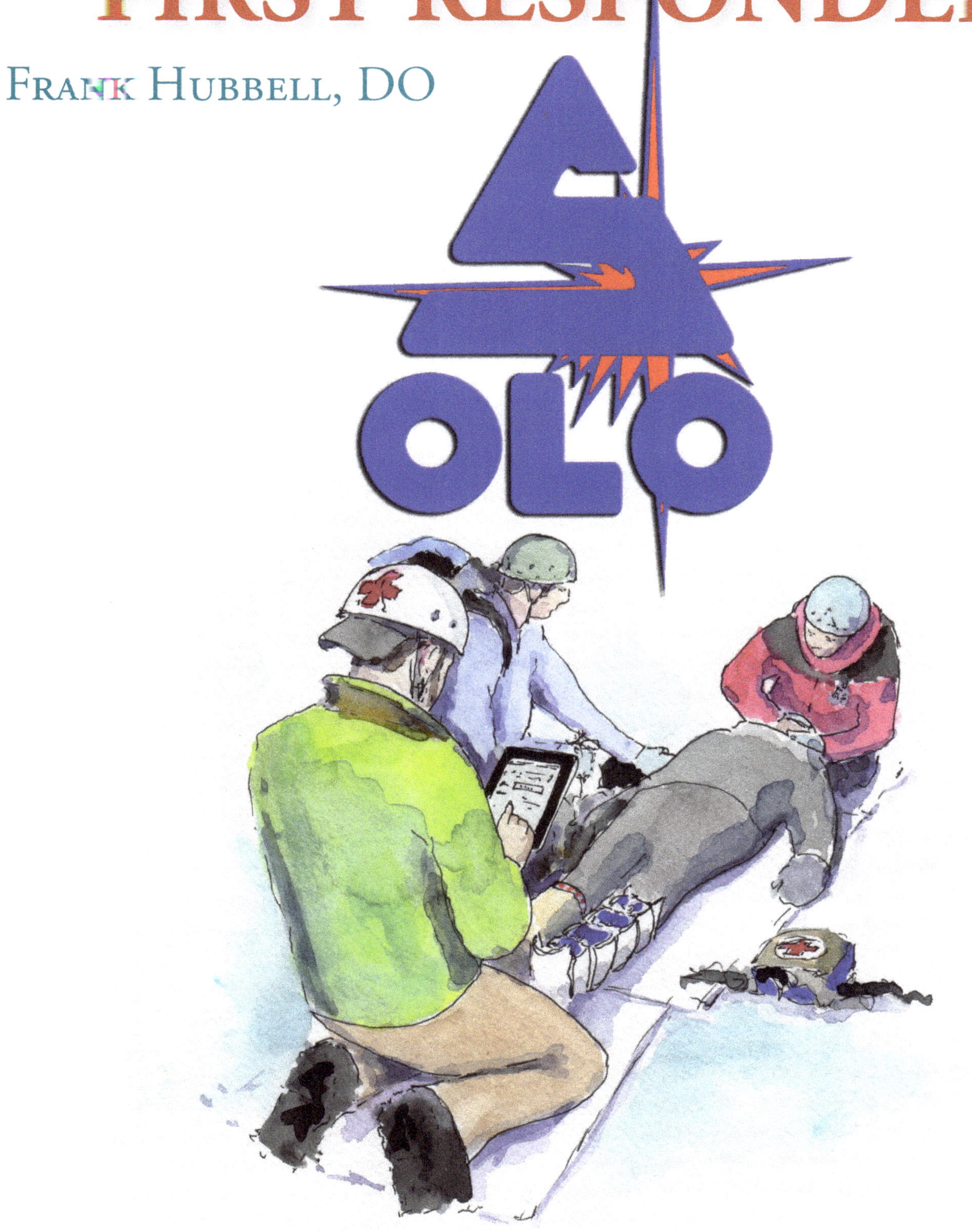

Illustrations by T.B.R. Walsh

Photographs by S. Peter Lewis

CONTENTS

INTRODUCTION
OVERVIEW: THE 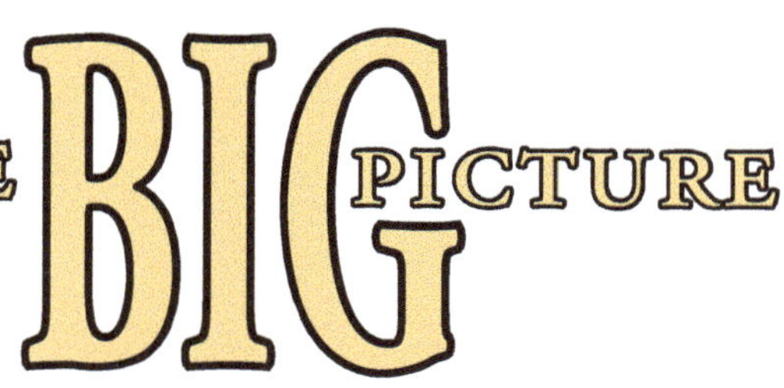 PICTURE

RESPONSE

Wilderness medical emergencies, by definition,
happen fast—at least initially. Something bad happens, unexpectedly, without warning, just when things are going so well:

- A hiker slips and their ankle snaps.
- An ice fisherman falls through the ice, and their core temperature begins to plummet.
- A bird watcher is stung by a bee and in minutes is having trouble breathing.
- A camper cutting firewood cuts an artery instead.
- Response is simple: it's what you do, and when you do it. In wilderness medicine we break response down as follows:
  - **FIRST RESPONSE**—the first 5 minutes.
  - **EMERGENCY CARE**—the first 60 minutes (the Golden Hour).
  - **EXTENDED CARE**—the first day (the first 24 hours).
  - **REMOTE CARE**—the days and weeks that follow (think disaster or remote medicine).

PATIENT ASSESSMENT SYSTEM

The Patient Assessment System (PAS) is the initial step-by-step process that the responder to an emergency goes through in order to evaluate a patient's physical condition and identify the nature and extent of their injuries or illness. The principles of PAS are:

- **SCENE SAFETY**—ensure that no one, including responders and bystanders, are in danger.
- **BODY SUBSTANCE ISOLATION**—put on clothing or equipment (e.g., gloves, goggles) to protect responders from exposure and contamination.
- **GENERAL IMPRESSION**—your first reaction: is this really bad (obvious life-threatening trauma or medical emergency), not so bad (no one is going to die, but we still have to act quickly and decisively), or minor (just a sprained ankle)?
- **LEVEL OF CONSCIOUSNESS (LOC)**—Conscious or unconscious? Responsive or unresponsive?
- **PRIMARY ASSESSMENT**
  - **A—Airway**: Does the patient have an open, functioning airway?
  - **B—Breathing**: Are they breathing? If so, how well?
  - **C—Circulation**: Do they have a pulse? Is there any obvious bleeding?
  - **D—Deformity**: Are all the patient's limbs intact, and in proper anatomical alignment?
  - **E—Environment**: Are they in a safe place? Can they stay where they are?
- **SECONDARY ASSESSMENT**
  - **Vital signs**: How well is the patient doing?
  - **Patient exam:** What are the patient's specific injuries?
  - **AMPLE History**: What is their past medical history?
  - **SOAPnote**: How should we record their medical data?
- **RESCUE PLAN** How are we going to get help?

CRITICAL CARE ASSESSMENT

Critical care refers to the treatment of immediate life threats that are discovered in the first few minutes of Patient Assessment. These are conditions that must be addressed **_NOW_**, or the patient will likely get worse or die.

- **CHANGE IN LEVEL OF CONSCIOUSNESS**—can indicate traumatic brain injury, drug overdose, or other major medical emergencies.
- **A COMPROMISED AIRWAY**—you've got about six minutes.
- **SHORTNESS OF BREATH**—has many causes and can indicate a serious condition.
- **SEVERE BLEEDING**—must be controlled immediately or the patient will develop hypovolemic shock and die
- **CHEST PAIN**—without a trauma mechanism, must be assumed to be a cardiac emergency; may lead to cardiac arrest.
- **ANAPHYLAXIS**—a severe allergic reaction (e.g., from a bee sting) that can cause death by asphyxia.
- **SHOCK**—a serious condition indicating an external or internal circulatory system compromise, which can kill in minutes.

Urban versus Wilderness Medicine Distinctives

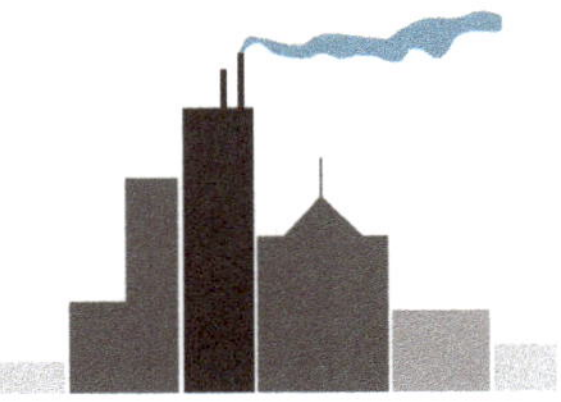

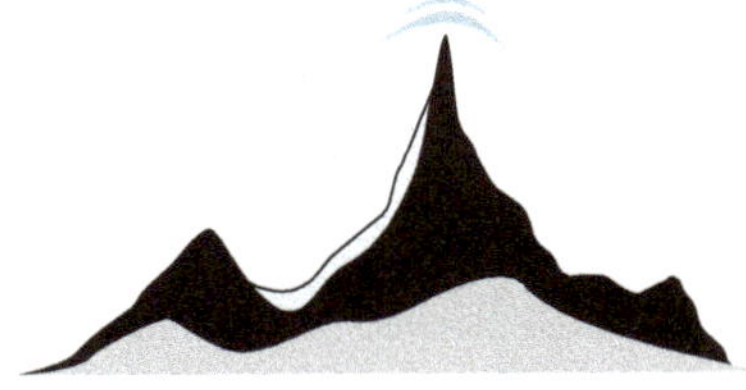

1. **We treat things** that in the urban world would be left for ER docs in the hospital:
   - Straightening angulated fractures
   - Reducing dislocations
   - Clearing the spine
   - Cleaning wounds

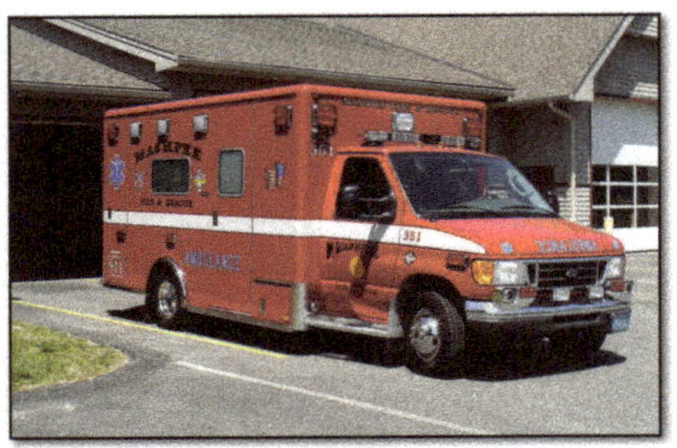

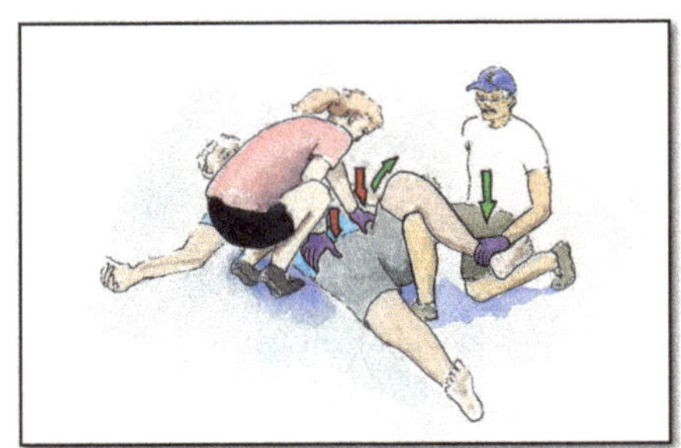

2. **We improvise equipment** typically found on ambulances and in hospitals:
   - Splints/bandages
   - Litters
   - Compression dressings
   - Cervical collars and spinal immobilization

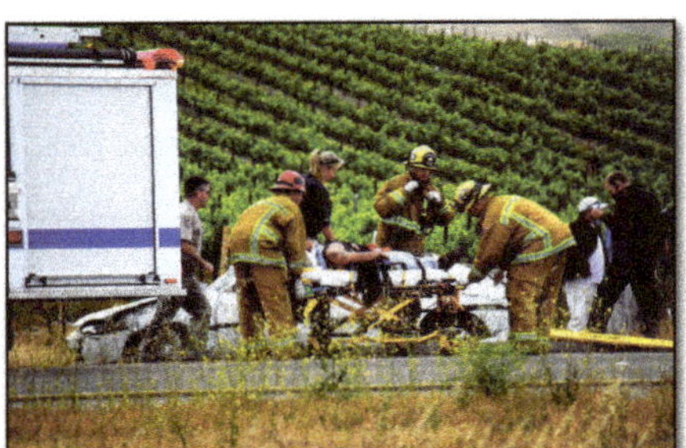

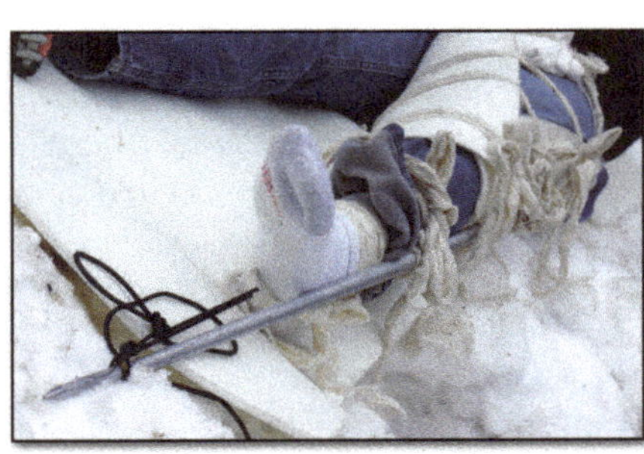

3. **We provide extended care** (beyond the Golden Hour) not only for injuries and illness, but for day-to-day needs:
   - Food/water/pee/poop
   - Protection from the elements
   - Long-term injury/illness treatment
   - Emotional support

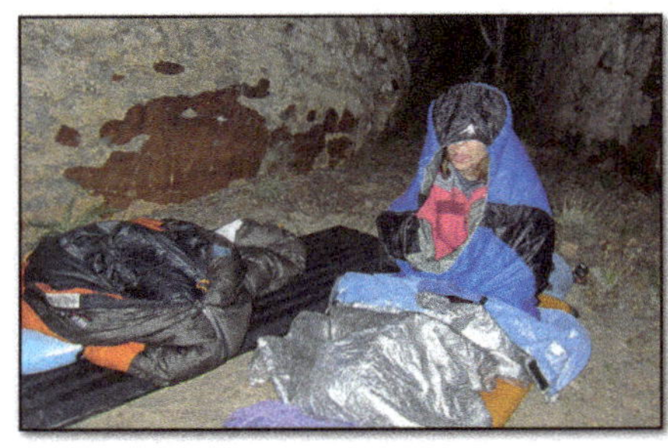

4. **We evacuate the patient**, which often requires improvisation:
   - Technical rescue/extrication
   - Litter carries
   - Survival skills (e.g., navigation, weather forecasting)

5. **Documentation**
   - Urban: run forms
   - Wilderness: SOAPnote

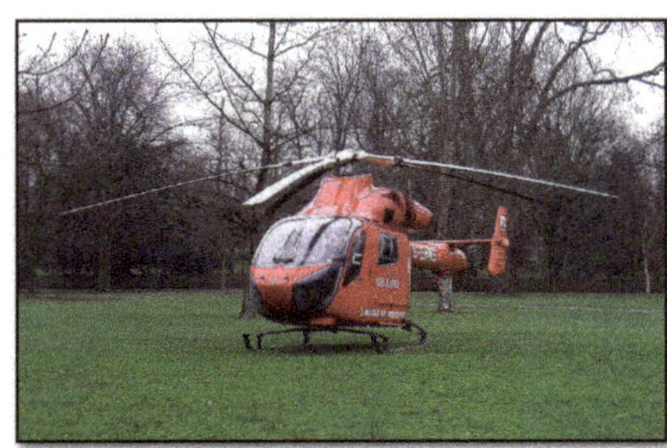

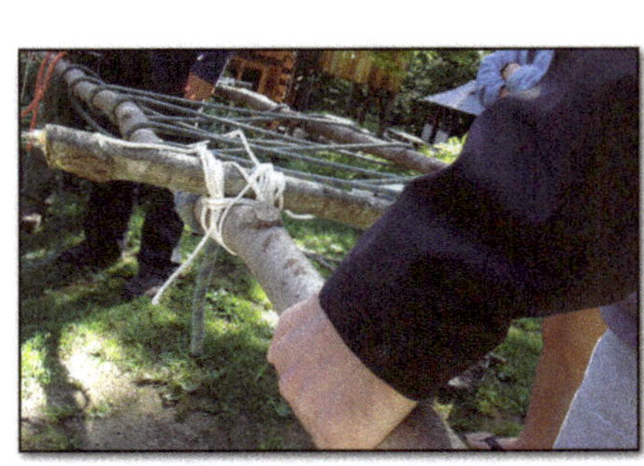

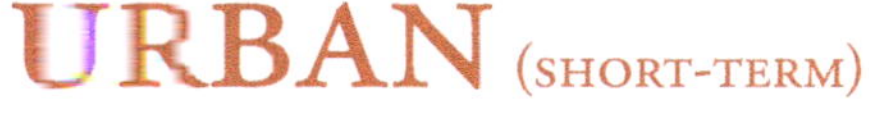

URBAN (SHORT-TERM)
VERSUS WILDERNESS CARE (LONG-TERM OR EXTENDED)

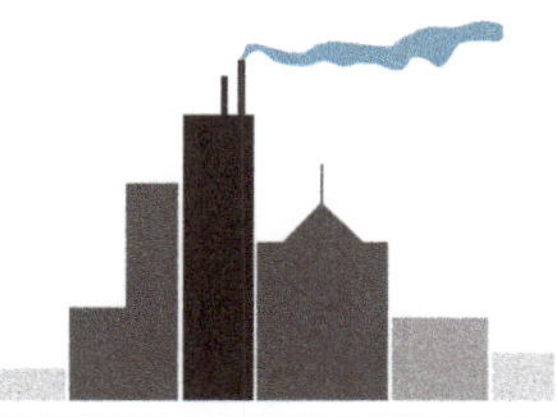

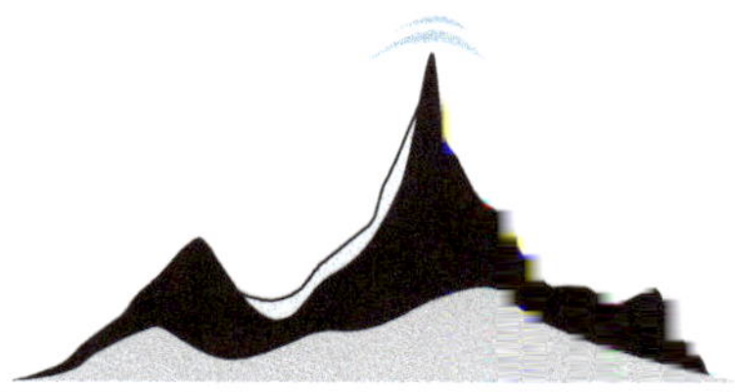

	Urban	*Wilderness*
TIME AND DISTANCE	Within the Golden Hour Rapid notification via technology—usually via 911 Rapid response and evacuation time, usually within minutes	Beyond the Golden Hour Very delayed notification—often via foot, which may take hours Very delayed response and evacuation time, usually hours
ENVIRONMENTAL CONCERNS	Short-term exposure; minimal weather concerns Little or no impact on patient care and rescuers Night/inclement weather/cold add few if any difficulties	Long-term exposure and weather concerns Potentially dramatic impact on patient care and rescuers Night/inclement weather/cold add to problems

DIFFICULTY OF TERRAIN	Terrain risks are usually minimal and easily controlled (an exception would be disaster situations with collapsed structures)
	
	Scene safety is almost always easy to manage
	
	Abundant resources are typically available quickly
		Scene safety for rescuers may be difficult to manage
		
		Technical or semi-technical terrain adds risk
		
		Frequent, unavoidable, rough handling of patient (a jostling, uneven litter ride during evacuation is inevitable—especially on uneven terrain)
		
		Difficult footing for rescuers (dangerous)
		
		May require specialized equipment and technical skills
		
		    Climbing equipment
		
		    Specialized litters
		
		    Lowering/raising skills
		
		Semi-technical terrain may require litter passing—which will require more personnel (at least 12 people) than is typical for an evacuation

IMPROVISATION OF EQUIPMENT AND RESOURCES	Easy access to state-of-the art equipment; many other resources readily available	Have to carry emergency gear on your back, minimize weight to maximize efficiency Specialized rescue/medical equipment is typically unavailable The need to improvise equipment is common (cravats, splints, litters) Limited access to other resources

SPECIALIZED SKILLS	The need for specialized skills is rare
	
	If specialized skills are necessary (e.g., confined space/high-angle rescue), there are experts to call
	
	If unsure, call Medical Control
		Providing long-term patient care and team management
		
		Reducing angulated fractures and dislocations and clearing the spine
		
		Managing environmental emergencies
		
		Expert outdoor skills
		
		    Using map and compass
		
		    Search and rescue skills
		
		    Forecasting weather and surviving severe weather conditions
		
		    Bivouac and survival skills
		
		    Food and water

MEDICOLEGAL ISSUES AND TERMS

MEDICOLEGAL: "of or relating to both medicine and the law." Laws differ slightly from state to state, and certifications and licenses may not transfer. Some organizations have their own rules and regulations to follow, in addition to state laws. Laws vary greatly from country to country.

CERTIFICATION—Upon the successful completion of a training course, a certification is awarded for that specific level of training.

- Certification is not a license to practice medicine—each state regulates licensure and governs scope of practice for each level of training.

LICENSURE—A license to practice medicine is issued by each state's office of emergency medicine (or equivalent).

- A license gives permission to provide patient care; a certification from a course does not.

STANDARD OF CARE—Acceptable level of care based on level of certification.

- Duty to perform
- Duty to inform
- What is prudent and reasonable
- Helps determine negligence

PROTOCOLS—A set of standing orders produced by an authoritative body, e.g., a state, that establishes the levels of licensure and the standards of care.

- Protocols give permissions for various aspects of providing patient care.

GOOD SAMARITAN LAWS—Protect and grant immunity to anyone who has acted in good faith to provide care, within their level of training.

- These laws were created to protect either volunteers or professionals in situations where they do not have a "duty to act."
- They do not protect volunteers on an organized rescue team or ambulance corps (they have a team name and advertise their ability to help; therefore, they are considered professionals, not Good Samaritans).

INFORMED AND EXPRESSED CONSENT—is received from an adult (or emancipated minor) who is mentally competent to make a rational decision.

- You are obligated to get consent to provide patient care.

- You inform the patient about the care you intend to provide and why that care is appropriate; the patient then either agrees or refuses to receive your care (See Right to Refuse Care).

IMPLIED CONSENT—If the patient is unconscious or irrational, the law assumes that they would want appropriate care, and you do not need their permission to provide care.

CONSENT FOR MINORS—In situations of life-threatening injury or illness, consent becomes implied.

- Parents and guardians may give consent before an injury or illness occurs via a pre-activity form.
- These forms do not fully negate the child's rights.
- Parents can also sign an assumption of liability for any lawsuits brought on behalf of or by the child.

RIGHT TO REFUSE CARE—The patient must be legally able to refuse (they are either an adult or an emancipated minor).

- The patient must be mentally competent and rational.
- The patient must be fully informed.
- The patient should sign a release form.

ABANDONMENT—The premature abandonment of care.

NEGLIGENCE—The failure to act or provide care as a reasonably prudent person would in the same conditions and with the same knowledge, experience, and background as you. Elements of negligence include:

- Duty to act: You were required to help due to a prior relationship or an offer to render aid.
- Breach of duty or standard of care: You did not help, or you provided care below or above the standard to which you are trained.
- Proximate cause: Your breach caused a patient's condition to worsen.

MEDICAL RECORD—In wilderness medicine, a SOAPnote records the events and medical care provided.

- Patient Care Report (PCR)
- It is confidential and legal.
- It allows for continuity of care as the patient is passed on to other providers.
- It provides legal protection, a record of what happened, what problems were found, and how those problems were treated.
- A SOAPnote can be used by programs for quality improvement.

CONFIDENTIALITY—Any information you obtain about the patient must be kept confidential, and it can only be passed on to others directly involved in patient care.

ADVANCE DIRECTIVES—A legal document that allows a person to state their choices for medical treatment before they actually need such care (e.g., a Do Not Resuscitate order—see below).

- They are used by emergency medical personnel to delineate the care a patient wants to receive.

DNR (Do Not Resuscitate) ORDERS—A type of advance directive in which a person requests no cardiopulmonary resuscitation in the event their heart or breathing stops.

- Patients may have a legal form requesting no CPR or that no "heroic" measures be taken.
- Patients may wear a DNR tag or bracelet.
- Check for this (and for medical alert tags, e.g., a blood type or diabetes tag) during patient assessment.

REPORTABLE CASES—Some emergencies must be reported to the police or other authorities.

- Possible child, elder, or spouse abuse or neglect
- Apparent homicide or suicide
- Injuries sustained during a felony
- Animal attacks

INFECTIOUS DISEASE CONTROL

Like all living organisms, we engage in a constant battle against invading microorganisms. We have defense mechanisms to help protect us from these constant threats of invasion, but once our defenses are breeched and the offending organisms are living in us (and often) we develop an infection. Our primary defense against infectious organisms is the integumentary system, our skin, a waterproof and pathogen-proof barrier. (For an in-depth look at skin, see the discussion at the front of the soft tissue injury section). Our second line of defense is the immune system, in particular, our white blood cells (WBCs). White blood cells are constantly scouring our body, seeking and destroying invading pathogens.

Illness

DISEASE—An interruption, alteration, or cessation of normal body system or organ function.

- It has a recognizable etiological or causative agent.
- It has an identifiable set of signs and symptoms.
- It has consistent anatomical alterations.

INFECTIOUS DISEASE—A disease caused by or resulting from the presence and activity of microbiological agents.

PATHOGEN—A disease-producing organism that causes infectious disease. (See details in the Appendix.)

BLOOD-BORNE PATHOGEN—Pathogenic (disease-causing) microorganisms present in infected human blood that can cause disease in another person.

COMMUNICABLE DISEASE—A disease that can be transmitted from one person to another by one of the modes of transmission (described later in this section).

Types of infectious organisms

PRION—A proteinaceous infectious particle (causes deadly brain diseases).

VIRUS—A small infectious agent that can replicate only inside the living cells of organisms.

- Genetic material, RNA or DNA, surrounded by a protective protein coat
- Obligate intracellular parasites
- Unable to reproduce on their own
- Examples: hepatitis A, B, C, HIV, common cold, rabies, viral meningitis

BACTERIA—A large group of single-celled microorganisms, typically a few millimeters in length, exhibiting a wide range of shapes, and which grow in every habitat on earth.

PROTOZOA—A unicellular heterotrophic protist, such as an amoeba. Like bacteria, they are unicellular, but protozoa have some form of locomotion.

MYCOSES—Fungal infections are single-celled organisms that reproduce by budding.

HELMINTHS—Multicellular intestinal worms that are usually parasitic.

Relationships

SYMBIOSIS—The biological association of two or more species for their mutual benefit

COMMENSALISM—A relationship where one organism benefits from another, but not at any cost to the other (e.g., a barnacle attached to a clam shell)

HOST—The organism in or on which an infectious agent lives and causes symptoms, and which the agent is dependent upon for its energy

PARASITE—An organism that lives on or in a host at the expense of that host

RESERVOIR—Living or nonliving material on which an infectious agent multiplies and develops and is dependent upon to survive in nature

VECTOR—The method or vehicle by which infectious disease is transmitted: e.g., water, food, insects, fomites (inanimate objects), coughs, sneezes, etc.

Defenses

INTEGUMENTARY SYSTEM—Skin, a waterproof, pathogen-proof barrier

IMMUNE SYSTEM—Responsible for recognizing self from non-self and destroying and eliminating anything that is non-self.

- Cellular immunity: the action of white blood cells to surround and kill any non-self entity
- Humeral immunity: the production of antibodies to help destroy invading pathogens and to create a memory of those microorganisms, thus preventing any future illness that could by caused by a re-infection with the same organisms

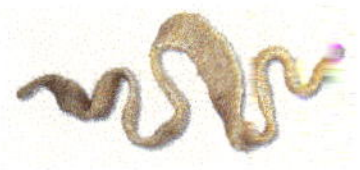

Modes of transmission of infectious disease

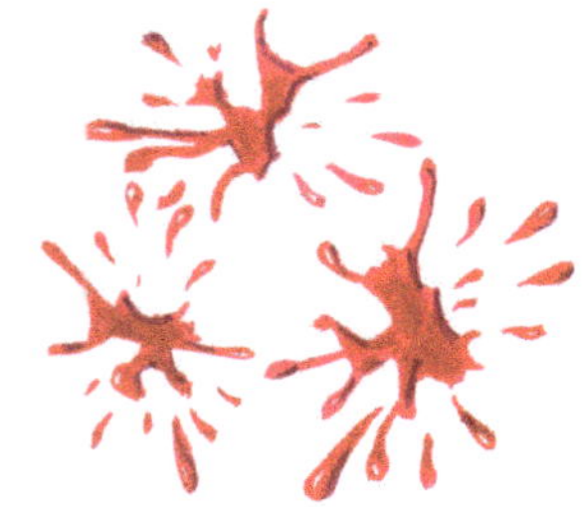

DIRECT CONTACT—Disease is spread by direct contact with the blood or other body substances (saliva, sputum, urine, feces, secretions) of an infected individual.

- These include blood-borne pathogens and sexually transmitted diseases (STDs).

AIRBORNE—Disease is spread through the air by coughing and sneezing.

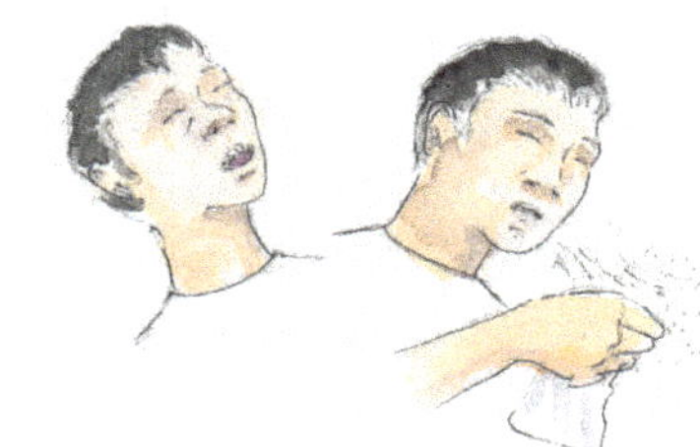

- Minimize this by containing coughs and sneezes, and by washing hands frequently.
- Do not allow contagious people to help with food preparation.

INDIRECT CONTACT—Disease is spread through indirect contact when someone touches a contaminated inanimate object (referred to as a fomite, e.g., clothing, a doorknob, stretcher, countertop, food, etc.) and then transfers the pathogen to their eyes or mouth with their hands. Alternately, indirect contact also includes airborne contamination, which occurs when someone inhales infected droplets of saliva or sputum expelled into the air by the coughing or sneezing of an infected person.

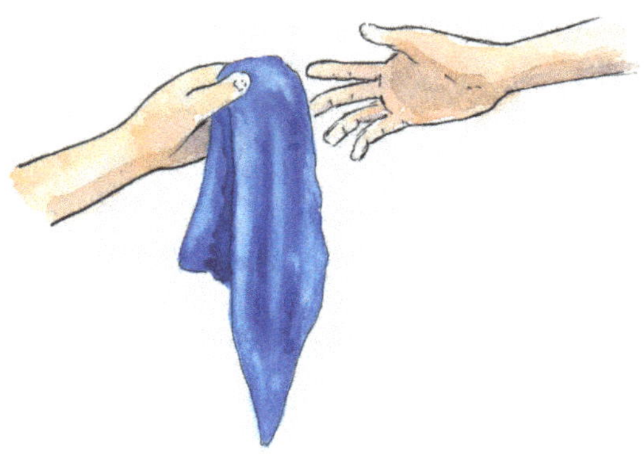

- Sharps containers—Always dispose of sharps, such as needles, appropriately. To prevent accidental needle sticks, never re-cap a needle.
- Surfaces—Clean surfaces appropriately after each patient contact to prevent the spread of pathogens by indirect contact.
- Clothing and linen disinfection—Minimize handling to reduce the spread of pathogens by indirect contact. Launder appropriately.
- Infected waste—Expendable materials that have become contaminated, such as gauze and dressings, must be disposed of properly (usually at the hospital) in a red bag labeled "Contaminated Human Waste." In the wilderness—double-bag infected waste and carry it out.

INSECT VECTOR—Disease is spread from one person to another by blood-sucking insects such as mosquitoes, fleas, black flies, or ticks. (See Bites and Stings in the Environmental Emergencies section.)

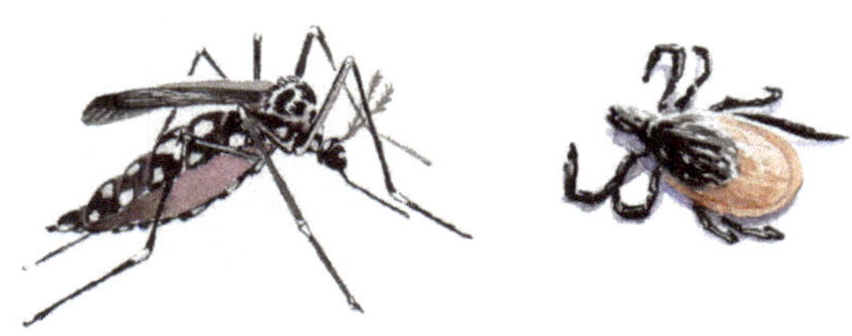

- After the insect has had a blood meal from an infected person, the infectious agent migrates to the insect's salivary glands.
- When the insect takes a subsequent blood meal from another person, it transfers the infectious agent to the bite site through its saliva.

WATERBORNE AND FOOD-BORNE—Disease is spread by the consumption of contaminated water or tainted food. When tainted by human waste, this is called oral-fecal contamination. Here are some basic guidelines for preventing this kind of contamination when traveling in the backcountry or in developing countries.

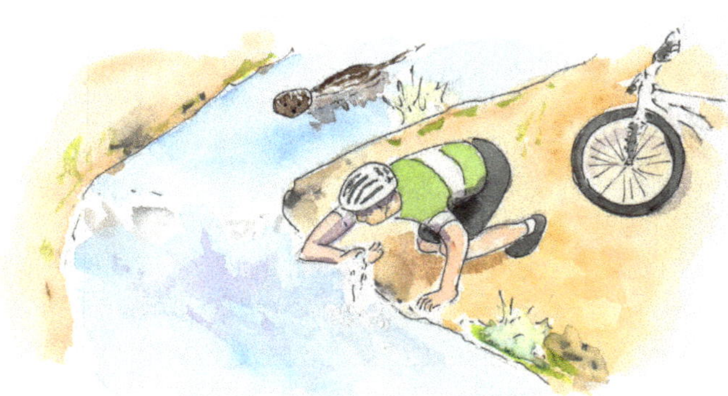

- Don't take ice in your drinks (freezing doesn't kill all the bugs).
- Purify your water.
- Don't eat raw or undercooked meat or vegetables (just say no to salad).
- Wash your hands frequently and follow that with chemical hand sanitizer.

Total Body Substance Isolation (BSI)

and Universal Precautions

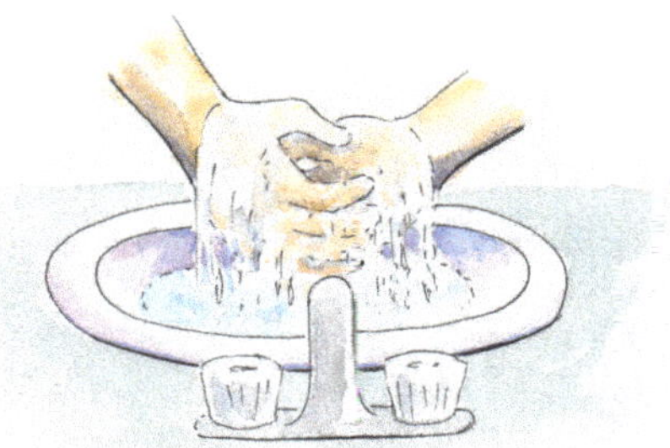

GLOVES
- To prevent **direct contact**, put gloves on before any potential exposure to body fluids.

HAND WASHING

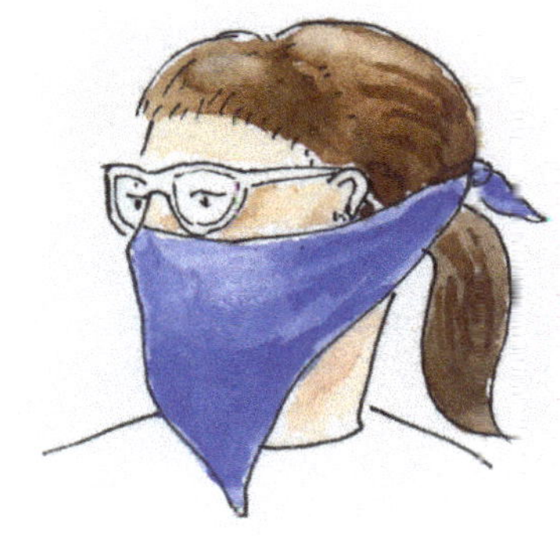

- To prevent patient-to-patient and hand-to-mouth transfer of pathogens by **indirect contact**, wash your hands frequently, especially after contact with any person, substance, or object that may be contaminated.
- Wash your hands before and after any patient contact.
- Use hand sanitizer frequently.

MASKS
- Masks prevent the **airborne** spread of disease by creating a barrier between you and droplets suspended in the air.
- Wear a mask or improvise one, before any potential exposure to airborne pathogens, especially tuberculosis and influenza.

COVER UP
- Whenever it is appropriate to wear gloves, it is also appropriate to wear waterproof clothing or rain gear to protect yourself from the splashing of potentially infected fluids, including bodily fluids.
- In the non-hospital setting, use turnout gear, rain gear, garbage bags, etc.
- Clean or dispose of all protective clothing after use.

EYE PROTECTION
- Protect your eyes—pathogens can be absorbed though the mucosa of the eyes.
- Wear eye protection or glasses to avoid splashing fluids into your eyes.
- Clean after use.

NETTING, CLOTHING, INSECT REPELLENTS
- Use mosquito netting while sleeping and bug head-nets while working outside.
- Wear long-sleeved shirts and pants (tuck pants into shoes) and avoid open-toed shoes, sandals, flip flops, etc.
- Use insect repellents. (See Bites and Stings in the Environmental Emergencies section.)

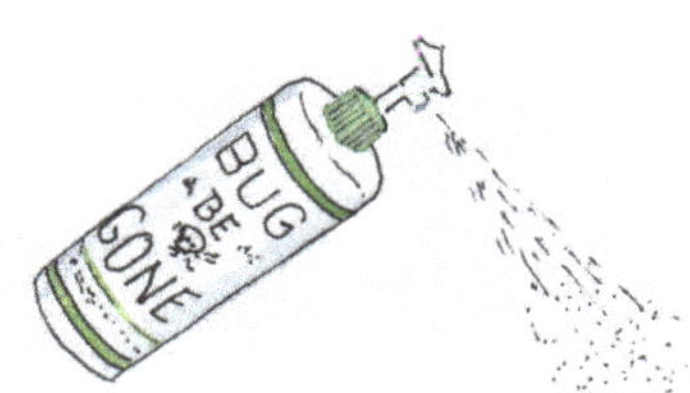

An ounce of prevention...
Vaccinations

A vaccine is used to pre-educate your immune system to recognize a pathogen before exposure. The vaccine contains killed or inactivated live pathogen which act as an antigen (from "antibody generator"). The immune system reacts to the antigen, producing antibodies against the disease-producing pathogen. If future exposure to that pathogen occurs, the immune system already has the antibodies needed to destroy the invading pathogenic organism before it can cause disease.

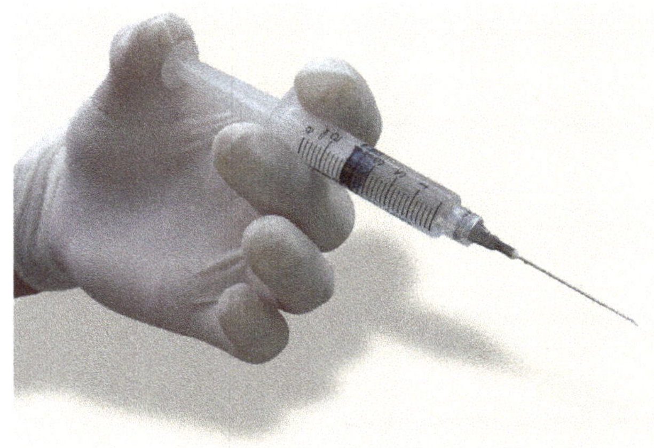

COMMON CHILDHOOD VACCINATIONS

- **DTap**: diphtheria, tetanus, and acellular pertussis (require boosters every 10 years)
- **MMR**: mumps, measles, and rubella (given during childhood)
- **OPV**: oral polio vaccine (given during childhood)
- **IPV**: inactivated polio vaccine (given to adults and travelers)
- **HAV**: hepatitis A virus vaccine (2 shots, 6 – 12 months apart)—see sidebar, below
- **HBV**: hepatitis B virus vaccine (3 shots: day 1, at 1 month, and at 6 months)—see sidebar, below
- Varicella: Prevents chickenpox
- Hib: Prevents haemophilus influenza B infections (which cause epiglottitis)
- Influenza: Decreases the likelihood of contracting the flu

TRAVEL VACCINATIONS

- Rabies: Both direct antibodies, Human Rabies Immunoglobulin (HRIG) for rabies exposure, and killed virus to develop antibodies over time (IMOVAX); rabies vaccines for both pre-exposure and post-exposure prophylaxis
- Typhoid: Prevents this tropical diarrheal disease
- Meningococcal vaccines: Prevents bacterial meningitis
- Yellow fever: Prevents the lethal viral yellow fever illness

HEPATITIS—VITAL VACCINES

- The hepatitis vaccines are essential for all healthcare workers.
- Having hepatitis A virus will make you sick for several weeks with 100% recovery.
- Having hepatitis B virus will make you very sick for 2 – 3 months; it can kill you or leave you in a permanently weakened state.
- But, even with a 100% recovery from HBV, you will remain at risk for developing liver cancer.
- Hepatitis viruses have no treatment: vaccination equals prevention.
- Hepatitis C, another common form of the disease, currently has no vaccine.

The Patient Assessment system

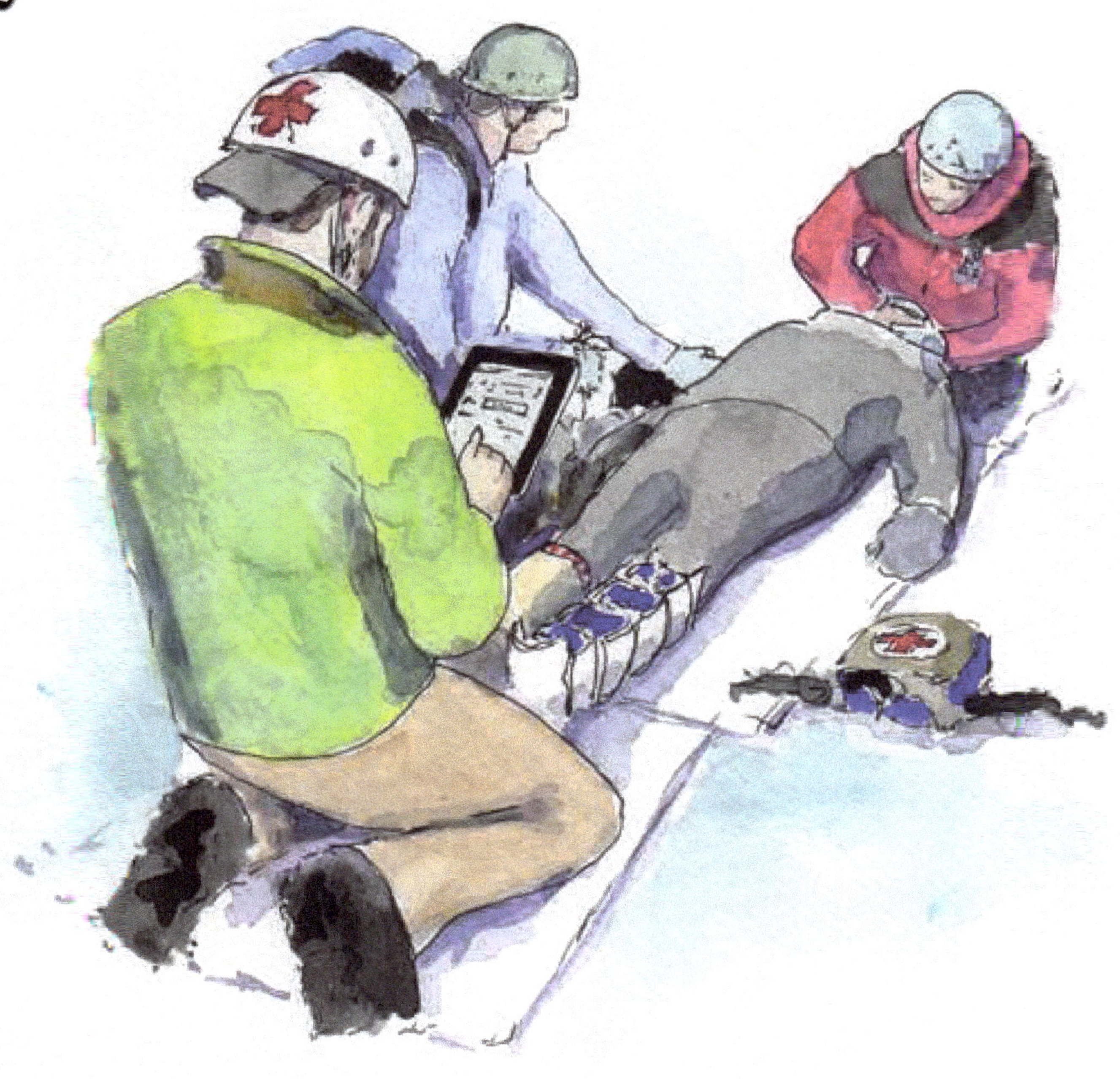

8

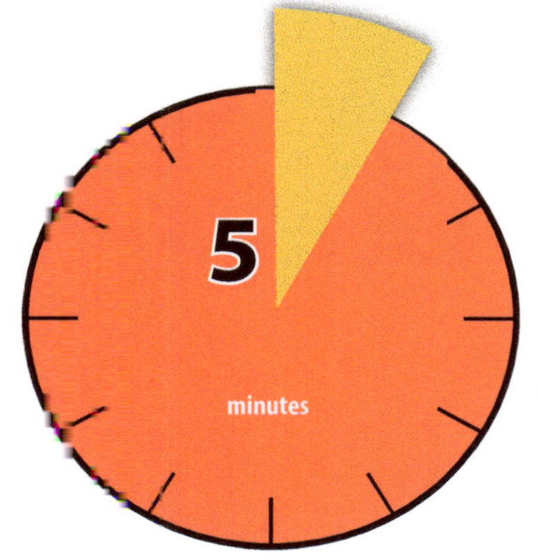

Nothing matters more than what you do in the first 5 minutes.

If a person's airway is blocked

or they stop breathing

or their heart stops beating

or they are bleeding profusely...

...we're going to teach you how to fix these things

While it's rewarding to learn how to build splints, or cobble a rescue litter together out of branches, or create a cozy bivouac site, or understand the ways to pull someone back from the edge of hypothermia, these and many other wilderness medical skills only matter *if your patient is alive*.

The way you handle the first five minutes of an emergency can make the difference between life and death. During these first fleeting moments you must discover all the potentially life-threatening problems and solve them as quickly as possible. The solution can be as simple as repositioning a patient's head to open their airway or applying direct pressure to control bleeding, or as complex and dramatic as rescue breathing, inserting an airway, or doing CPR.

To find and treat the most basic life-threats requires a logical approach to response and assessment—the Patient Assessment System (PAS), which consists of a list of questions that need to be answered and corresponding tasks that need to be performed, all during those first **precious** minutes.

We have arranged these questions and tasks by priority and they *must be done in order*. Short-cutting the system can make things worse—don't move on until you have successfully completed the task you're on.

This section deals with first response (the first five minutes) and emergency care (the Golden Hour), in order:

Survey the Scene
Assess overall site dangers.

Primary Assessment
Identify and treat immediate life threats.

Secondary Assessment
Identify other problems, take vital signs.

Rescue Plan
Implement the evacuation.

Survey the scene

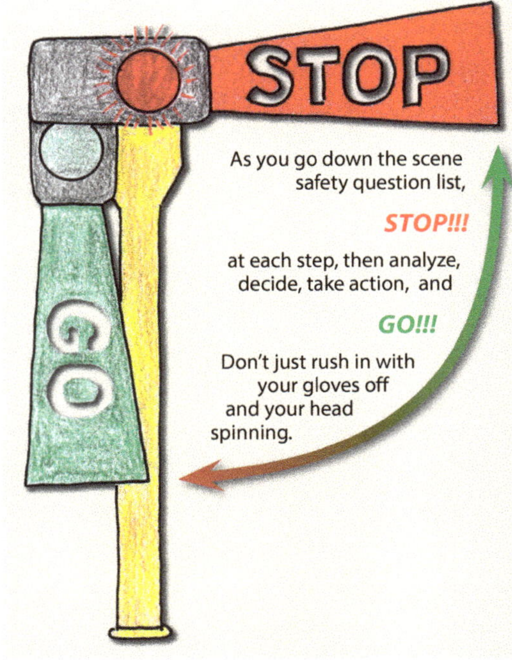

Scene safety: The overall safety of an accident scene is of primary importance to the victim, the rescuers, and any bystanders. Ensuring the safety of the scene keeps bad things from getting worse.

1. Am I safe and am I going to stay safe?

2. Is the group safe and will they stay safe?

3. Is the victim safe and will he or she stay safe?

   - When you approach an accident scene, stop when you can see and communicate with the victim but before you are so close that you risk missing obvious dangers. The answers to these first three questions should be obvious, and they should come quickly—seconds count. Consider the following:
     - Look for obvious objective hazards: danger from falling rocks, avalanche, rushing water, and other terrain threats.
     - Consider environmental dangers: approaching severe weather, darkness, extreme cold or heat, etc.
     - Assess issues with the group: more than one hurt person, unattended children, uninjured people in obvious distress (e.g., cold and hungry), etc.
     - Make immediate decisions to minimize any risks identified.
   - If you answer "No" to any of the three scene-safety questions, you must take action before continuing. Once you've assessed overall scene safety, made any critical immediate decisions and acted on them (e.g., someone will have to direct the uninjured people away from the edge of the cliff), swiftly continue with the next steps.

4. Take appropriate BSI precautions.

5. Form your general impression.

   - How serious is this? What happened? What is the Mechanism of Injury (MOI)—is it significant (see sidebar)? Will the victim have to be moved in order to be assessed? How will you safely approach the victim?

6. Attempt to communicate with the victim.

   - Before you approach the victim, shout: "Are you okay?" Do you get a response? (By doing this from a distance you can help minimize risk to yourself—imagine this response: "Help! There are bees everywhere!")
   - When you arrive, kneel and place a hand on the patient's forehead—this protects their cervical spine and provides the "human touch."
   - Are their eyes open? What position are they in?
   - If they are conscious, ask them what happened and where they hurt.

PRIMARY ASSESSMENT

The primary assessment is your initial physical exam. It takes just a few minutes and identifies any immediate life threats using a simple A, B, C, D, E system (*Airway*, *Breathing*, *Circulation*, *Deformity*, and *Environment*). Any compromise in the first three (the ABCs) can kill a person in just a few minutes; a significant deformity (femur or spine) that goes untreated can kill or paralyze a patient when they are moved; and the environment (freezing rain, avalanche) can be deadly.

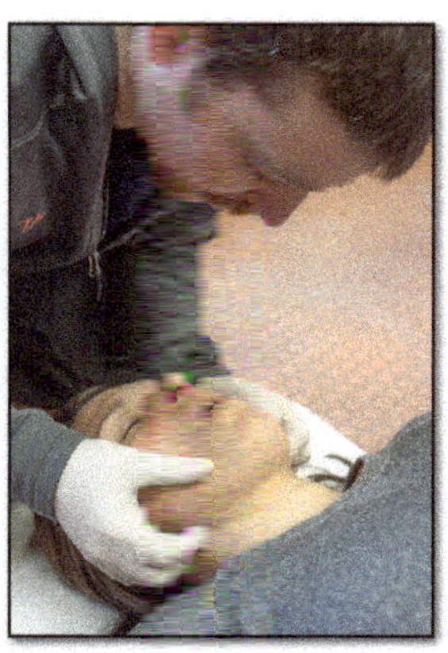

Visually inspect the airway.

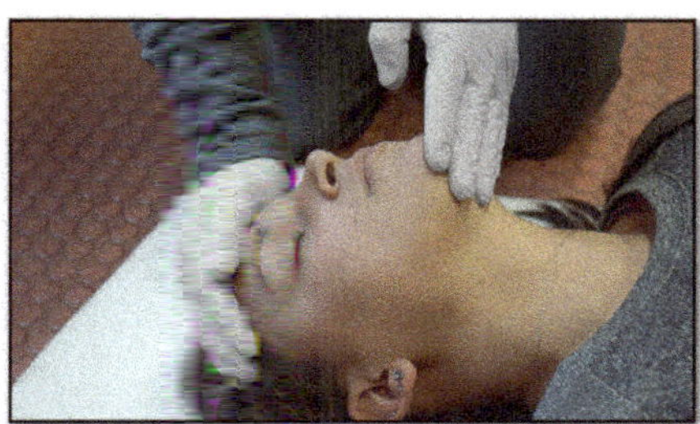

Perform a head-tilt/chin-lift.

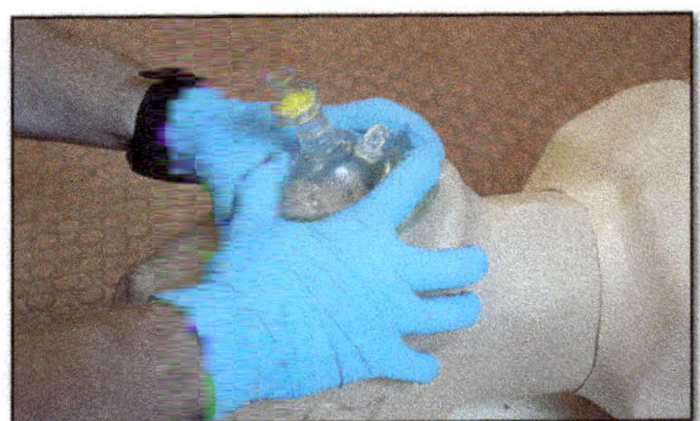

Give rescue breaths (mouth-to-mask).

A **APPROACH AND ASSESS**—Determine your patient's *level of consciousness*. Are they conscious and responsive or unconscious and unresponsive?

- **Look**: Are their eyes open, and do they track movement?
- **Listen**: Ask, "Hey, how are you doing?" Do they respond to you?
- **Feel**: Pinch the skin on the back of their hand or give them a sternum rub. Do you get a response?
- Talk to the patient—they may be able to hear even if they cannot respond.

AIRWAY—Assess the quality of your patient's airway. If they responded verbally during your initial contact or when you determined their LOC, then their airway is open and functioning. If they are unresponsive, your first job is to open their airway.

- **Look**: Open and visually inspect their airway. Is it clear? What color is it?
- **Listen**: Can you hear air moving in and out?
- **Feel**: Put your ear to their mouth—Can you feel air moving in and out?

If you answered YES to all of the airway questions, *move on to B.*

If you answered NO to any of the airway questions, *take airway actions.*

AIRWAY ACTIONS

1. To open the airway, perform a head-tilt/chin-lift (this moves the musculature of the tongue forward and opens the airway):
   - Move the head into proper anatomical position.
   - Tilt it slightly back (extension).
   - Gently pull the lower jaw (mandible) forward.
2. Is the airway clear? If not, log roll the patient into the recovery position. This allows any blood, fluid, or vomitus to drain.
3. Is the patient spontaneously breathing?

   If the patient is breathing, *move on to B.*
   If the patient is not breathing, *begin rescue breathing.*

RESCUE BREATHING

1. Give two rescue breaths and check for a pulse.
2. If they have a pulse, continue to give rescue breaths every 4 – 5 seconds until they begin breathing.
3. If the patient has no heartbeat, initiate CPR (see next spread).
4. If the patient does not respond within 30 minutes, stop all resuscitation efforts.

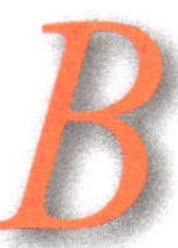

BREATHING—Assess the quality of your patient's breathing—are they breathing often enough and deeply enough to get an adequate supply of oxygen?

- **Look**: Do you see their chest rising and falling?
- **Listen**: Is their breathing clear and without adventitious breath sounds (wheezing, gurgling, or snoring)?
- **Feel**: Can you feel the patient's chest rise and fall as they breathe? Is the rate normal:10 – 30 breaths per minute (bpm)?

If you answered YES to all of the breathing questions, *move on to C.*
If you answered NO to any of the breathing questions, *take action.*

BREATHING ACTIONS

1. Log-roll your patient into the *recovery position* to help clear and maintain an open airway—gravity will help drain fluids and allow the tongue to fall forward and open the airway. Swipe their mouth, if necessary.
2. If their breathing does not improve sufficiently, or it is too fast (>30bpm) or too slow (<10bpm), control their respirations with a pocket mask using mouth-to-mask ventilation at a rate of 12 – 20bpm.

Now *move on to C.*

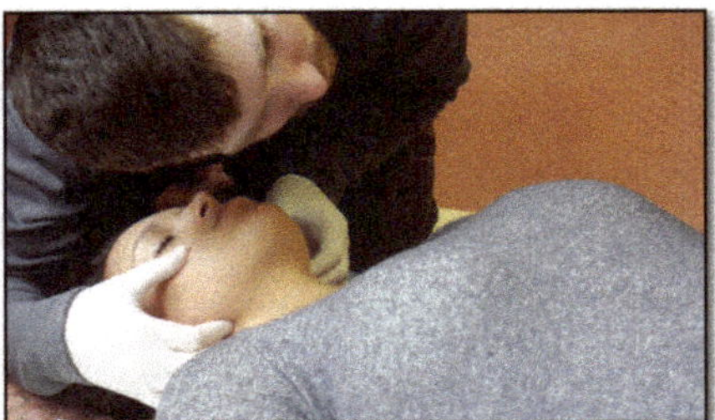

While holding the airway open, check for chest rise—which demonstrates that the patient is breathing.

RESPIRATORY RATE AND EFFORT (RR)

The respiratory rate and effort shows you how well the respiratory system (the airway and lungs) is exchanging oxygen, in particular, in supplying the brain with oxygen. Look, listen, and feel air move in and out of the lungs.

- **RESPIRATORY RATE**: Count the number of breaths per minute (breaths in 15 seconds x 4).
  - The typical rate is 10 – 30 breaths/minute (BPM).
  - If the rate is slower than 10 or faster than 30, the patient needs assisted ventilations via mouth-to-mouth, mouth-to-mask, or a bag valve mask (BVM) at a rate of one breath every 4 – 5 seconds (12 – 15 breaths per minute) to make sure they are getting enough oxygen into their lungs.
- **RESPIRATORY EFFORT**: In addition to how many breaths per minute your patient is taking, you also need to assess how hard they are working.
  - **Look:** Do they look like they are having difficulty breathing? Are they complaining of shortness of breath or difficulty breathing?
  - **Listen:** Are the patient's breath sounds normal and quiet?
  - **Feel:** Is the patient's chest moving normally as they breathe? Breathing should be easy and effortless. It should not take any noticeable effort to breathe or take a deep breath.

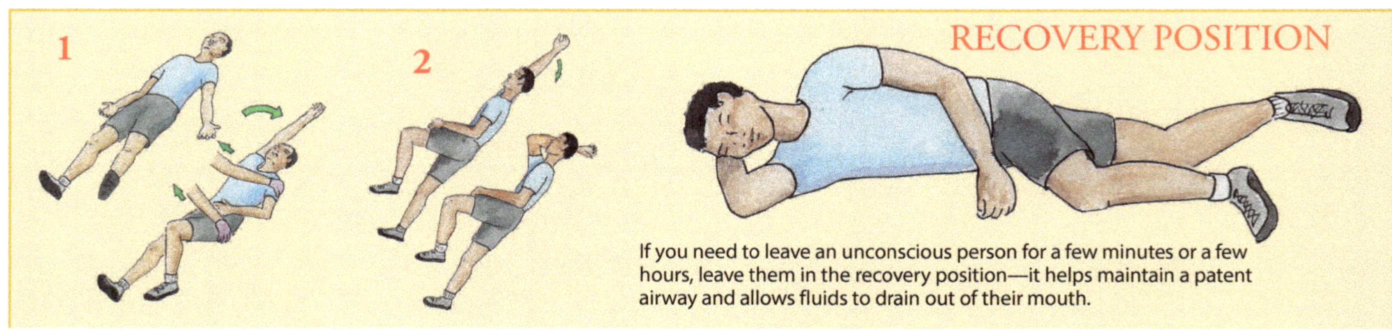

If you need to leave an unconscious person for a few minutes or a few hours, leave them in the recovery position—it helps maintain a patent airway and allows fluids to drain out of their mouth.

SOLO Wilderness First Responder

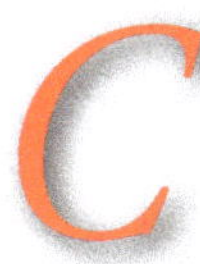

CIRCULATION (PULSE)—Assess your patient's circulatory system.
- **Look**: What is their skin color? Are they bleeding, and is it controlled?
- **Listen**: Put your ear to their chest—can you hear a heartbeat?
- **Feel**: Palpate their carotid artery—do you feel a pulse?

If the patient has a pulse, note quality (fast, slow, weak, strong) and *move on to bleeding*.
If the patient has no pulse, *perform CPR* and continue until successful, exhausted, or until 30 minutes have passed.

CPR

1. 30 compressions to 2 ventilations
2. 5 cycles (about 2 minutes)
3. Compression rate of 100 per minute (about 1.5 compressions per second)

CIRCULATION (BLEEDING)—Assess for bleeding.
- **Look and feel**: Visually scan and use your hands to check for bleeding (make sure to check underneath the patient)—if you find any bleeding, is it under control (i.e. not clotted/ not pooling)?

If the patient is not bleeding, or the bleeding is controlled, *move on to D*.
If the patient has uncontrolled bleeding, *take action*.

BLEEDING ACTIONS

1. Find the source(s) of the bleeding by scanning down the body and reaching under the torso and limbs. If there is significant mechanism of injury (MOI)—e.g. a fall greater than three times body height, consider the possibility of spinal injury and do not compromise the spine while searching for bleed(s).
2. Apply direct pressure until the bleeding stops.
3. Apply pressure dressing(s) as necessary, or if that does not work, apply a tourniquet. (see page 14)
4. When the bleeding has been controlled, move on to D (or get someone else to control the bleeding while you move on with the exam).
5. Hemostatic clotting agents and tourniquets are generally not available in remote settings.

Once bleeding is controlled, *move on to D*.

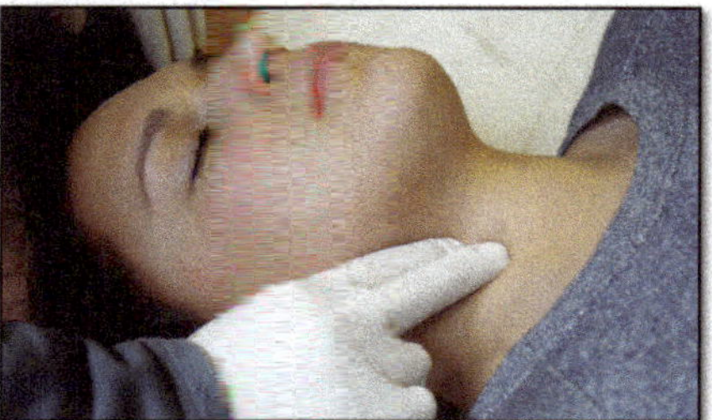

Check the carotid pulse.

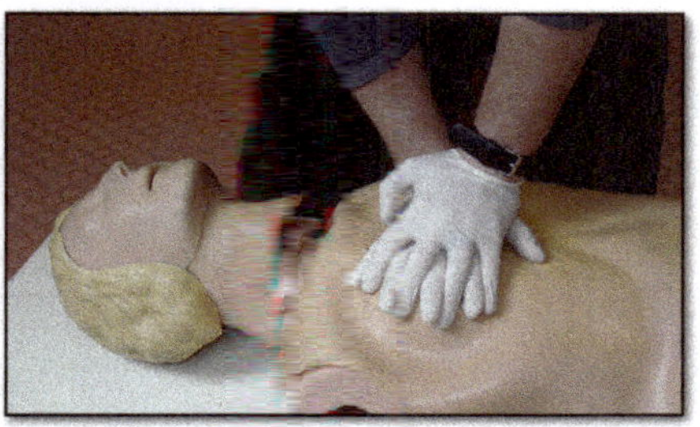

Perform CPR.

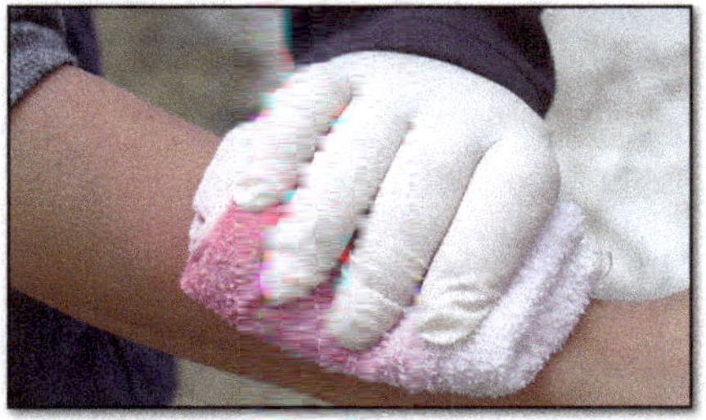

Control bleeding.

AFTER THE ABCs

You have a good idea of how injured or sick your patient is. If this is a life-threatening situation, then you may be breathing for your patient and/or performing CPR; get whatever information you can about the patient from bystanders, and call 911, or send someone for help. If your patient is not critically injured or ill, move on to D.

CONTROLLING BLEEDING

CONTROLLING BLEEDING This is a primary concern with any wound—try to keep as much of the "red stuff" in the vasculature as possible! And before you start treating any wound, ***put on your BSI***.

1 DIRECT PRESSURE

- Apply pressure directly to the wound with your gloved hand.
- If possible, place some absorbent material, such as gauze pads, on top of the wound before applying pressure—it will act as a sponge and help hold the blood in place.
- Because the vast majority of bleeding is venous, it is under low pressure, and can usually be controlled with gentle direct pressure.
  - It may take 10 – 20 minutes to completely stop the bleeding.
- Once the bleeding has stopped, maintain direct pressure for ten additional minutes to allow blood clots to form.

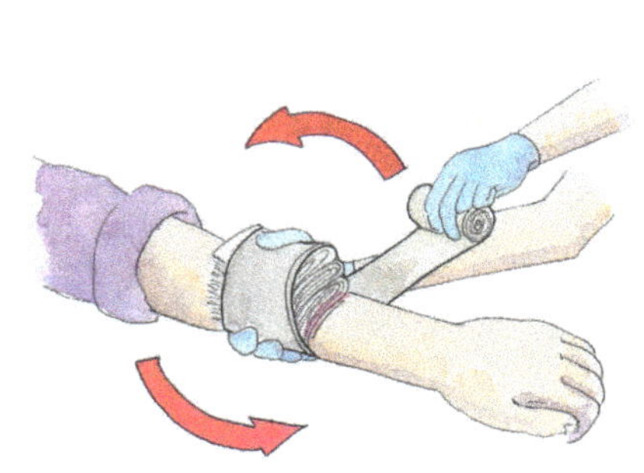

2 PRESSURE DRESSING

- If a wound bleeds stubbornly, or you need to do other things for your patient, you can apply a pressure dressing, which will maintain light pressure for you.

3 WOUND PACKING

- For a life-threatening bleed where a tourniquet can not be used, pack the wound with bleeding control gauze (hemostatic gauze), plain gauze, or a clean cloth and then apply pressure with both (gloved) hands.
- Apply steady pressure with both hands directly on top of the bleeding wound. Press down hard on the bleeding would and continue to press down.

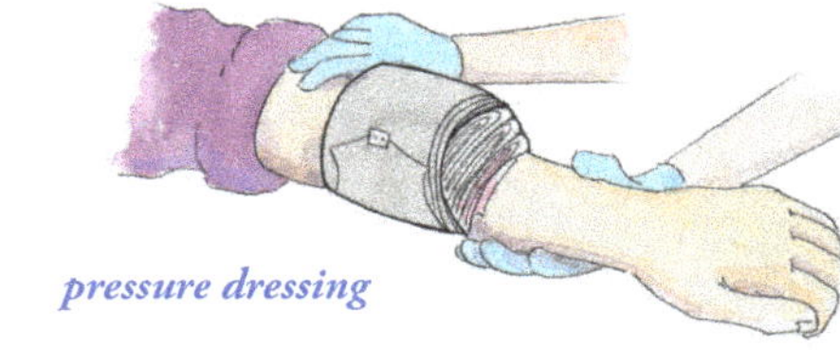

pressure dressing

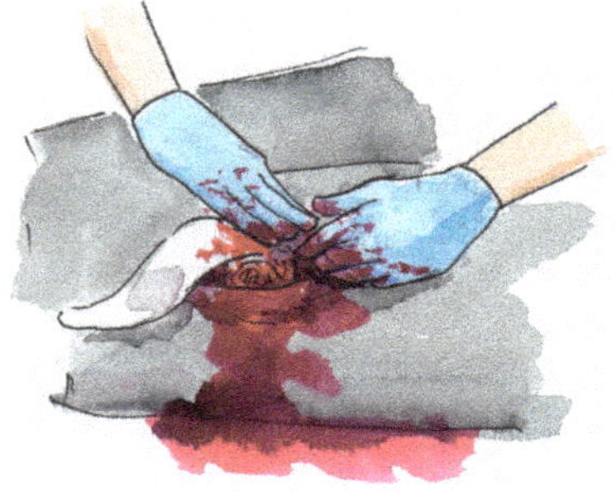

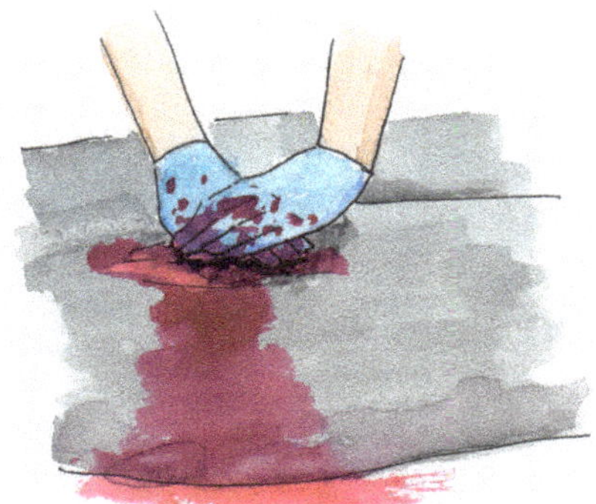

wound packing

more on HEMOSTATIC AGENTS

- These are chemical substances that act by inhibiting fibrinolysis (the body's natural tendency to prevent blood clots from growing too large) and/or promoting coagulation (clotting).
- Hemostatic agents are use primarily for severe junctional bleeds where bleeding cannot be controlled with direct pressure, pressure dressings, or toourniquets.
- Most hemostatic agents are incorporated into gauze rather than being used granulated or as a powder—the loose agent could be blown into the rescuer's eyes, causing significant vision problems or reacting with other bodily fluids.
- To maximize effectiveness, Gauze-style hemostatic agents should be applied with 3 minutes of sustained direct pressure over the bleeding site, followed by the application of a pressure dressing for an additional 20 minutes.

15

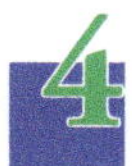

TOURNIQUETS

If your efforts to stop the bleeding fail, you may have to use a tourniquet and you've determined that the patient may die without it.

Tourniquets have been used for at least 2,000 years—the Romans used tourniquets (straps of bronze over leather) to control bleeding, especially during amputations. Throughout the 1700s, 1800s and 1900s, many advances and refinements were made, and by the 1980s microprocessor-controlled tourniquets were in use. Modern automatic tourniquet systems are self-calibrating and self-contained and offer much greater safety than the older mechanical systems. There are two types of tourniquets: 1) surgical tourniquets, which provide a bloodless environment for increased precision, safety, and speed in the operating room, and 2) emergency tourniquets, which are limited to extreme emergency situations (e.g., combat) to control bleeding in the most severe injuries.

In wilderness emergency situations, it is unlikely that you will have a high-tech, microchip-driven tourniquet with you. Likely you will be forced to improvise. Please bear the following in mind.

- A tourniquet is very rarely needed—do not apply it to simple wounds involving only venous bleeding; virtually all bleeding can be controlled with direct pressure and and a pressure dressing. An example of a situation where a tourniquet may be needed would be a laceration of an artery (e.g., femoral or brachial) in a leg or arm.
- A tourniquet should only be used for extreme life-threatening arterial bleeding in an extremity that cannot be controlled any other way—for instance, if an arm or leg has been mangled or severed.
- Tourniquets are used on extremities only.

Improvised Tourniquet

1. Wrap a wide band around the extremity not over clothing, at least 2" to 3" proximal to the bleeding and not over the elbow or knee.

Locate the tourniquet above, or proximal, to the injury.

2. Tie a simple knot in the band.

3. Place a 6" stick or bar over the knot and tie a second knot over it to secure it.

4. Using the stick as a "Spanish windlass," twist it to tighten the band.

5. Tighten the windlass until both the bleeding and the distal pulse stop.

6. Secure the free end of the windlass in place with another band or tape.

7. Write a capital "T" and the time of application on the patient's forehead.

8. If possible, cold pack the extremity to increase the duration of survivability, just like an amputation.

9. Start the evacuation process immediately..

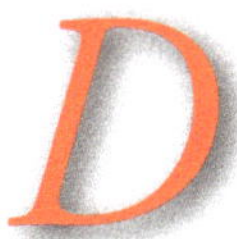

D

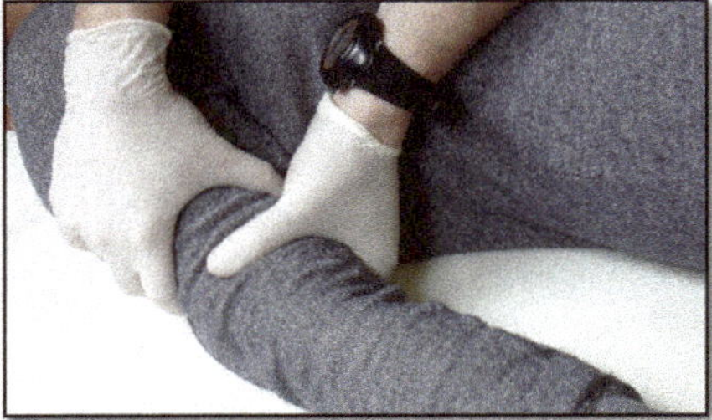

Check for deformity.

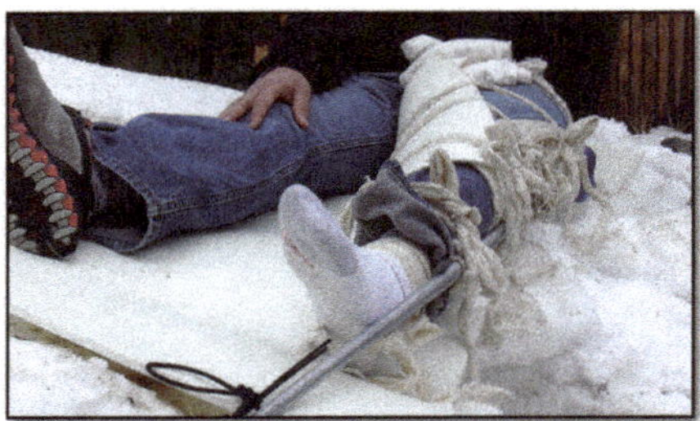

Splint unstable fractures right away.

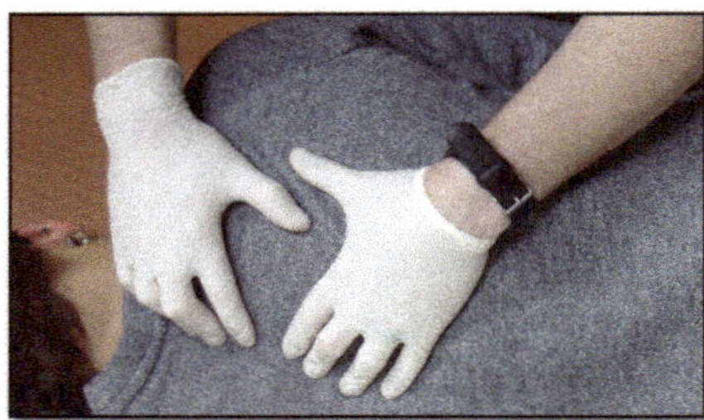

Assess the spine from neck to sacrum.

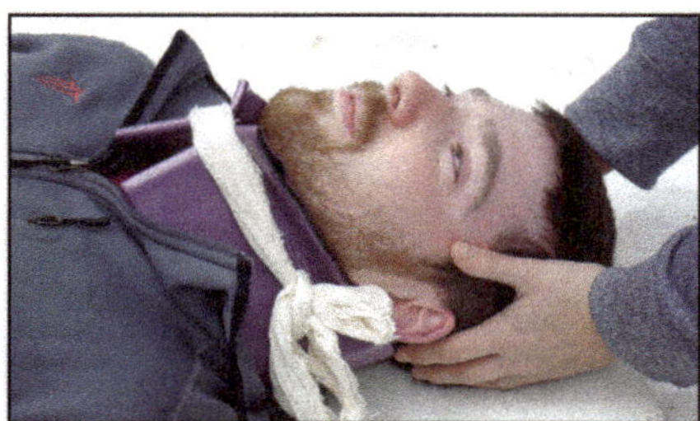

An improvised C-collar.

DEFORMITY—Assess your patient, checking for deformation, alignment, symmetry, and impaled objects.

- **Look**: Scan your patient's body—is it free from obvious deformities— angulated fractures (bone fragments out of alignment), compound fractures (bone ends poking through the skin), dislocations (joint deformities), or impaled objects?
- **Listen**: Is the patient pain-free?
- **Feel**: Do a "chunk check" by palpating major body parts: is your patient still pain-free? Are there signs of deformity or crepitus (bone fragments grating)?

If no major deformities are found, *move on to disability.*
If major deformities are found, *take action.*

DEFORMITY ACTIONS

1. If you find any skeletal injuries, inspect them to determine if there is anything you need to treat immediately.
2. Femur fractures are the most dangerous because they can pose grave internal bleeding risks. If found, traction must be applied as soon as possible. Bilateral femur fractures (both femurs broken) are considered life-threatening.

Once stabilized, *move on to disability.*

DISABILITY—Assess your patient for head and/or spinal injuries.

- **Look**: Was the MOI insignificant (see previous spread)? Is the patient able to move their extremities with ease? Do they appear free from injury or deformity?
- **Listen**: Is the patient free from neck or back pain?
- **Feel**: Does everything feel right? Does your palpation elicit no additional pain? Does the patient have normal sensations in their extremities?

If you answer yes to all of these questions, *move on to E.*
If you answer no to any question, *take action.*

DISABILITY ACTIONS

- Neck and spine fractures pose a risk of paralysis and death.
1. If the patient is unconscious and the MOI is significant, assume a risk of spine injury; if possible, have someone hold the patient's head still.
2. If the patient is conscious and the MOI is significant, keep them lying still.

Once stabilized, *move on to E.*

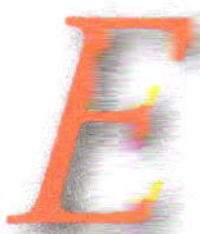

E

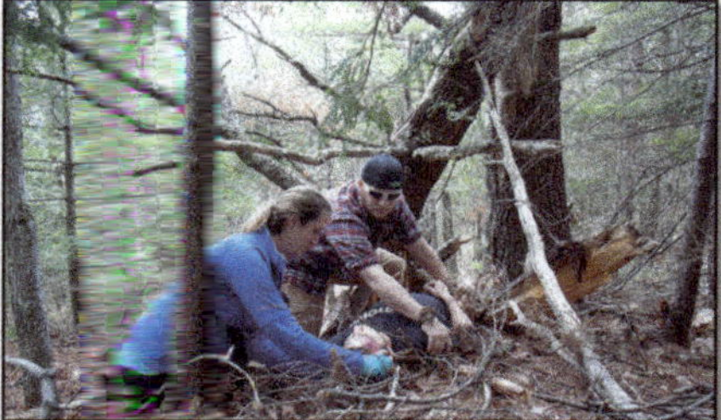

Assess the scene—is it safe? It's easy to get tunnel vision and focus on the patient while losing sight of obvious hazards (e.g., the overhanging and potentially unstable dead snag)

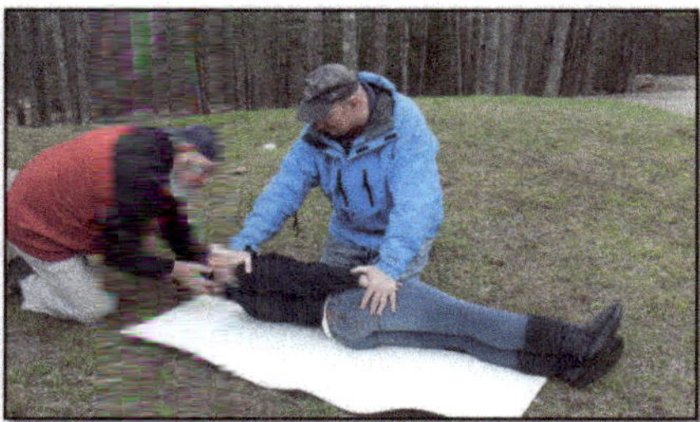

Moving a patient onto a foam pad.

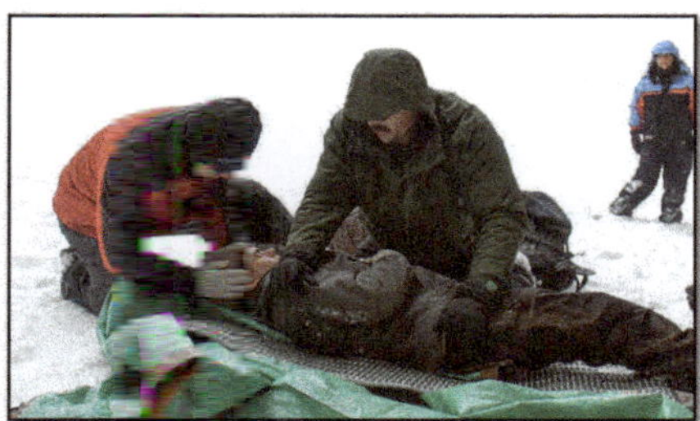

Don't get tunnel vision—there may be others in the group who need help (perhaps just reassurance and direction).

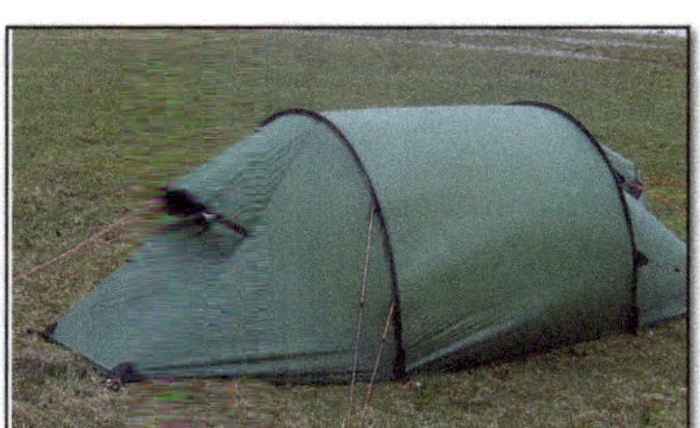

Sometimes the best shelter for your group is the one you bring with you.

ENVIRONMENT (THE PATIENT)—Assess the terrain, weather conditions, and the condition of your patient.

■ **Look**: Consider where your patient is lying: are they safe and comfortable where they are (e.g., they're not lying in water)? Are they protected from cold, heat, sun, or objective hazards? Is the weather good and is darkness far off?

■ **Listen**: Are they telling you that they are comfortable—not too hot, cold, or wet?

■ **Feel**: Do they feel normal (not hot, cold, or wet)?

If you answered yes to all the above questions, *move on to everyone else.*

If you answered no to any question, *take action.*

ENVIRONMENTAL (THE PATIENT) ACTIONS

1. Whenever possible, keep the patient lying still where you found them until you complete the entire patient assessment.
2. If you must move the patient, decide where and how they can be relocated (see the lifting and moving section).
3. At a minimum, as soon as you can, get them on a foam pad to protect them from the ground.
4. You may need to surround them with insulating material (see hypo-wrap) and move them into a shelter (e.g., a tent).

Once the patient's environment is stable, *move on to everyone else.*

ENVIRONMENT (EVERYONE ELSE)—Assess the terrain, weather conditions, and the condition of the rest of the group.

■ **Look**: Does everyone else look okay? Are they going to stay okay?

■ **Listen**: Is everyone verbalizing that they are okay, with no complaints about being cold, wet, hungry, or scared?

■ **Feel**: Is your general impression that the group doesn't need any immediate attention?

If you answered yes to all the above questions, *your Primary Assessment is complete.*

If you answered no to any question, *take action.*

ENVIRONMENTAL (EVERYONE ELSE) ACTIONS

1. Take whatever actions are necessary to protect yourself, your patient, and the group from environmental challenges and hazards.
2. Ensure everyone's safety and comfort and see to their basic needs (food, shelter, warmth, emotional support).
3. Direct someone in the group to take charge and keep everyone safe, fed, hydrated, sheltered, warm, and busy.

Once the group's environment is stable, *your Primary Assessment is complete.*

SECONDARY ASSESSMENT

At this point—assuming things are either not critical or that others are taking over any necessary life-saving procedures (e.g., ventilations or CPR), you have likely spent less than five minutes at your patient's side, and your physical examination of them has been limited to the basics—finding and treating major problems. You have an overall understanding of their condition (ABCDs), are aware of the group dynamics (the patient, anyone with the patient, and you and your group) and any environmental (E) challenges (terrain, weather, darkness) that must be dealt with. You now have the luxury of time.

Once the primary assessment has been completed, it's time to take a much closer look at your patient. During the Secondary Assessment, you will explore your patient's body with your eyes and hands, palpating virtually every inch of them, uncovering, identifying, and diagnosing their injuries and/or illnesses. You will measure data about their basic body systems and collect information about their past and present medical history. You will make specific treatment decisions and begin to take (or direct) specific treatment actions. The secondary survey consists of four parts.

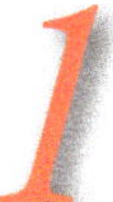 ## Vital Signs

Measurements of basic body functions:
- Level of Consciousness (beyond merely responsive/unresponsive)
- Respiratory rate and effort (RR)
- Heart rate (HR—pulse)
- Heart effort (BP—blood pressure)
- Skin color, temperature, and moisture (SCTM)
- Pupil size and reaction to light (PERRL)

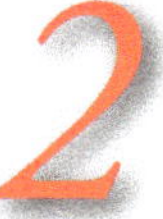 ## Patient Exam

A detailed physical examination that helps you locate and determine the extent of injuries and make treatment decisions

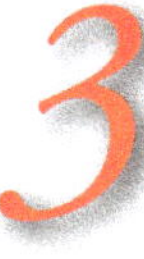 ## AMPLE History

Information about the patient's medical history gathered using a simple mnemonic:
- **A**: Allergies
- **M**: Medications
- **P**: Past medical history
- **L**: Last in (food) and last out (poop and pee)
- **E**. Events leading up to the accident/crisis (the short history of what happened)

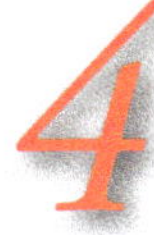 ## SOAPnote

The wilderness medicine equivalent of a patient's medical chart

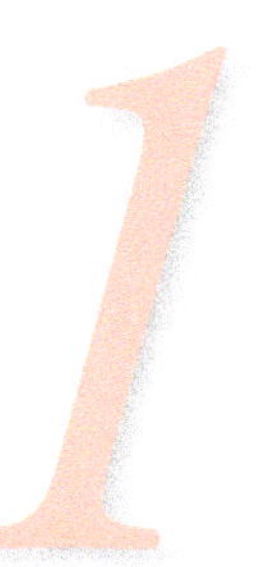 ## VITAL SIGNS

The collection of data that forms a patient's vital signs (you will often hear EMS personnel talk about "getting a set of vitals") tells you how the patient is doing *right now*. And, when the "vitals" are updated regularly (every 5 – 15 minutes, depending on the circumstances) they tell you how your patient is doing *over time*. Knowing which way your patient is headed (improving or deteriorating) helps you adjust your treatment and evacuation plans on the fly. Vital signs don't tell you what the specific injuries or illnesses are—the patient exam does this—but they do tell you how your patient is responding to their injuries and illnesses, as well as to your treatment.

Level of consciousness is a measure of a person's arousability and responsiveness to stimuli. You made a basic determination of their alertness when you called to the victim—if they answered you coherently, then you know three things:

- They are conscious.
- They have an open airway.
- They are breathing.

In wilderness medicine, we differentiate a person's level of consciousness by using the **AVPU** scale.

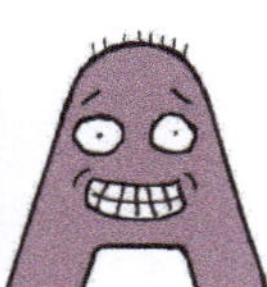

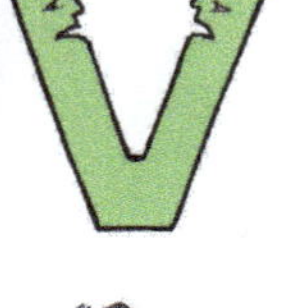

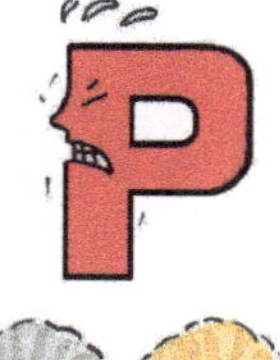

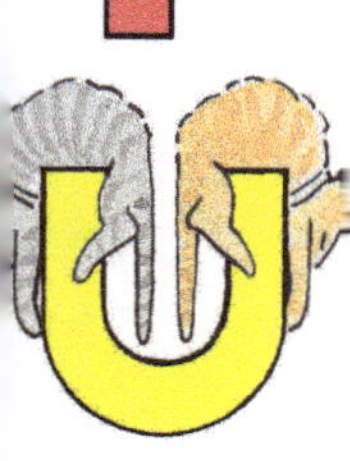

AWAKE: This person is spontaneously responsive and completely aware of their surroundings. They shouted back when you first hailed them, and now that you are by their side they are talking freely. If they answer the following diagnostic questions correctly, they are said to be Alert and Oriented Times Three (AOx3): alert as to person, place, and time.

1. What is your name?
2. Where are you?
3. What is the date?

If they respond appropriately to those three questions, then ask them what happened.

VERBAL: This person is not spontaneously responsive, but does respond to verbal stimuli. They are lethargic. They likely did not give you a hearty reply to your shout—although they may have groaned in response. When you talk to them, they do answer (which confirms an open airway), but they may not make complete sense. Ask them the same three diagnostic questions to determine how altered their mental status is.

PAINFUL: This person does not respond to verbal stimuli. They are stuporous and will likely appear to be asleep. Even shouting right in their ear elicits no response. Pinch the skin on the back of their hand or give them a sternum rub. If this arouses them, then they are deemed to be painfully responsive (if they groan, this also confirms at least a partially open airway).

UNRESPONSIVE: This person appears comatose and they make no purposeful response to any stimuli: you speak, shout, and pinch to no avail. Unresponsive people are often in serious trouble, but they still may be able to hear and comprehend—talk to them, encourage them; don't pretend they're not there.

A change in level of consciousness indicates that there is something wrong with the brain—a potentially life-threatening problem. If the patient's LOC deteriorates over time, assume their condition is getting worse. To survive and thrive, the brain needs:

oxygen

glucose

proper temperature

proper intracranial pressure

appropriate neuronal (electrical) activity

The heart rate (pulse) and effort (blood pressure—see next) tell you how well the circulatory system (heart and blood vessels) is doing.

- **RATE**: Palpate the pulse at the wrist and count the beats per minute (beats in 15 seconds x 4).
- **QUALITY**: based on palpation, determine if the pulse is normal, weak, strong, pounding, or thready (eg., weak, hard to palpate, often rapid—characteristic of hypovolemia, such as occurs with severe hemorrhage).
  - **Look:** What is the skin color? It should be normal for their race.
  - **Listen:** Does your patient have normal heart sounds ("lub-dub:)?
  - **Feel:** Do they have a radial pulse?

BLOOD PRESSURE (BP)

Blood pressure tells you how hard the heart is working—the effort it takes to pump blood around the body. There are two measurements of arterial pressure, systolic and diastolic, and they are both typically taken via a blood pressure cuff with an accompanying pressure gauge (called a sphygmomanometer) and a stethoscope. The measurement units are millimeters of mercury (mmHg).

- **SYSTOLIC**: This is the pressure in the arteries while the left ventricle of the heart is contracting. The acceptable systolic pressure range is 90 – 140mmHg.
- **DIASTOLIC**: This is the residual arterial pressure when the heart is relaxed and the left ventricle is refilling. The acceptable diastolic pressure range is 60 – 90mmHg.

MEASURING BLOOD PRESSURE VIA AUSCULTATION (LISTENING)

The traditional method used in a doctor's office or hospital, this requires a sphygmomanometer (BP cuff) and a stethoscope.

1. Remove the clothing from one arm, if possible.
2. Locate the brachial artery at the elbow.
3. Place the cuff with the "artery" tag pointing at the brachial artery above the elbow and position the pressure gauge so that you can read it easily.
4. Place the diaphragm of the stethoscope over the brachial artery distal to the cuff—you will not hear any pulse yet.
5. Tighten the valve on the cuff and inflate it to 200mmHg.
6. Slowly deflate the cuff while listening carefully.

   - When you first hear a pulse through the stethoscope, it means that the blood pressure has overcome the constricting power of the cuff and is forcing blood through the artery—this is the systolic pressure.

   - When the sound of the pulse disappears, it means that the cuff is no longer restricting the blood flow at all—this is the diastolic pressure.
8. Remove the cuff and record your findings.

MEASURING BLOOD PRESSURE VIA PALPATION (FEELING)

With only a BP cuff but no stethoscope, you can still determine the systolic pressure.

1. Do steps 1 – 4, and 6, above.
2. Deflate the cuff slowly and note the pressure at the point where you feel a pulse—this is the systolic pressure.
3. Record this finding as "systolic by palpation."

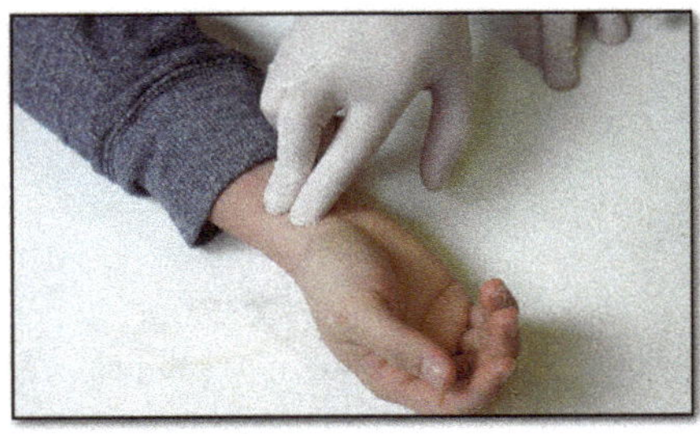

Taking radial pulse.

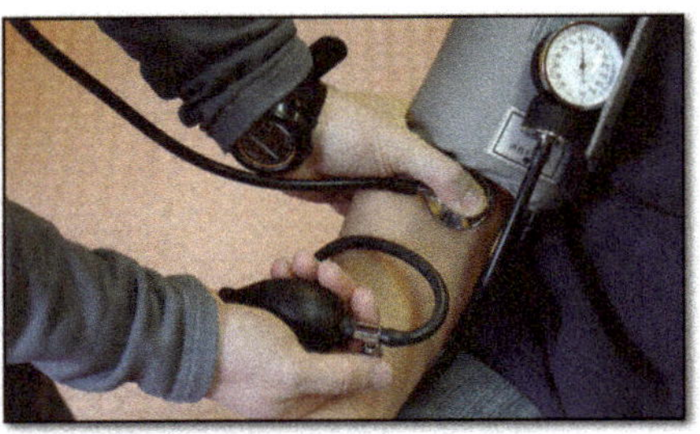

Checking blood pressure with a BP cuff (sphygmomanometer) and stethoscope.

GOING CUFF-LESS IN THE WILDERNESS

If you do not have a BP cuff, the presence or absence of pulses at different locations on the body can be used to estimate the minimum systolic pressure, and can help determine if the patient's blood pressure is changing over time.

- If a pulse is present in the carotid artery in the neck, the minimum systolic pressure is 60mmHg—which is only enough to perfuse the brain, but not the other vital organs.

- If a pulse is present in the radial artery at the wrist, the minimum systolic pressure is 90mmHg—enough to perfuse the entire body.

- If a pulse is present in the femoral artery in the leg, the minimum systolic pressure is 80mmHg—enough to perfuse the vital organs and the brain.

SKIN COLOR, TEMPERATURE, AND MOISTURE (SCTM)

The skin (the integumentary system) is the largest organ in the human body, accounting for about 10% of a person's total body weight. It is durable, self-repairing and very sensitive to internal changes. A healthy person at rest in a benign environment (neither hot nor cold) will have skin that is normal in color, warm, and dry. Any deviation in any of the three characteristics indicates some compromise in health. When you are looking at a patient's skin, keep two points in mind:

1. Skin color varies by race. For Caucasians, the normal skin color is pink. For darker races, non-pigmented areas such as the fingernail beds, under the eyelids, or inside the mouth should be checked—these areas are non-pigmented and should be pink.
2. When evaluating your patient's skin, consider their recent physical activity—vigorous exercise will cause skin to become reddish, warm, and sweaty.

SKIN COLOR AND CAPILLARY REFILL

- Loss of color (pallor) or cyanosis (bluish or purplish coloration) of the skin or mucous membranes indicates that the person's brain has perceived that there is a crisis and is shunting blood away from the skin to the vital organs: the brain, heart, lungs, liver, and kidneys.
- How quickly the capillaries refill is easy to test by looking at a person's fingernails.
    - Squeeze the blood out of a fingertip by pinching it until the skin underneath the fingernail turns white—then release it.
    - In a healthy person, the capillary bed beneath the nail should refill and turn pink within two seconds—a delay indicates a compromise in circulation.
    - This test works in people of all races because there is no pigment in the skin beneath the fingernails.

SKIN TEMPERATURE AND MOISTURE

- Touch the patient's abdomen—are they hot or cold to the touch? Temperature gives you a good indication of whether a person is hyperthermic or hypothermic, and to what degree.
- Is their skin dry or sweaty (clammy)? Excessive moisture can indicate sweating associated with exercise or a fever, and can be associated with anxiety, shock, or an acute myocardial infarction (heart attack).

PUPIL SIZE AND REACTION TO LIGHT

Our pupils are extremely sensitive to changes in light and their reaction to these changes are good indicators of how well a person's brain is functioning. In a healthy person, their pupils should be PERRL: Pupils Equal, Round, and Reactive to Light.

- Look at both of your patient's pupils—are they equal in size?
- Are they both round?
- Use a light source such as a penlight or headlamp and swipe it past your patient's eyes—do both pupils contract immediately and equally?
- If your patient is awake and alert, ask them to keep their head still and track your finger with their eyes as you move the light back and forth and up and down—do both eyes track smoothly and in unison?
    - Unequal pupil size, sluggish or unequal reaction to changing light intensity, and tracking problems can indicate increased intracranial pressure (ICP), nerve damage, drug interference, or other problems.

Note: If your patient's pupils are fixed (they do not react to light at all) and fully dilated (as big as they can get), the situation is extremely serious—brain injury is likely. Evacuate as quickly as possible.

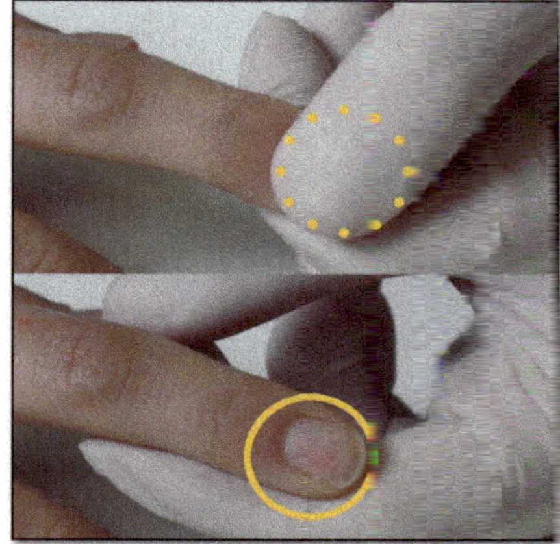

Testing for capillary refill: (top) squeeze the blood out from under a fingernail for five seconds (top), then quickly release the finger and observe how long it takes for the nail bed to pink-up again (bottom)—it should take two seconds or less in an adult and three seconds or less in an infant. (Note: colored nail polish will make this test impossible.)

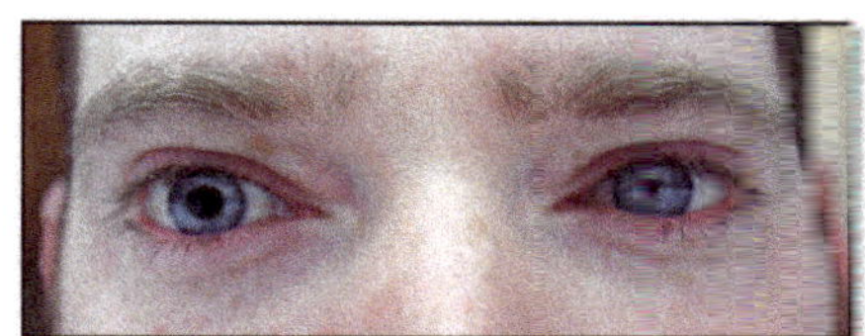

Unequal pupil size means something bad is going on inside your patient's head—even if there are no obvious injuries, unequal pupil size indicates a true emergency and evacuation should begin immediately.

2 PATIENT EXAM

In the Primary Survey you examined your patient, you touched them, albeit briefly and superficially. You held their head still, especially if you suspected significant MOI. You may have performed a jaw thrust, done a quick chunk check to look for deformity and disability, logrolled them to clear their airway, or even moved them out of the way of an environmental hazard. You were looking for life-threats, and you were in a hurry. Now it's time to settle down and go over things an inch at a time.

The detailed physical exam outlined here is designed to help you determine everything that is wrong with your patient, to identify both surface injuries (e.g., contusions, lacerations) as well as underlying musculoskeletal and soft tissue injuries (fractures, tenderness). It is done *efficiently*, *deliberately*, and *systematically*.

The critical first five minutes have passed and your patient is still alive (and, if you're fortunate, stable). What you do in the next 5 – 10 minutes will determine what you need to treat, how you need to treat it, and how (and how quickly) to evacuate your patient. In the numbered list that follows, when we write "examine," we mean with your eyes and your hands.

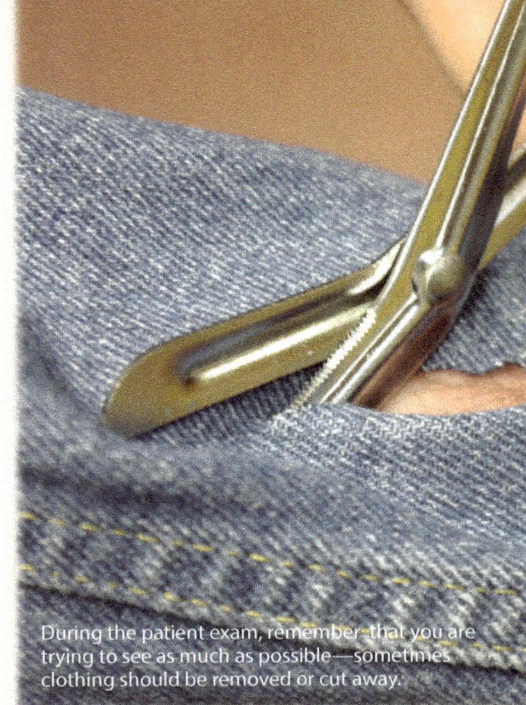
During the patient exam, remember that you are trying to see as much as possible—sometimes clothing should be removed or cut away.

PRINCIPLES OF THE PATIENT EXAM

- **LOOK**
  - Inspection: Be observant—look for bleeding, impaled objects, and deformities.
  - Comparison: compare the symmetry of body parts (arms to arms, legs to legs); if symmetry is compromised, determine why.
- **LISTEN**
  - Is the patient complaining of pain or tenderness? What are their symptoms?
- **FEEL**
  - **Palpation**: palpate the muscles, bones, and joints—is there deformity, crepitation (the sound of grating bone ends and fragments) or tenderness? (See palpation sidebar on the next page for tips on doing this.)
  - **Circulation (C)**: are there pulses in all four extremities?
  - **Sensation (S)**: is there normal sensation (pressure, temperature, pain) in all four extremities?
  - **Movement (M)**: is there normal range of motion in all four extremities?

    Note: These last three points are referred to as a patient's CSMs—get used to hearing the term; you will be checking CSMs regularly.

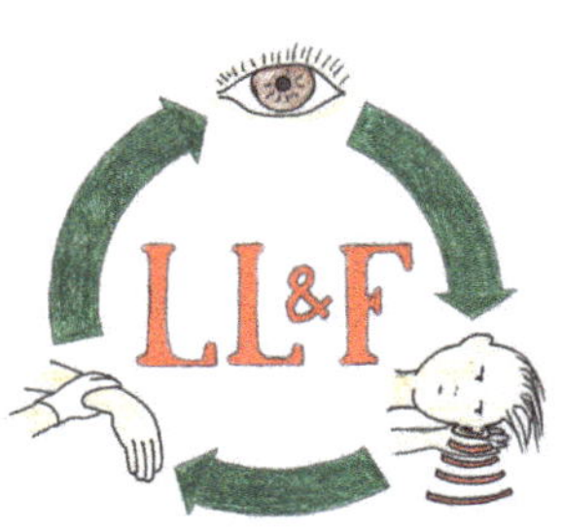

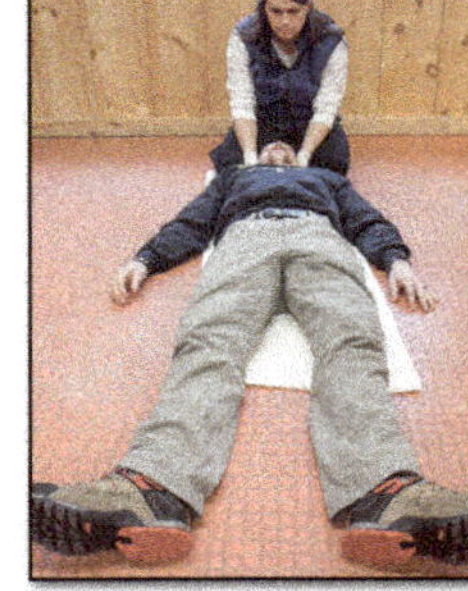

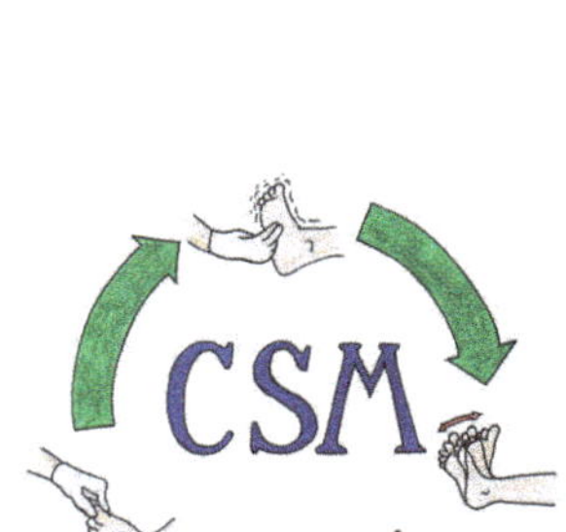

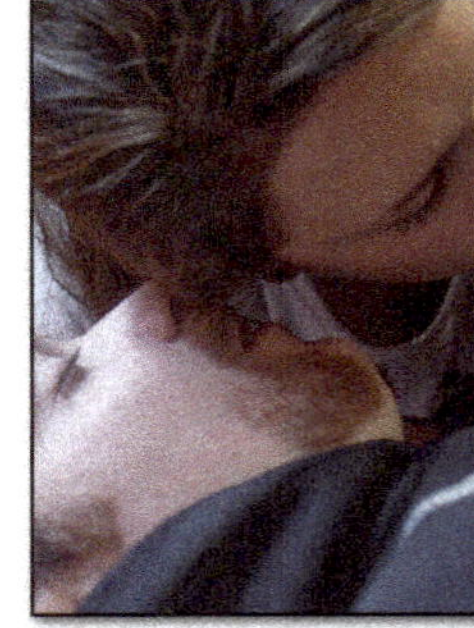

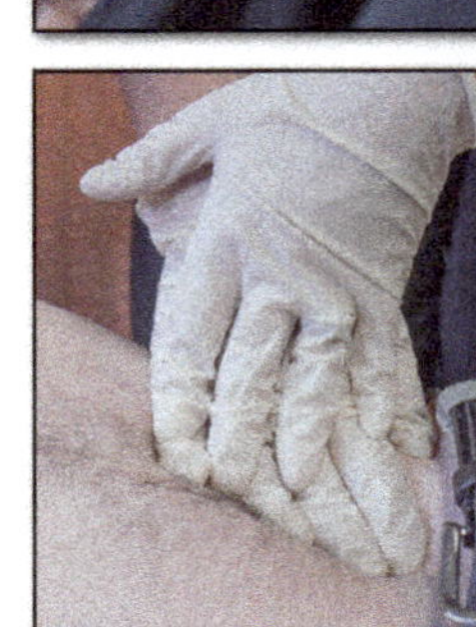

- **THINGS TO REMEMBER**
  - Talk to your patient; explain what you are doing.
  - If you elicit pain, ask the patient to describe it.
    1. Precisely where does it hurt?
    2. What kind of pain is it (dull, sharp, etc.)?
    3. How much does it hurt (0 – 10 scale with 0 being no pain and 10 being the worst pain they have ever experienced)?
  - Move the patient only as much as is necessary to complete the exam—needless movement of the head, neck, spine, or limbs can cause further injury.
  - Conduct the patient exam in the order described.

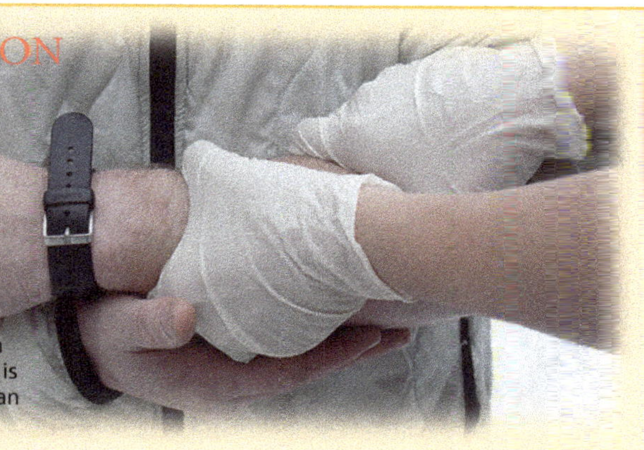

THE NOT-SO-GENTLE ART OF PALPATION

- Use light-to-firm pressure (like a good massage).
- Assess everything from soft tissue to bony structures.
- If unconscious, monitor for pain response.
- Evaluating levels of pain is part of the assessment.
- Hands, fingers, and finger tips are three different tools to use during assessment.

Good palpation is not difficult, but it is as much an art as a science. Use enough pressure—remember, you are trying to identify broken bones. Squeezing hard is necessary, and causing momentary pain is diagnostically useful. If working on an appendage, squeeze circumferentially so you do not risk additional deformity.

1 HEAD

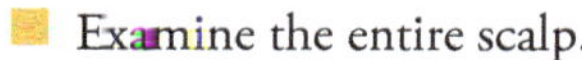

- Examine the entire scalp.
- Examine the face, including the facial bones: cheeks, jaw, and the area around the eyes.
- Examine the ears, nose, and mouth (including teeth). If you know or suspect significant MOI for trauma, look for bruising behind the ears (Battle's Sign) and around the eyes (raccoon eyes), and for clear fluid (cerebral spinal fluid—CFS) coming from the ears or nose—any of these things indicate serious head injury (and a life-threatening emergency).

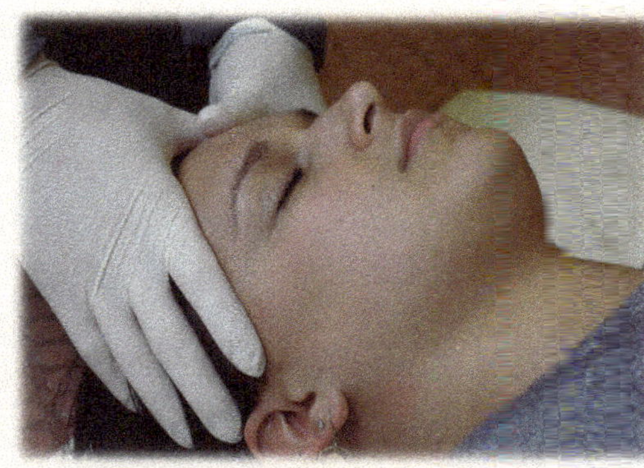

2 NECK

- Examine the cervical spine and trachea.
  - With your fingers, walk the spine from the base of the skull to between the shoulder blades, palpating for tenderness—if you find it, you must immobilize your patient's C-spine with a cervical collar.
  - When you examine the trachea, look for two things: 1) Note if the trachea has shifted from its normal, center-line position (called tracheal shift) and, 2) look to see if either jugular vein is swollen, called jugular vein distension (JVD)—either or both of these signs often point to lung damage.

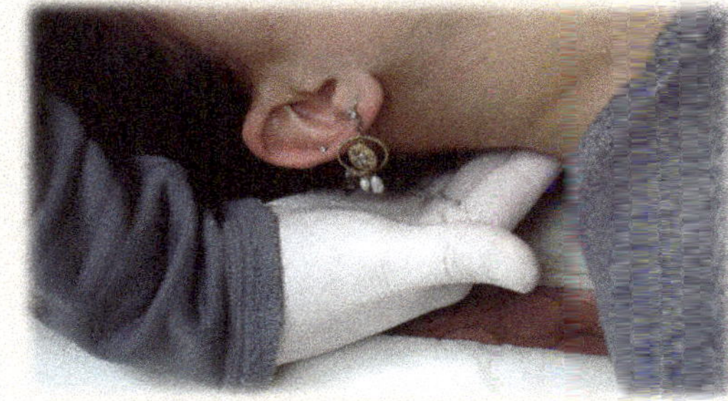

3 SHOULDER

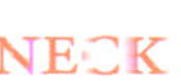

- Examine the shoulders by compressing each one in your hands—palpate for tenderness and deformity.

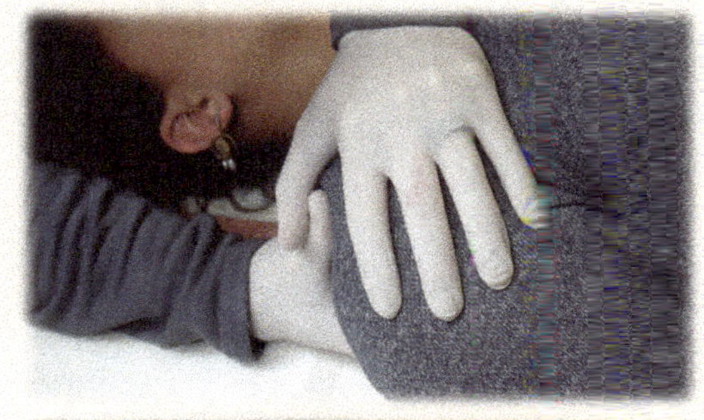

4 CHEST

- Examine the clavicles.
- Examine and gently compress the rib cage.
  - Severely broken ribs (e.g., a flail chest), puncture wounds involving the lungs, holes with air moving in and out, and other major injuries will need immediate attention.

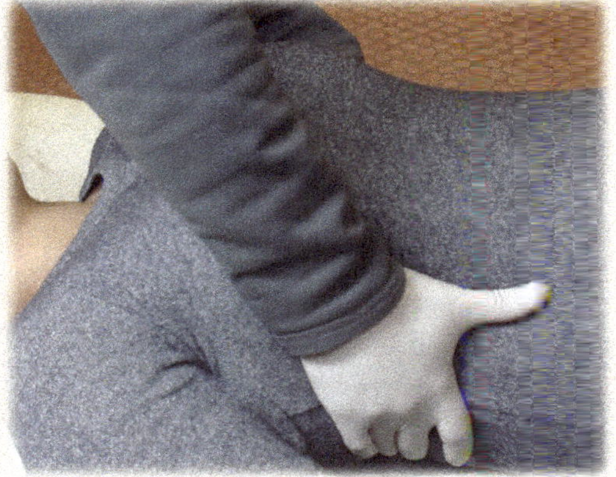

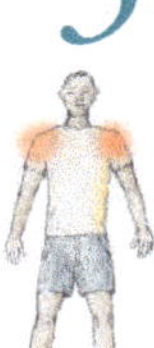
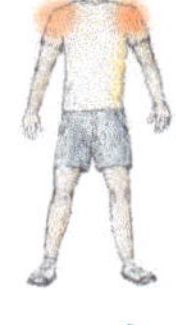
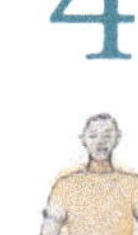

ABDOMEN

5

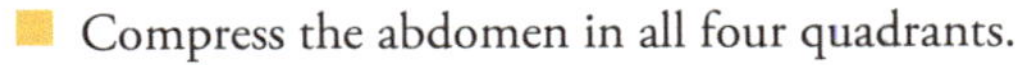

- Compress the abdomen in all four quadrants.
  - Push hard enough to determine if there is any rigidity (which can indicate internal bleeding).
  - If your palpation elicits pain, note its type (e.g., sharp, dull, etc.) and position—there may be severe internal damage or a problem such as appendicitis.

PELVIS

6

- Compress the pelvis both front-to-back (like opening a book) and outside-to-inside (like closing a book).
  - If you find instability during either of these tests, it indicates a pelvic fracture, which is potentially extremely serious—the pelvic girdle is laced with major blood vessels and severe internal bleeding is a real risk. The pelvis will have to be immobilized.

  Note: An unstable pelvis should be moved only once; otherwise you risk damage to its vast vasculature.

LEGS

7

- Palpate both legs from hip to ankle (there is a lot of muscle here, so squeeze hard).
- Check for Circulation, Sensation, and Movement (CSMs).
  - Check for a pedal (on the foot) pulse and capillary refill (toes).
  - If the patient is conscious, grab a toe and ask the patient to identify it.
  - Flex the knees and ankles, looking and feeling for abnormal movement or crepitation—stop if you elicit pain.

ARMS

8

- Palpate both arms from shoulder to wrist.
- Check for Circulation, Sensation, and Movement (CSMs).
  - Check for a radial pulse (at the wrist) and capillary refill (fingers).
  - Flex the elbows and wrists.

BACK

9

- Palpate the spine along the length of the back from the base of the skull to the coccyx (tail bone), walking your fingers, feeling for tenderness and deformity.
- You may need to logroll your patient to gain access to their back.
  - If there is significant MOI, you must keep the entire spine in line and immobilized while you perform the log roll—this may take more than one person.
  - If you find any injuries, logroll the patient onto their uninjured side to avoid further injury and pain.

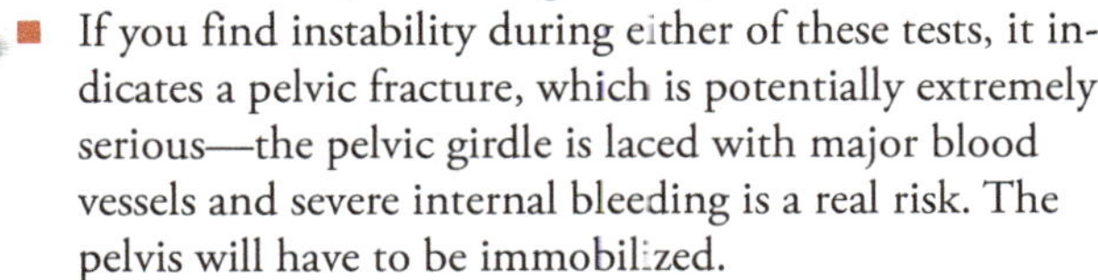

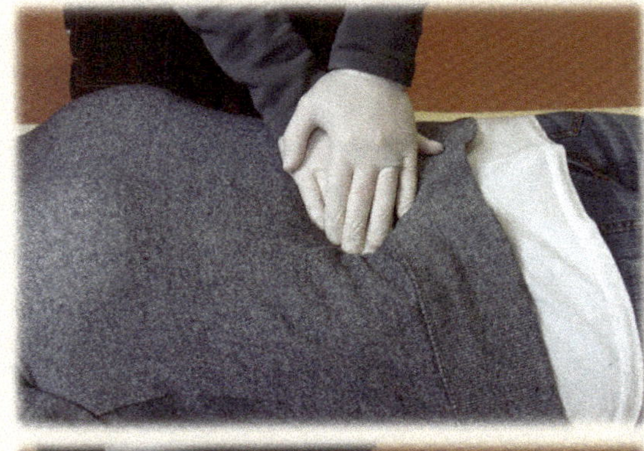

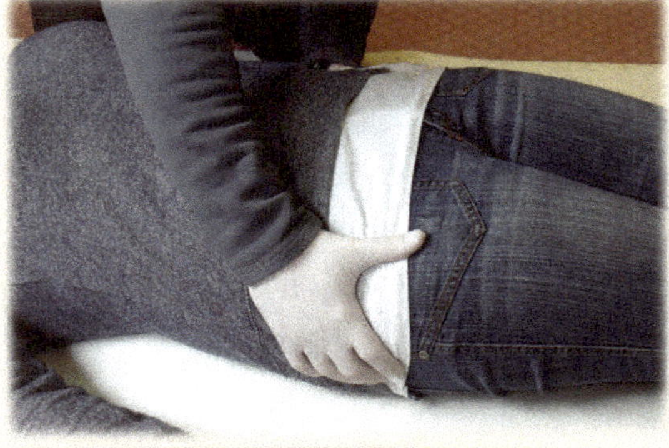

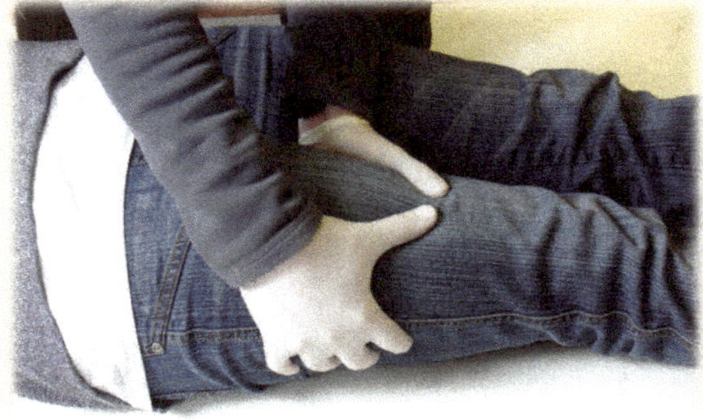

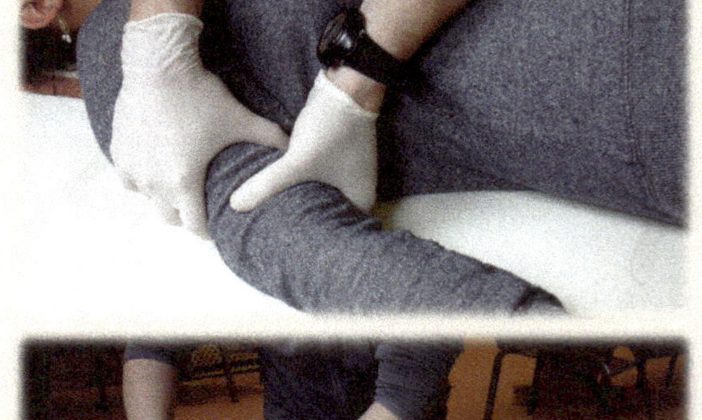

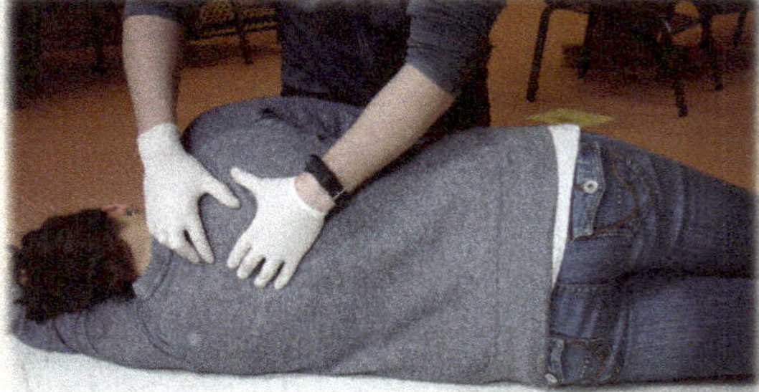

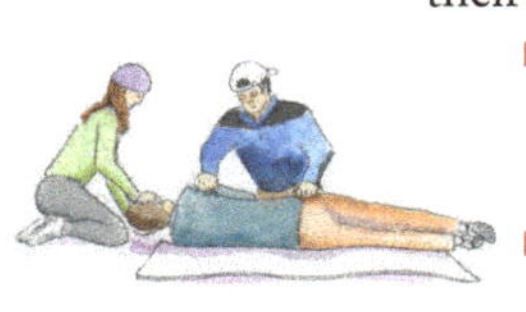

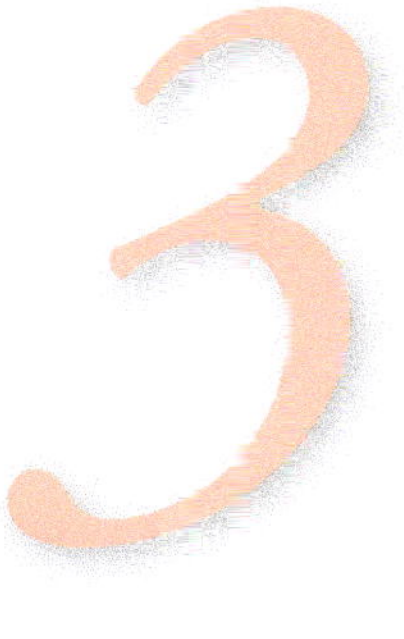

3 AMPLE HISTORY

For anyone having a medical emergency, their past medical history—both the distant past and the recent past—as well as their recent behavior and actions, can have great bearing on the situation and help you make both diagnostic and treatment decisions. To remind us of the appropriate questions to ask our patients, we use the simple mnemonic *AMPLE*. Talk to your patient, or others in the group, to gather the following information.

A: ALLERGIES

- Is your patient allergic to any medications or foods?
- Do they have any environmental allergies (e.g., bee stings)?
- If they have any allergies, find out what happens when they have a reaction, and what treatment should take place (Do they have an EpiPen?).

M: MEDICATIONS

- Is your patient taking any prescription or over-the-counter (OTC) medications? It's easy to forget these.
- If so, what, how much, how often, and when did they take it last?
- What happens if they don't take their med?

P: PAST MEDICAL HISTORY

- Has your patient ever had any previous major medical problems or surgeries? If so, what and when?
- Have they ever been hospitalized overnight? If so, for what and when?
- Is there any recent or past injury or illness that could contribute to the current problem? If so, what and when?

L: LAST IN, LAST OUT

- When did your patient last eat and drink? What did they last eat and drink? And how much?
- When did they last have a bowel movement and void their bladder?

E: EVENTS LEADING UP TO THE ACCIDENT/ILLNESS

- What led up to the accident or illness? (What was the specific trigger?)
- What occurred prior to the event? (This may give you valuable insight into peripheral things—e.g., a 15-mile hike in a cold rain without much to eat may account for someone seeming "out of it" and point to hypothermia).

Ask your patient to name the thing that is bothering them the most.

- Sometimes it's obvious—that broken femur really hurts.
- Sometimes it's not obvious; in fact, it may take you by surprise—your patient may have a dramatic injury (e.g., a compound fracture), but when asked, they say, "I have the worst headache that I've ever experienced." Pay attention to this—it may be the most medically relevant thing going on!

EXPLORE THE HISTORY OF PRESENT ILLNESS (HPI)

The next set of questions seeks to gather all the information about the patient's current illness or injury, specifically as it relates to the pain they are feeling.

- **TIMING**
  - **Onset:** *When did the pain begin?* The timing of the onset of pain gives you an idea of how serious the problem may be.
  - **Duration:** *How long have you had the pain?* Someone with an acute onset of pain or a sudden worsening of pain is much more concerning than someone who has had pain for the past several days or weeks and is just not getting any better.
  - **Frequency:** *How often does it occur and how long does it last?* The nature of the pain's frequency can give you valuable clues regarding its cause—especially if the chief complaint is vague or the injury/illness isn't obvious.

- **LOCATION**
  - *Where does it hurt?* Have them verbalize this and point to the location (or locations) if possible.
  - Sometimes the places the patient tells you they feel pain are not obvious or consistent with their apparent injuries.

- **DESCRIPTION and SEVERITY**
  - **Quality:** *What does the pain feel like?* Let the patient describe it in words—you're looking for adjectives like sharp, dull, throbbing, etc. If they have trouble, ask the question in different ways (but don't lead them).
  - **Quantity:** *How bad is the pain?* Ask them to rate the pain on a 0 – 10 scale, with 0 being no pain at all and 10 being the worst pain they have ever felt.

- **EXACERBATION and RELIEF**
  - *What makes the pain feel worse?*
  - *What makes the pain feel better?*

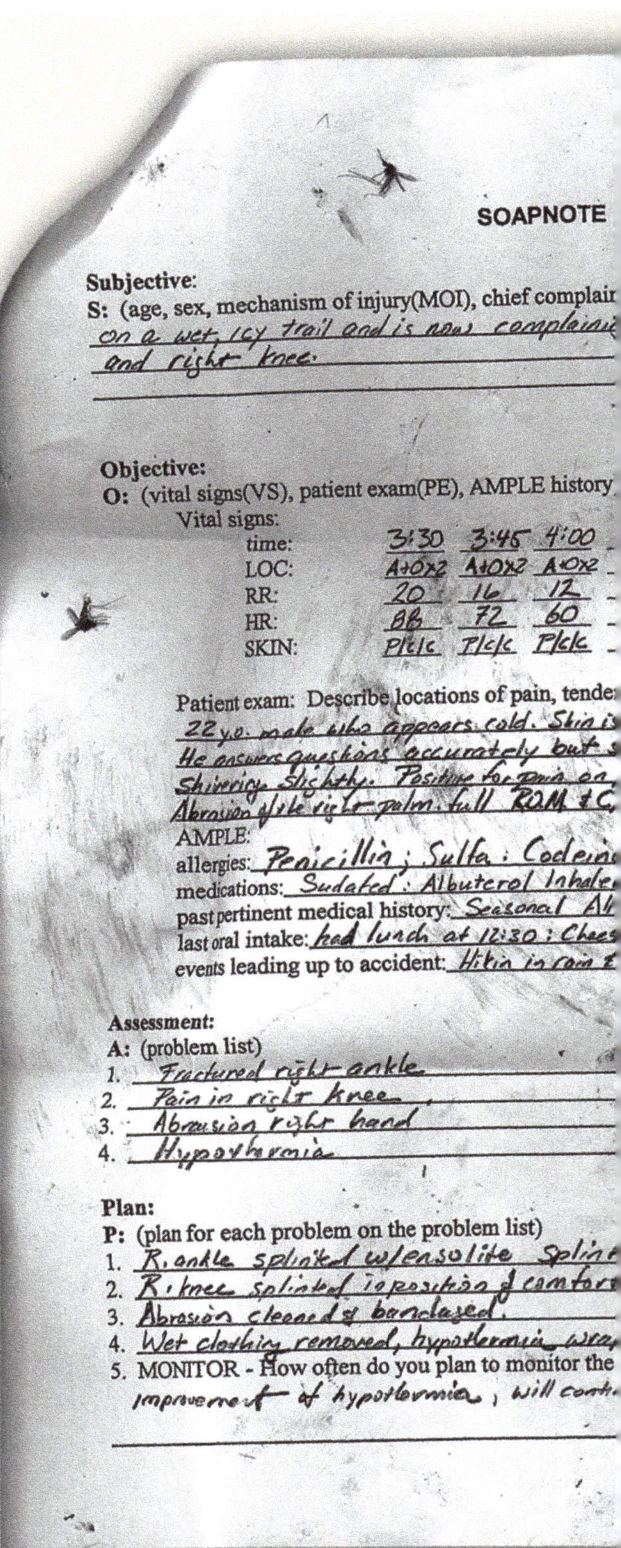

SOAPNOTE

Subjective:
S: (age, sex, mechanism of injury(MOI), chief complain
on a wet, icy trail and is now complainin
and right knee.

Objective:
O: (vital signs(VS), patient exam(PE), AMPLE history
Vital signs:

time:	3:30	3:45	4:00
LOC:	A+O×2	A+O×2	A+O×2
RR:	20	16	12
HR:	88	72	60
SKIN:	P/c/c	P/c/c	P/c/c

Patient exam: Describe locations of pain, tender
22 y.o. male who appears cold. Skin is
He answers questions accurately but s
Shivering slightly. Positive for pain on
Abrasion of the right palm. Full ROM & C
AMPLE:
allergies: _Penicillin; Sulfa; Codein_
medications: _Sudafed; Albuterol Inhaler_
past pertinent medical history: _Seasonal All_
last oral intake: _had lunch at 12:30; Chees_
events leading up to accident: _Hikin in rain t_

Assessment:
A: (problem list)
1. _Fractured right ankle_
2. _Pain in right knee_
3. _Abrasion right hand_
4. _Hypothermia_

Plan:
P: (plan for each problem on the problem list)
1. _R. ankle splinted w/ensolite splint_
2. _R. knee splinted i position of comfort_
3. _Abrasion cleaned & bandaged._
4. _Wet clothing removed, hypothermia wrap_
5. MONITOR - How often do you plan to monitor the
improvement of hypothermia, will cont.

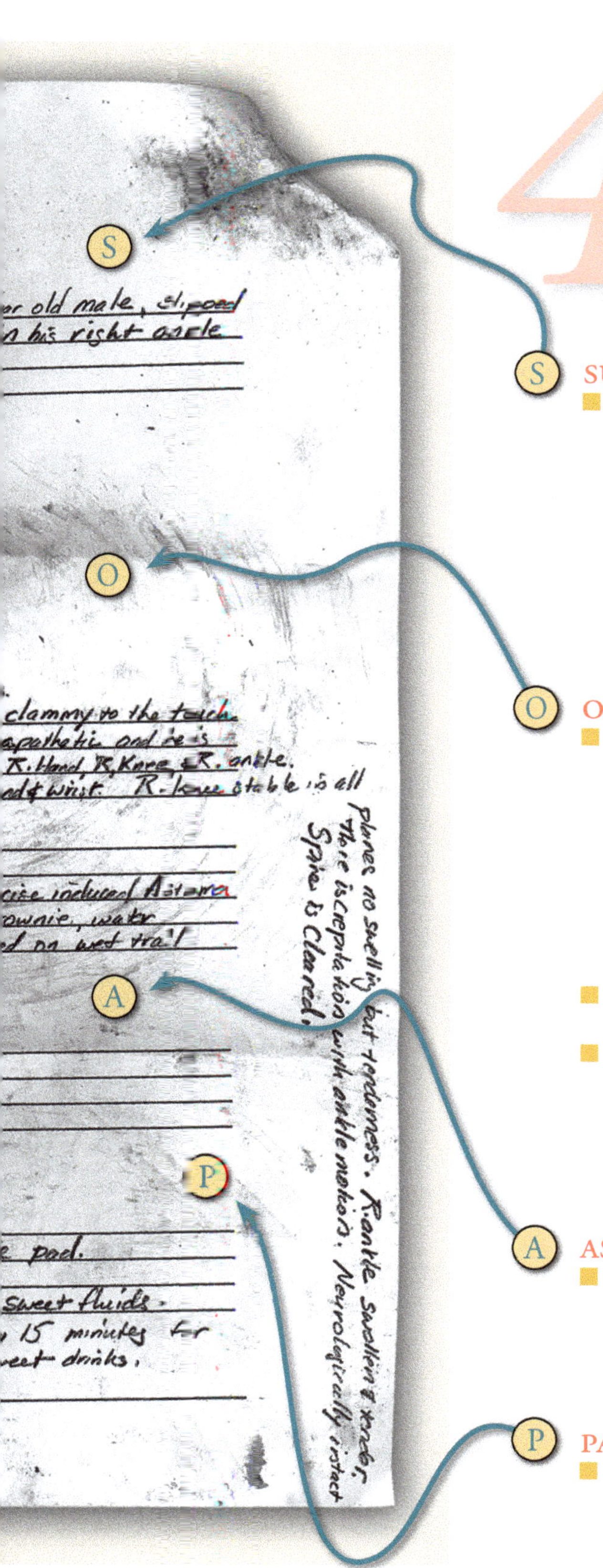

4 SOAPnote

At this point in the patient assessment system, you have obtained a fair amount of information that needs to be organized and recorded—it's time for the wilderness version of the ubiquitous medical chart. But unlike on TV, where a clipboard dangles from the foot of every hospital bed, out here in the howling wilderness we may need to improvise by scribbling on a scrap of paper, the back of a map, or even a bandanna. So, what's a SOAPnote? It's a simple record of the following info—and it always travels with the patient.

SUBJECTIVE INFORMATION

- This is the information you get from the patient or others in the group.
  - The age and gender of the patient
  - The Mechanism of Injury (MOI)—what happened? "I was running from a bee and tripped over that log"
  - The Chief Complaint (CC—what hurts?) "My forearm hurts bad"
  - The History of Present Illness (HPI, see previous page) e.g., (O) it began when she fell and has been steady since; (P) support makes it feel better; motion makes it worse; (Q) it is described as "sharp"; (R) it does not radiate; (S) on the pain scale it is 4/10; (T) it hurts pretty much all the time

OBJECTIVE INFORMATION

- The baseline vital signs (first set), and subsequent sets (every 5 – 15 minutes depending on circumstances)
  - Level of Consciousness (LOC)
  - Respiratory Rate and effort (RR)
  - Blood Pressure (BP)—remember, without a BP cuff, you will have to estimate BP based on which pulses are present: carotid, radial, medial, or femoral
  - Skin color, temperature, and moisture (SCTM)
  - Pupils equal, round, and reactive to light (PERRL)
- The results of the Patient Exam (PE)
  - Locations of pain, tenderness, and injuries
- AMPLE History
  - Allergies
  - Medications
  - Past Medical History
  - Last oral intake, last bowel movement and bladder void
  - Events leading up to the accident/illness

ASSESSMENT

- This is where you write down what you think is wrong—your problem list. Using the example from the HPI (above):
  - The MOI and CC indicate a possible broken forearm
  - Possible dehydration
  - Possible allergy to bee sting

PATIENT CARE PLAN

- This is where you outline your treatment and evacuation plans
  - Splint lower right arm; check CSMs distal to splint
  - Hydrate and feed patient
  - Evacuate to definitive care by walking, if PT is able
  - Continue to monitor vitals and CSMs every 15 minutes

Patient lifting and moving techniques

At some point during any backcountry rescue, the patient will have to move themselves or be moved by others. Unless scene safety or patient/rescuer safety is a concern, the patient should be kept lying still until the extent of their injuries is determined.

WHEN TO MOVE YOUR PATIENT FIRST

In situations when objective hazards pose an immediate danger, consider moving your patient before beginning your assessment. These hazards include, but are not limited to, the following:

- Cold water
- Rockfall
- Icefall
- Avalanche
- Proximity to a drop off

Other reasons to move the patient early may include:

- To assure and maintain a patent airway
- To better splint injuries or stabilize the spine
- To get the patient off the cold ground or protect them from the environment

The cardinal rule of moving hurt people...

It is always safe to move someone from the position of injury to the position of function.

...but

Avoid flexion of the head and neck.

- May move the head & neck into neutral position, but do not flex forward.

Avoid rotation of the pelvis out of alignment with the shoulders.

- May line up the shoulders and the pelvis, but do not rotate out of alignment.

POSITIONS:

SUPINE: Lying flat on your back.

PRONE: Lying flat on your chest & stomach.

RECOVERY POSITION: 3/4 prone position used to maintain the airway.

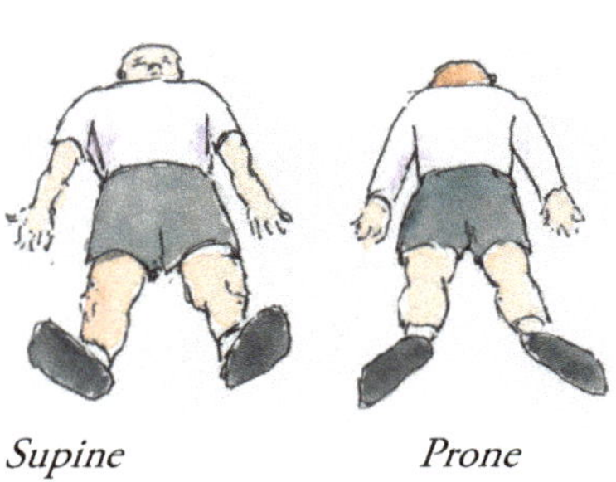

Supine   *Prone*

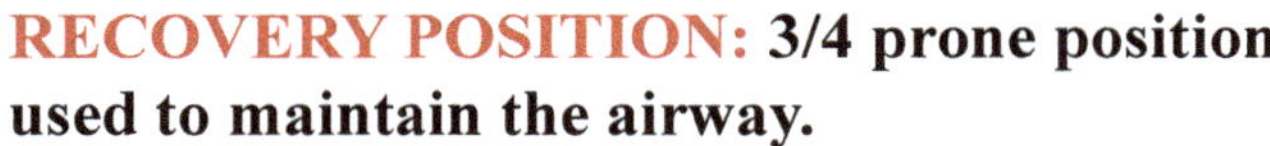

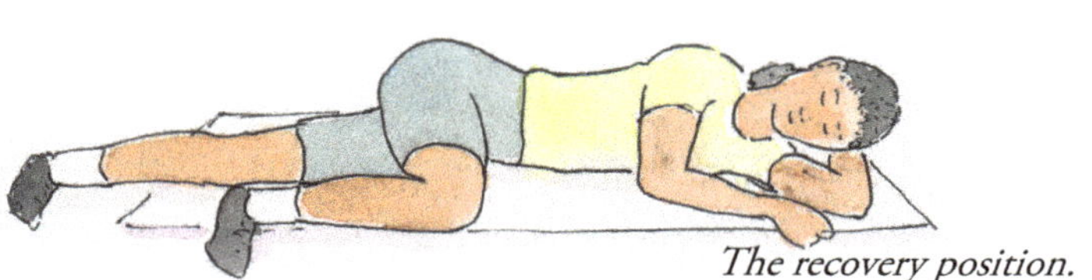

The recovery position.

When lifting, use proper body mechanics:

- Lift with your legs.
- Keep your back straight and your butt down.
- Try not to overreach or twist.
- Keep the weight as close to your body as possible.
- Use assists such as blankets, rain flies, or ensolite pads.

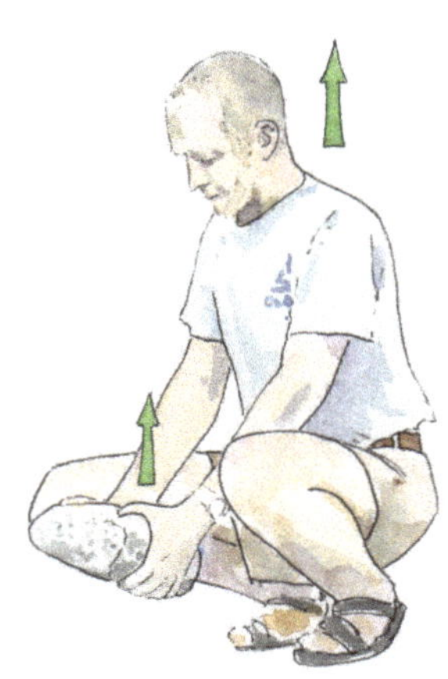

- Know your own strength and physical limitations—do not put yourself (or your back) in danger.
- Work together—many hands make light work.
- Plan your moves.
- The person at the patient's head always directs the team's movements (counting "one, two, three, lift" is the usual method)
- Logroll the patient to assess their spine or get them onto a pad.
    - Keep their head, shoulders, and pelvis in line while rolling them onto their side (avoid rolling them onto an injury, eg , broken ribs).
    - Although one person can do it, two or three make it much easier
- Body Elevation and Movement (BEAM).
    - Use many hands (5 – 7 people) to support the body and spine.
    - With good spinal immobilization, you can move the patient short distances (<30 feet).

LIFTING AND MOVING:

LOG ROLL: **Keeping the head, shoulders, and pelvis in line, roll the patient onto their side.**

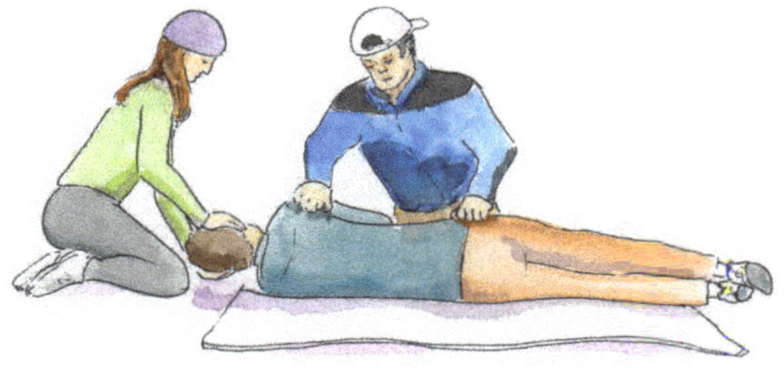

DRAGS: **Drag them by their clothing or on a pad. ONE-PERSON: Roll onto a pad to drag.**

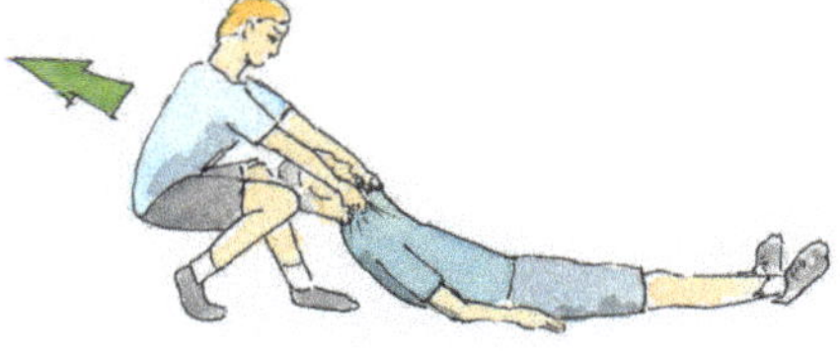

TWO-PERSON: May be able to carry or drag.

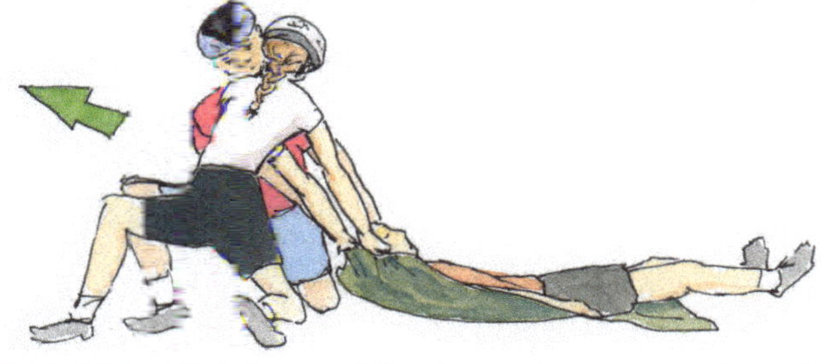

MANY PERSONS: Much easier, many hands on.

MOVE AS A UNIT: With many hands on, move the person as if they were frozen stiff.

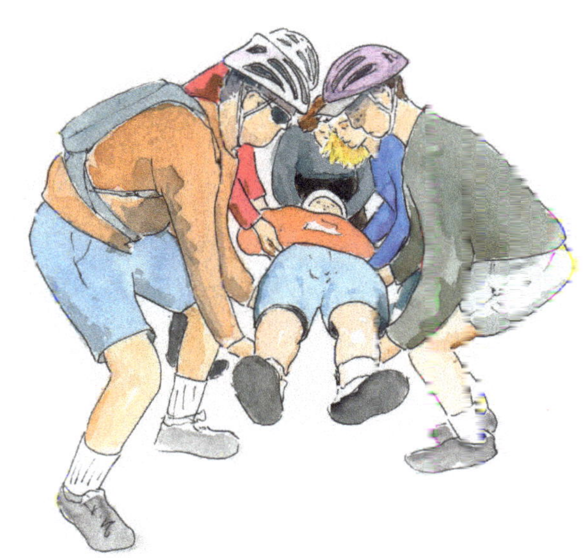

Some types of improvised litters

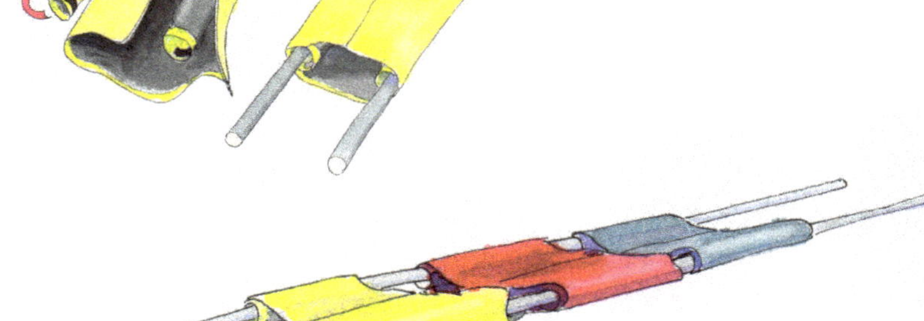

Turn sleeve inside the jackets and be sure to tuck in hood or any adjustment strings that might dangle down and catch on objects on the trail.

Tarp and poles 1

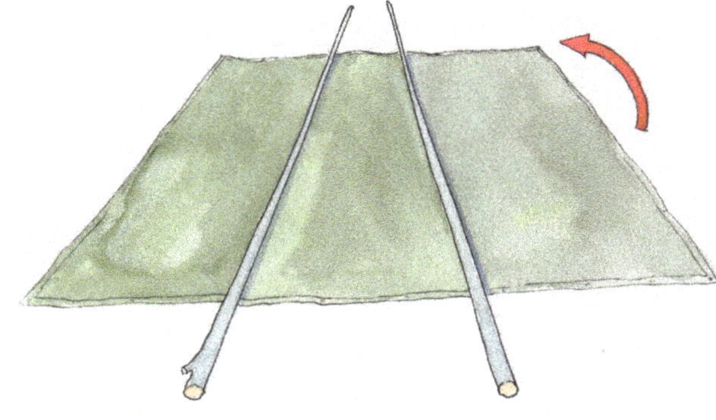

Tarp and poles 2

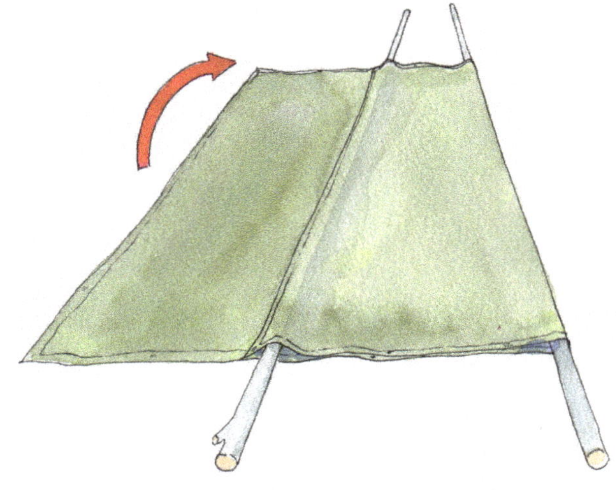

Tarp and poles 3

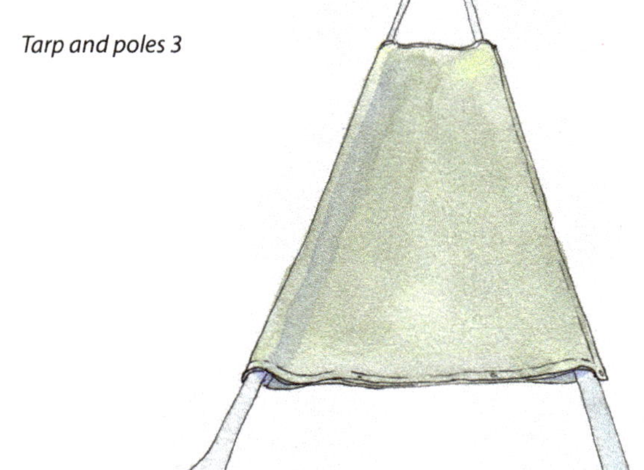

Rectangle with rope

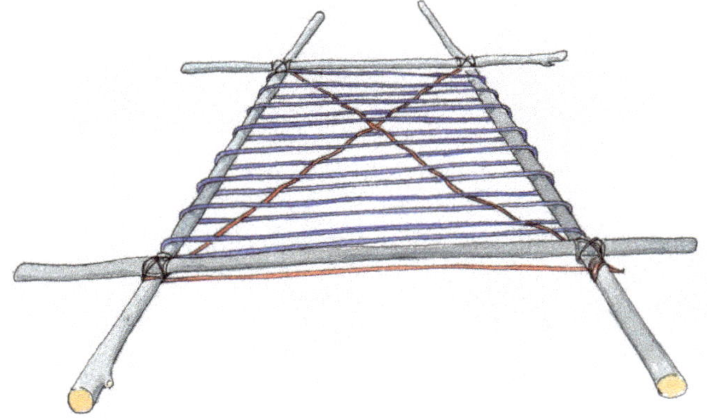

Ladder litter

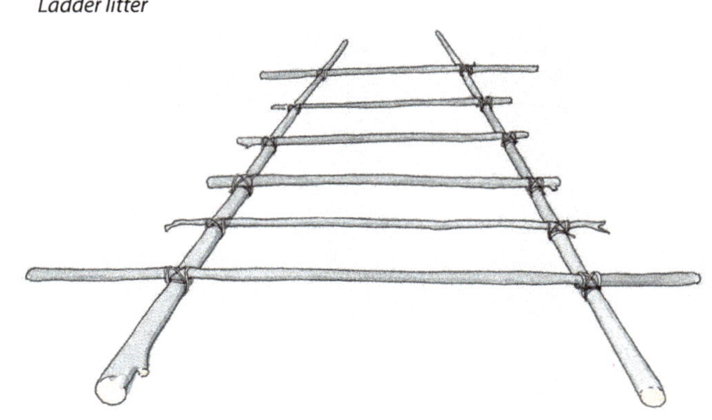

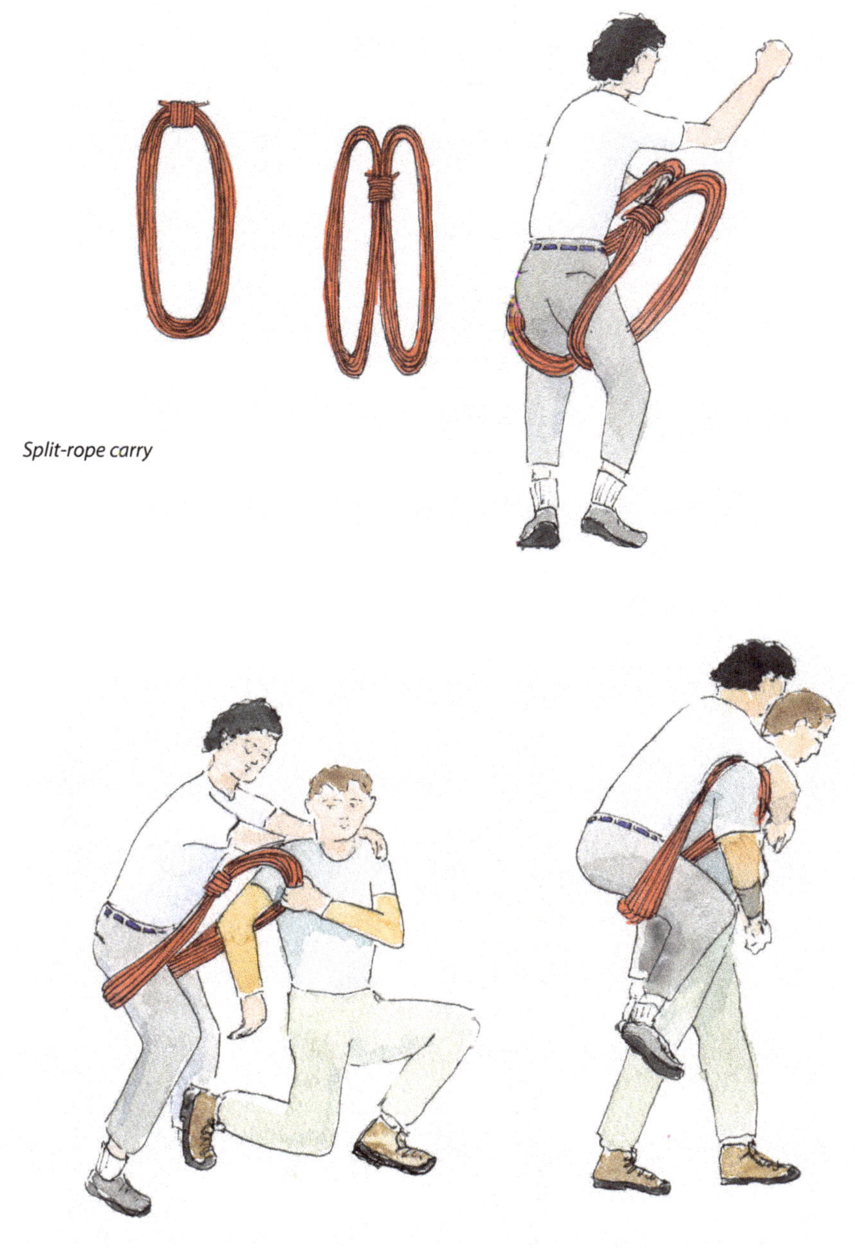

Split-rope carry

RESCUE PLAN

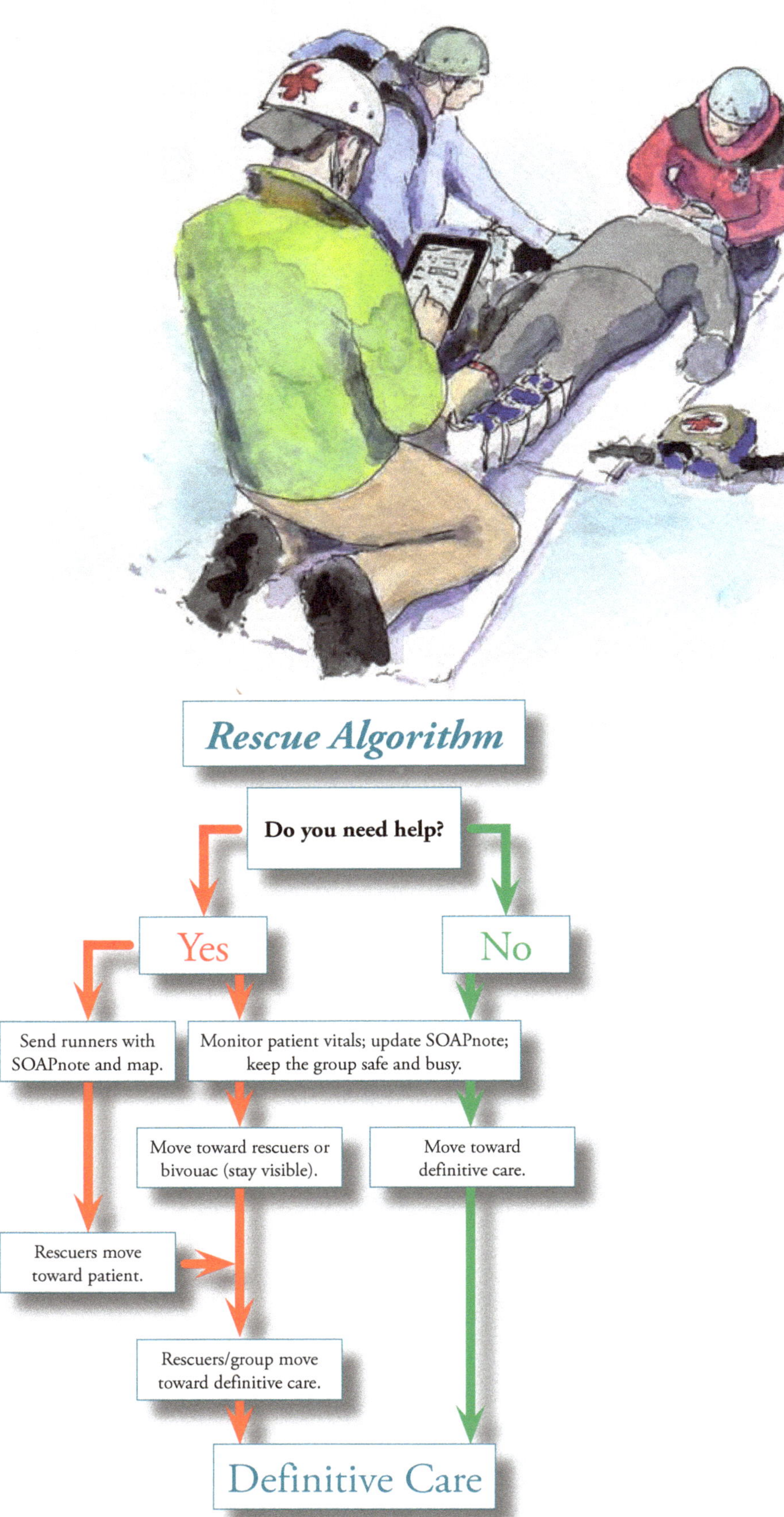

Congratulations!

1. The scene is safe.
2. The primary and secondary surveys are done.
3. You've checked on the group and ensured that they are comfortable, safe, and busy.
4. You've examined the patient from head to toe and taken their vital signs.
5. You've interviewed them, diagnosed and field-treated their injuries, and recorded everything on a SOAPnote.
6. Now you are ready to **consider the rescue options.**

Don't evacuate

Evacuate

Initiate rescue

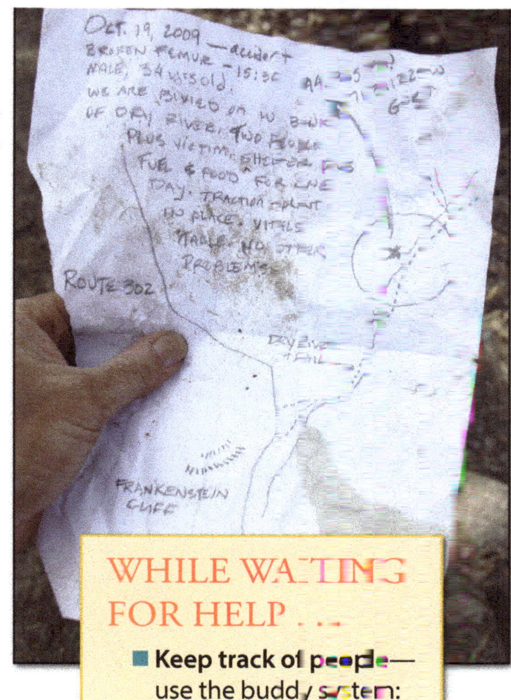

Don't evacuate: go—green light

You don't need to evacuate your patient if their problem is minor enough that they will recover quickly and can continue on their own.

- Minor musculoskeletal injuries (e.g., ankle strain, jammed finger)
- Minor soft tissue injuries (e.g., contusions, minor burns, muscle strain)
- Minor environmental emergencies (e.g., mild hypothermia or heat exhaustion)
- Resolved medical issues (e.g., hypoglycemia, a bee sting that doesn't evolve into anaphylaxis)
- If you decide evacuation is not necessary, be sure that the patient and each person in the group will remain safe until the group can carry on.
    - Ensure that they have shelter, food, water, etc.
    - If a bivouac is necessary, make sure that the group knows how to do this, or that you help them (especially important if you are going to leave the group on their own for any length of time).

Evacuate: yield—what are your options?

If your patient's injury or illness is severe enough that they need further treatment by a physician, you must evacuate—which raises additional questions, including two big ones:

1. Can you perform a self-rescue?
2. Do you need help (see below)?

- If you decide to self-rescue, you must:
    - Know how to do it.
    - Know when you can start and how long it will take.
    - Have the necessary personnel, skills, and equipment. For instance, can the patient walk with assistance? Will you improvise a litter, and are there enough people to carry it?
    - Do you know how to lift and carry the patient, if necessary (see the lifting and moving section on the next page)?
    - Can you be certain that the patient and each person in the group will remain safe until you get everyone out?

Initiate rescue: stop—you need help

Your patient needs definitive care, and you don't have the personnel, skills, or equipment to effect a rescue on your own. Okay...

- How will you get help? Via runners (send two people, if possible), cell phone, radio, or a combination?
- If you send runners, what will they have with them?
    - SOAPnote (also, begin a new SOAPnote for your patient after the runners leave)
    - A list of the people in your group
    - A map with your location (GPS coordinates), landmarks and the time you left clearly marked
    - Bivouac equipment, and food, if necessary
    - Communication devices, if available
- Will you bivouac and wait for the rescuers or move toward the rescuers as they respond to the scene? (See algorithm at left).
- What will you do to keep your patient stabilized while you wait or move?
- What things can you do to keep the group safe—sheltered, fed, hydrated, and busy?

WHILE WAITING FOR HELP . . .

- **Keep track of people**—use the buddy system: no one wanders off alone.
- **Keep everyone busy** (e.g., gathering wood, making shelters cooking, rubbing each other's feet, etc.
- **Create shelter for** everyone in the best location (e.g., safe, access to water, fuel for fire, etc.).
- **Get water** or melt snow and make something warm to drink (purify the water first).
- If food is available, **make a meal and eat.**
- **Keep spirits up,** be positive, reassure, make sure everyone has something to do.
- **Create light and warmth**—build a fire; hypo-wrap if necessary.
- **Make yourselves big** and easy to find: fire (light and smoke), whistle (three blasts), survey tape (string it everywhere to lead rescuers to you).
- **Continuously monitor** your patient.
- **Continuously monitor** everyone else in the group.

34

BODY SYSTEMS OVERVIEW

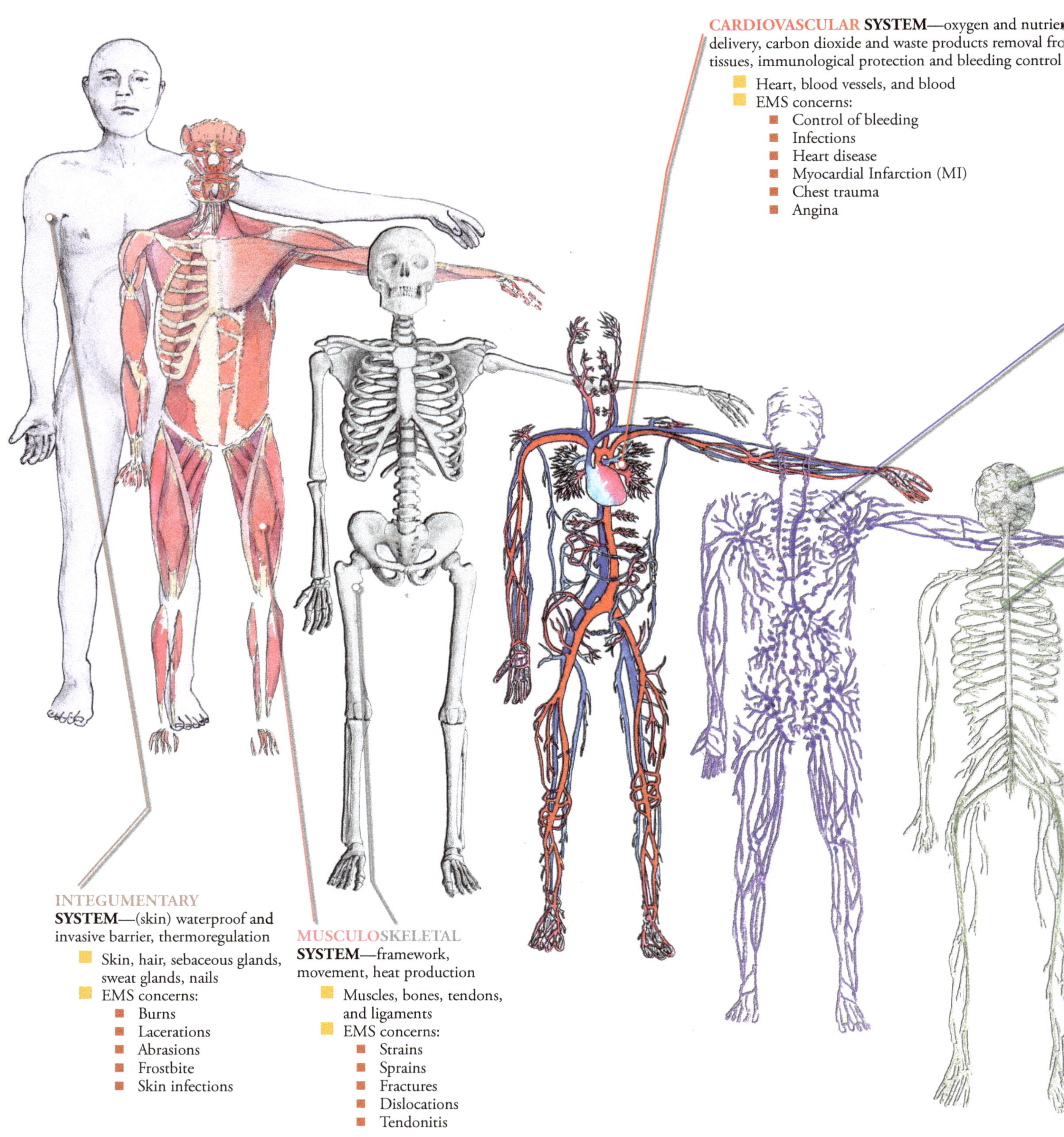

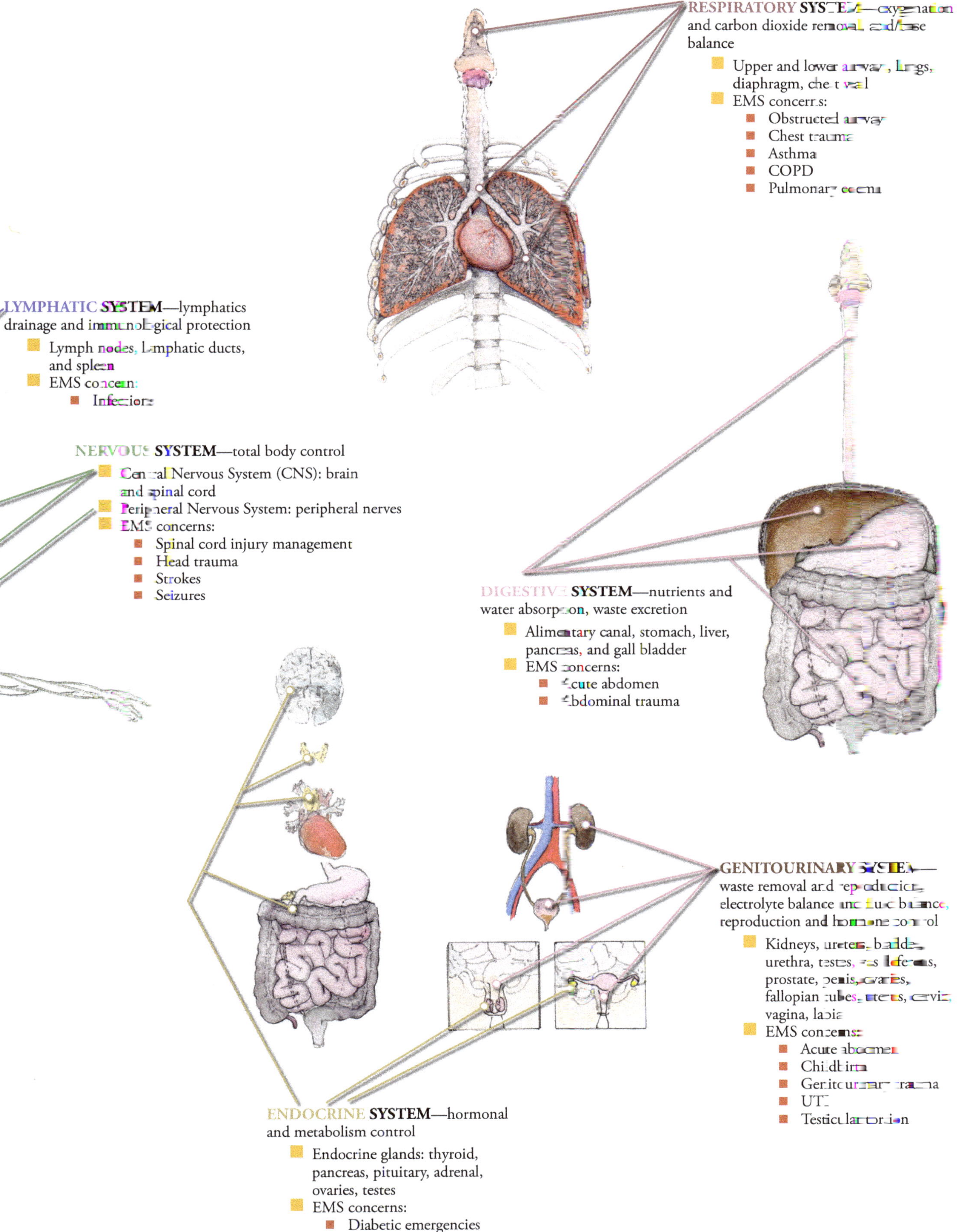

RESPIRATORY SYSTEM—oxygenation and carbon dioxide removal, acid/base balance
Upper and lower airway, lungs, diaphragm, chest wall
EMS concerns:
Obstructed airway
Chest trauma
Asthma
COPD
Pulmonary edema

LYMPHATIC SYSTEM—lymphatics drainage and immunological protection
Lymph nodes, lymphatic ducts, and spleen
EMS concern:
Infection

NERVOUS SYSTEM—total body control
Central Nervous System (CNS): brain and spinal cord
Peripheral Nervous System: peripheral nerves
EMS concerns:
Spinal cord injury management
Head trauma
Strokes
Seizures

DIGESTIVE SYSTEM—nutrients and water absorption, waste excretion
Alimentary canal, stomach, liver, pancreas, and gall bladder
EMS concerns:
Acute abdomen
Abdominal trauma

GENITOURINARY SYSTEM—waste removal and reproduction, electrolyte balance and fluid balance, reproduction and hormone control
Kidneys, ureters, bladder, urethra, testes, vas deferens, prostate, penis, ovaries, fallopian tubes, uterus, cervix, vagina, labia
EMS concerns:
Acute abdomen
Childbirth
Genitourinary trauma
UTI
Testicular torsion

ENDOCRINE SYSTEM—hormonal and metabolism control
Endocrine glands: thyroid, pancreas, pituitary, adrenal, ovaries, testes
EMS concerns:
Diabetic emergencies

The Cardiovascular System

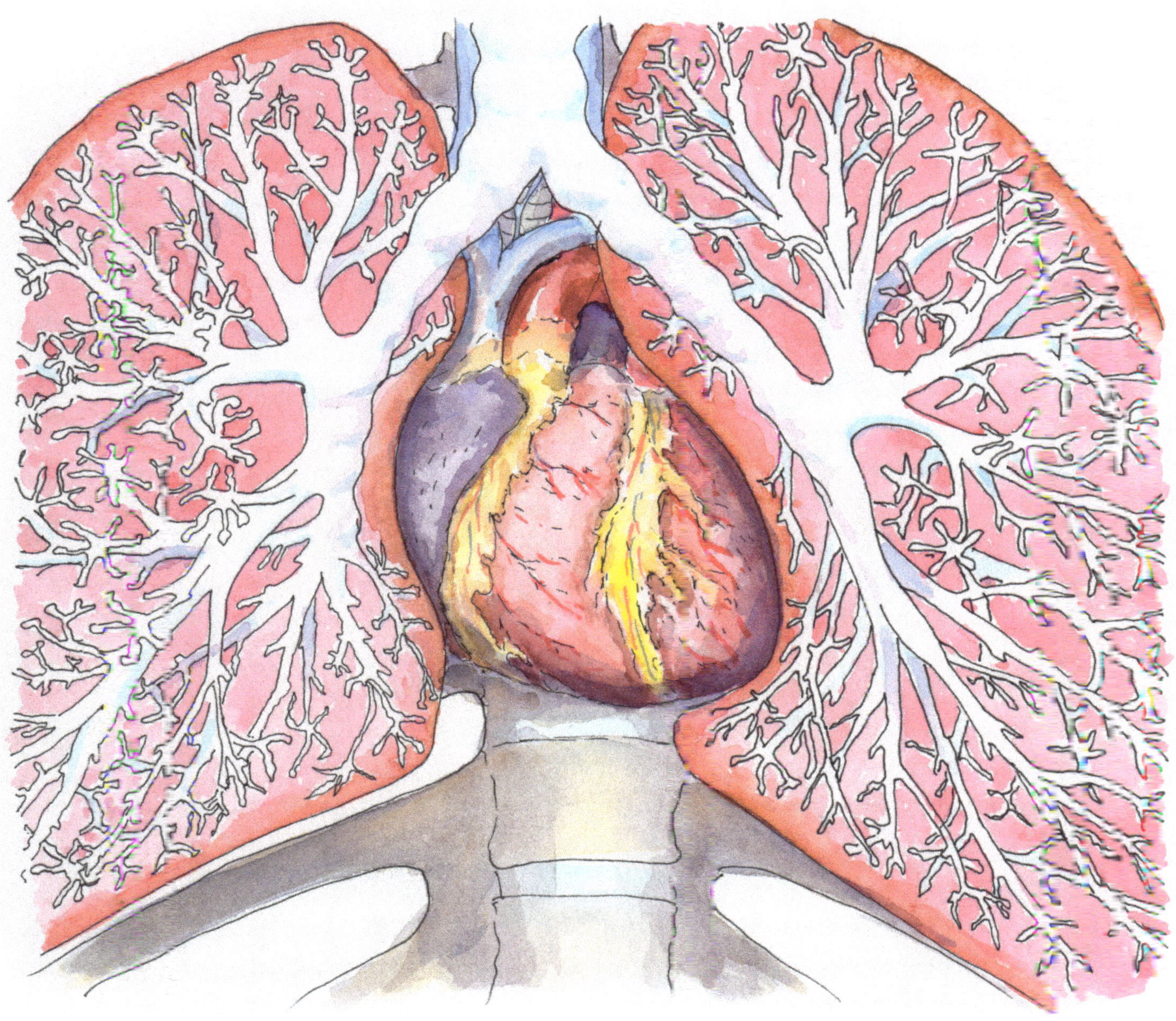

Chest Anatomy

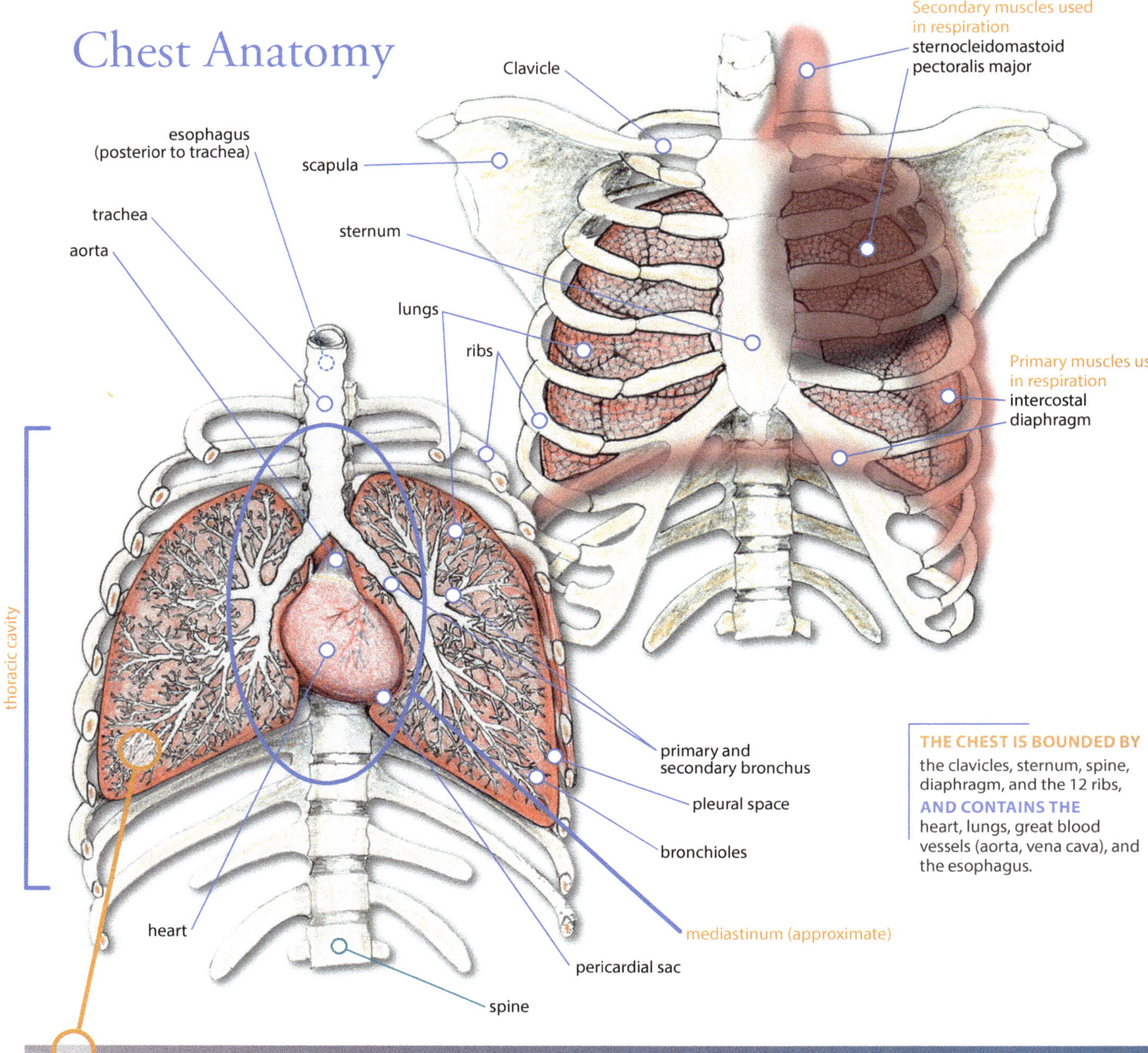

THE CHEST IS BOUNDED BY the clavicles, sternum, spine, diaphragm, and the 12 ribs, **AND CONTAINS THE** heart, lungs, great blood vessels (aorta, vena cava), and the esophagus.

Inhalation/Exhalation

THE INS AND OUTS OF RESPIRATION

Each lung is sheathed by a delicate serous membrane, the pleura, in the form of a closed invaginated (sheathed) sac. The portion of the membrane that covers the surface of the lung and follows the wrinkles and fissures between its lobes is called the visceral pleura, and it is attached directly to the lungs.

The parietal pleura is a similar membrane that is attached to the opposing interior surface of the thoracic cavity.

The potential space between these two membranes is known as the pleural space, and it can hold 2 – 3 liters of air in an adult if the lung collapses.

The diaphragm contracts and drops, and the intercostal muscles are brought into play through contraction, creating negative pressure in the pleural space, which causes the lungs to expand and air to rush in—this is active inhalation.

Exhalation is purely passive: the diaphragm and other muscles relax, and as the elastic lungs recoil, positive pressure pushes air out.

JUST IN CASE YOU WERE WONDERING . . .

The average person (at rest) breathes about: 16 times a minute

- 16 times a minute
- 960 times an hour
- 23,040 times a day
- 8,415,360 times a year
- that's 673,228,800 to age 80...
- Whew!

SOLO CARDIOPULMONARY RESUSCITATION (CPR)

THE HEART

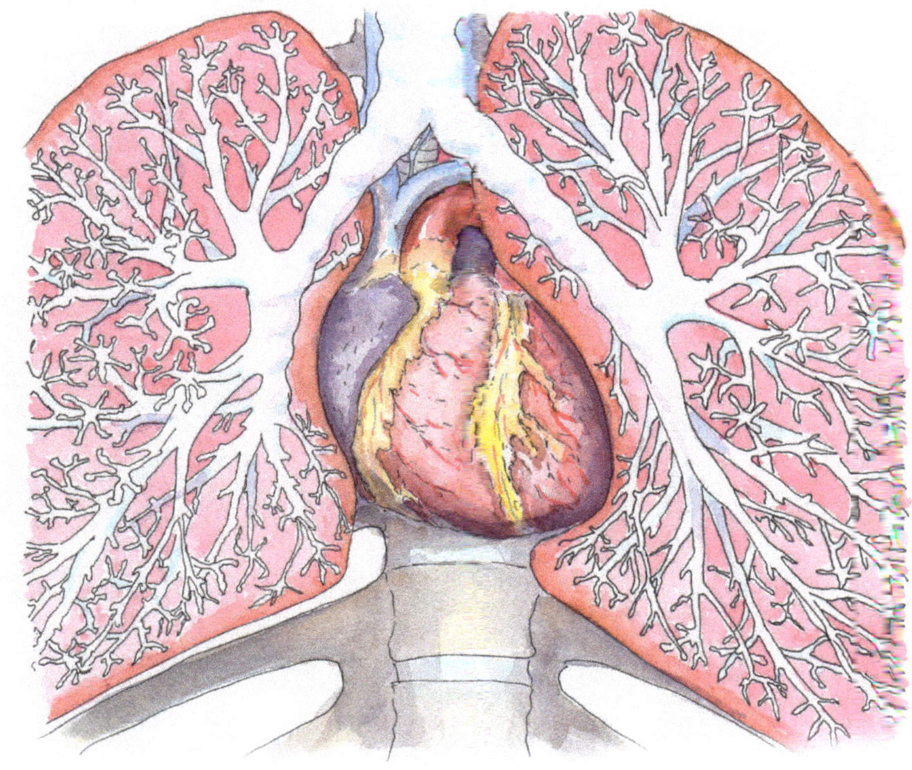

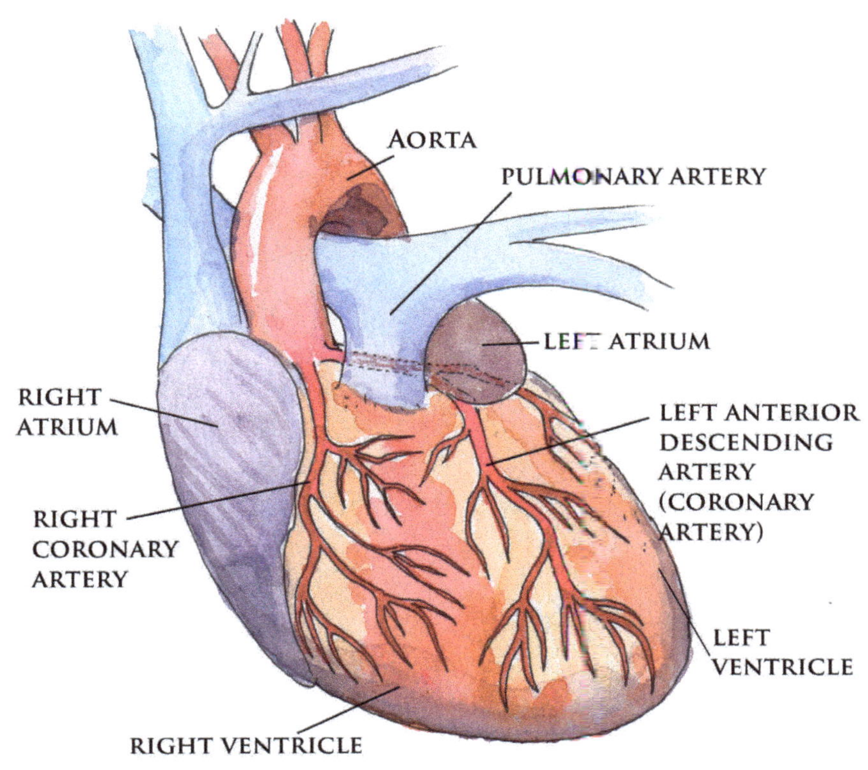

CPR AND HEART FACTS

DATA from AHA - Heart Disease and Stroke Statistics Update 2019

Cardiovascular Disease (CVD):

Includes: coronary artery disease (CAD)

hypertension (HTN)

congestive heart failure (CHF)

strokes (CVA)

- CVD is the #1 cause of death, 1 in 3 deaths, or 840,000 per year.
- 121.5 million Americans have some form of CVD.
- Men have higher incidence of CVD until age 65, then women have higher incidence.
- 43.2% of all deaths in US in 2000 were due to CVD.
- Since 1900, CVD has been the #1 killer in US except for 1918.
- CVD claims more lives than next 5 leading causes of death combined.

CARDIOVASCULAR DISEASE TERMS:

Arteriosclerosis: A disease of the arteries with thickening, hardening, and loss of elasticity in the arterial walls.

Atherosclerosis: The most common form of arteriosclerosis, marked by cholesterol-lipid-calcium deposits in arterial linings.

Coronary Artery Disease (CAD): Narrowing of coronary arteries sufficient to prevent adequate blood supply to the heart muscle.

Angina Pectoris: Pain around the heart caused by deficiency of blood supply to the heart.

Myocardial Infarction: Condition caused by partial or complete occlusion of one of the coronary arteries.

Clinical Death: Patient without a pulse.

Biological Death: Occurs within 10 minutes of clinical death due to lack of oxygen to the brain.

SUDDEN CARDIAC DEATH (SCD):

When the heartbeat stops abruptly and unexpectedly, unassociated with any illness or injury.

Most common underlying cause of SCD is a heart attack that results in Ventricular Fibrillation (V-fib).

70 % of SCD occur at home, 18% in public settings, and 12% in nursing homes.

Approximately 90% of SCD victims die before reaching hospital.

Without bystander CPR success rates decline 7-10% every minute defibrillation is delayed.

Approximately 250,000 people die of coronary disease each year without ever being hospitalized.

Causes of sudden death:

Sudden Cardiac Death – Cardiac Arrest

Trauma

Drowning

Asphyxiation

Electric Shock

Allergic Reactions

RISK FACTORS FOR CARDIOVASCULAR DISEASE THAT CANNOT BE CHANGED:

Heredity, Sex, Age, Race

RISK FACTORS FOR CARDIOVASCULAR DISEASE THAT CAN BE CHANGED:

CHOLESTEROL – LIPID PANEL:

Total Cholesterol, HDL, LDL, and HDL/LDL ratios.

10% decrease in total cholesterol may result in 30% decrease in incidence of CVD.

Risk of heart attack greatest with Low High Density Lipoproteins (LDL) and high total cholesterol count (low HDL, high LDL).

DIET AND OBESITY:

300,000 people die each year due to obesity-related problems.

129 million people in American are overweight or obese, > 20% over ideal body weight.

61.2 million are obese (30.0Kg/m2).

INACTIVITY:

38.3% of Americans over-20-years old report ZERO leisure time physical activity.

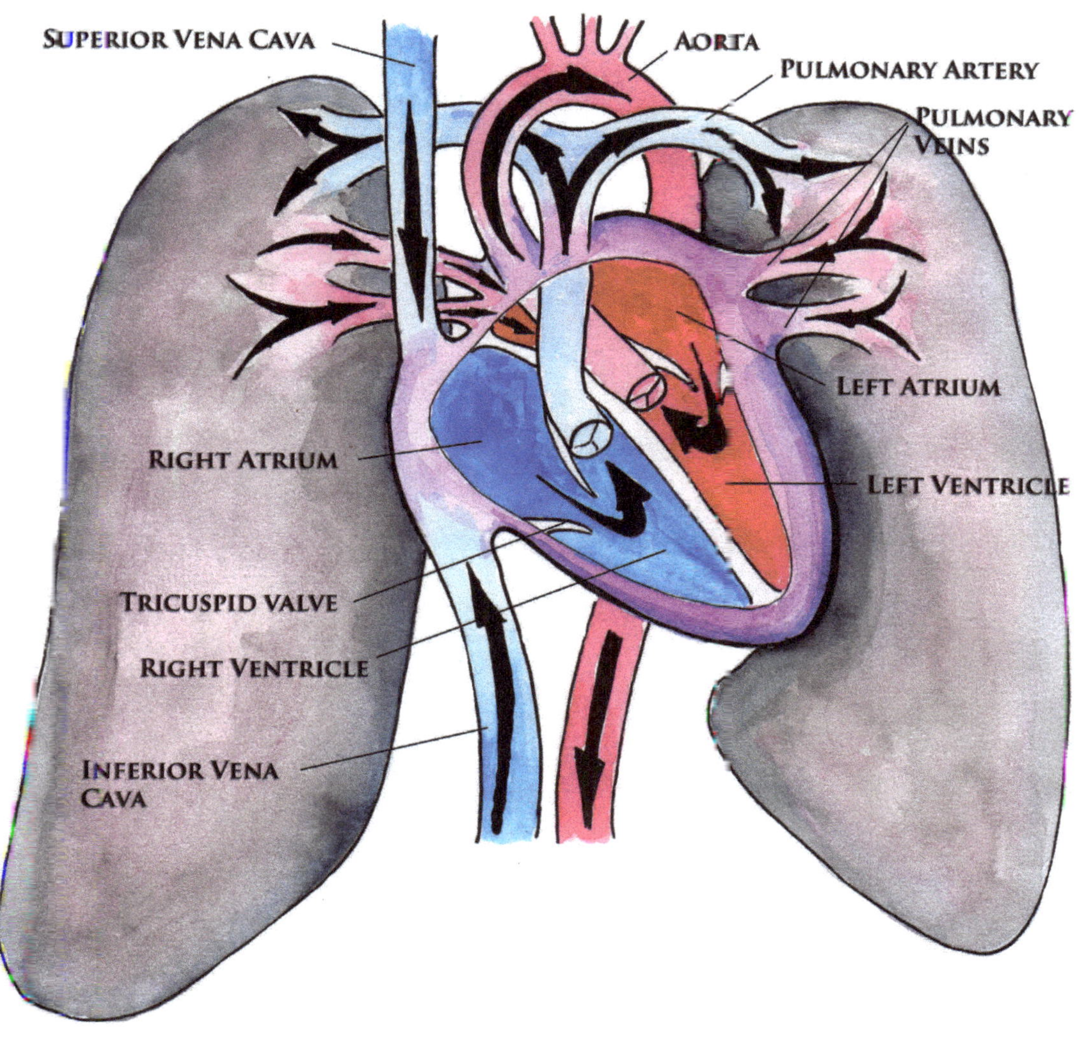

SUPERIOR VENA CAVA
AORTA
PULMONARY ARTERY
PULMONARY VEINS
LEFT ATRIUM
RIGHT ATRIUM
LEFT VENTRICLE
TRICUSPID VALVE
RIGHT VENTRICLE
INFERIOR VENA CAVA

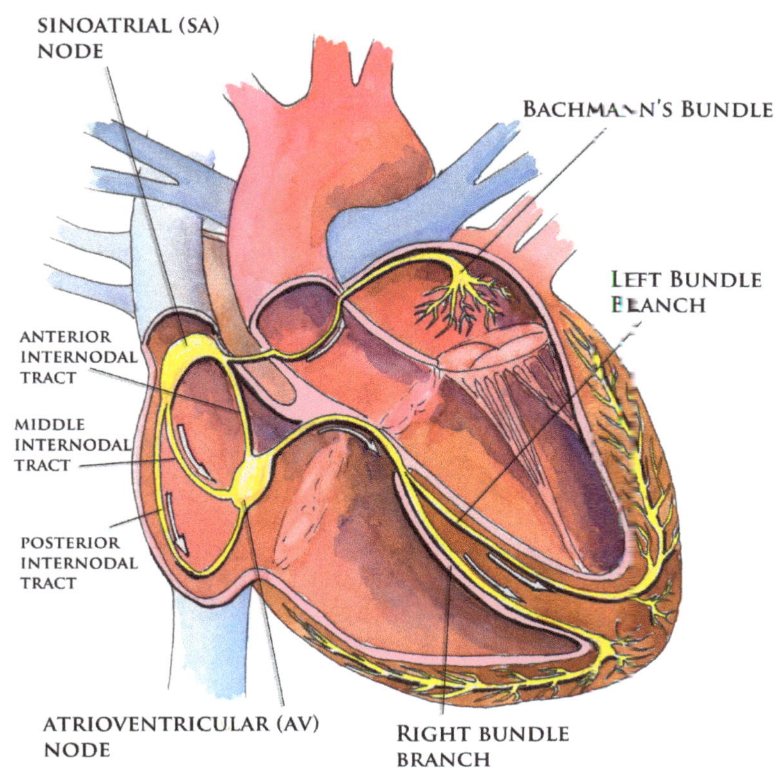

SINOATRIAL (SA) NODE
BACHMANN'S BUNDLE
LEFT BUNDLE BRANCH
ANTERIOR INTERNODAL TRACT
MIDDLE INTERNODAL TRACT
POSTERIOR INTERNODAL TRACT
ATRIOVENTRICULAR (AV) NODE
RIGHT BUNDLE BRANCH

SMOKING:

1995-1999 an average of 442,398 Americans died per year of smoking-related illnesses.

25.7 % of males, and 21% of females over 18 report current tobacco use.

Since 1965, smoking of people over 18 has decreased by over 40%.

DIABETES:

10.9 million Americans have physician-diagnosed Diabetes.

75% of people with Diabetes die of some heart or blood vessel disease.

HYPERTENSION (HTN):

Systolic pressure of 140 mmHg or greater, or Diastolic of 90 mmHg or greater.

50 million Americans over 6-years-old have HTN (1 in 5).

1 in 4 adults have HTN.

50% of people who have first heart attack, and 66% of those who have their first stroke have blood pressure of 160/94 or higher.

ALCOHOL AND RECREATIONAL DRUG USE

increase the risk of CVD.

HEART ATTACKS - Acute Coronary Syndrome (ACS):

May be Angina Pectoris or Acute Myocardial Infarction

Treat all chest pain as if it were a heart attack.

Signs and Symptoms of ACS - Angina Pectoris or Acute Myocardial Infarction:

Pain: Substernal chest pain or back pain; pain may radiate to jaw, neck, or left arm.

Patient may deny that anything is wrong.

They may be anxious with a sense of impending doom.

They may have Shortness of Breath which is made worse with exertion.

Weakness

Nausea

Indigestion

Vital Signs indicate Cardiogenic Shock:

LOC: Anxious

Skin: Pale, Cool, Clammy

Pulse: Rapid and weak

Respirations: Rapid and shallow

BP: Steady, then falling

Pupils: PERRL

The difference between angina and an acute MI, is that with angina the symptoms will improve with rest, but not with an acute MI.

Treatment:

Maintain ABCs.

Reassure.

Place in a Position of Comfort.

Encourage rest.

Assist the patient with their sublingual nitroglycerin.

You may give up to three doses of nitro, five minutes apart, as long as the systolic blood pressure is greater than 100 mmHg.

Give aspirin, unless otherwise contraindicated. Give them four 81mg chewable tablets or 1 adult aspirin, 325mg, as long as they do not have a severe allergy to aspirin (anaphylaxis). Do not use coated aspirin, as they are time-released.

Monitor.

Evacuate.

Cardiopulmonary Resuscitation (CPR)

Increases time between clinical death and biological death by oxygenating the brain.

Best results are from a combination of early CPR and early defibrillation.

Complications of CPR:

Aspiration of Vomit

Fractured Ribs

Complications of not doing CPR – DEATH

SOLO ADULT CPR Skill Sheet:

What to Check for:	Skill to be demonstrated:
1. ASSESSES: Check for Responsiveness Check for Breathing	Shout "Are you OK?" If no response, apply painful stimuli. Check for no breathing or normal breathing.

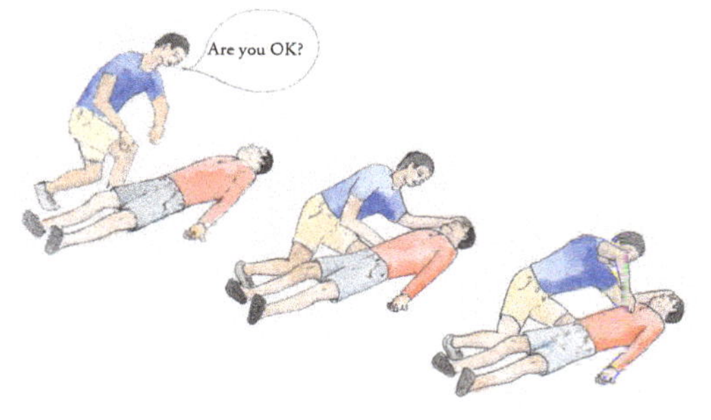

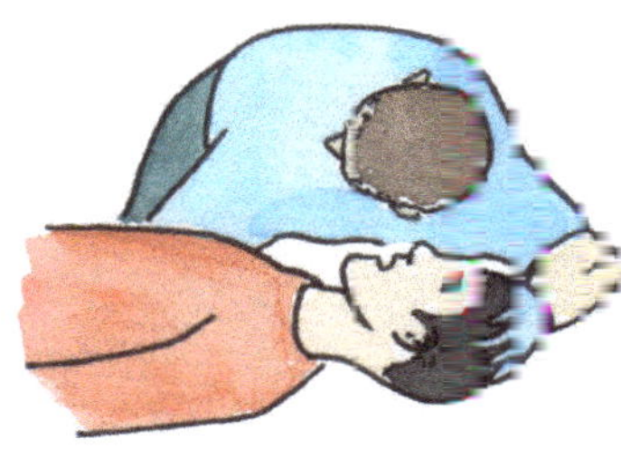

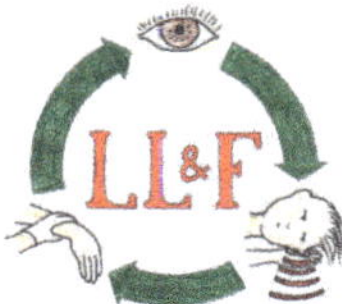

2. ACTIVATE: Emergency Response System. Can use your cell phone to call for help.	Shout for help; direct someone to call for help. Activate Emergency Response System and get an AED/defibrillator if available.
3. PULSE: Check for pulse	Check for carotid pulse (less than 10 seconds).
4. If there is a pulse but no breath sounds: Start rescue breathing	Ventilate Patient once every 6 seconds, 10 breaths per minute.

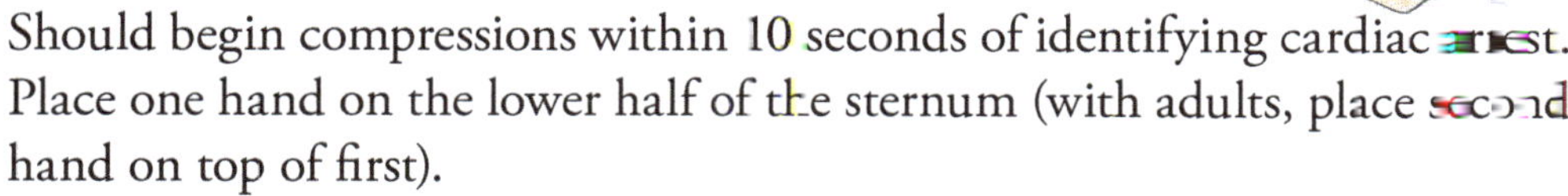

5. If there is no pulse: **Start CPR.** Check for correct hand placement Check for adequate rate. Check for adequate depth Allow for complete chest recoil Minimize interruptions	Should begin compressions within 10 seconds of identifying cardiac arrest. Place one hand on the lower half of the sternum (with adults, place second hand on top of first). Compress the chest at least 2 inches (5cm or 1/3 body depth), but not greater than 2.4 inches (6cm) 30 times in 20 seconds (1 1/2 times per second) allowing chest to fully recoil. Follow with 2 rescue breaths. (Each breath delivered over one second, each causing the chest to rise). Continue 30 compressions followed by 2 breaths (Use the same ratio for either one rescuer or two).
6. If no AED is available, continue CPR for 5 cycles of 30:2, stopping every five cycles to check for pulse.	

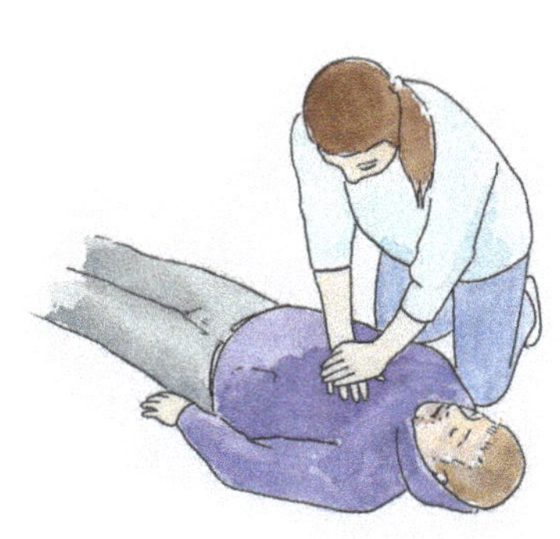

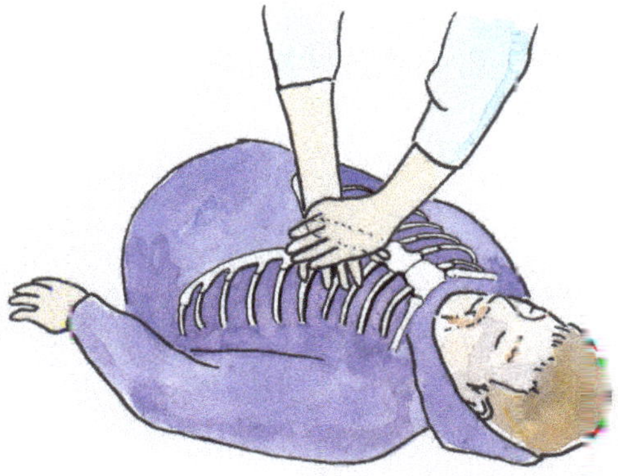

SOLO ADULT CPR Skill Sheet:

What to Check for:	Skill to be demonstrated:
7. AED and CPR	Apply and use AED as soon as it arrives.
8. AED	Turn on AED. Place proper size pads in correct locations. Clear patient and allow AED to analyze rhythm. If advised by AED, clear patient and deliver a shock. Resume CPR immediately after shock delivery. Do not turn off AED during CPR. **If shock not advised**, check for pulse. If no pulse, resume CPR, five cycles of 30:2
9. After 5 cycles (approximately 2 minutes) of 30 compressions to 2 breaths, stop CPR and let AED re-analyze.	After approximately 2 minutes the AED will tell you to stop CPR so it can analyze the rhythm. Follow prompts from the AED. If 'Shock advised," repeat step **8,** re-shock and continue CPR. If "no shock advised," reassess patient for pulse and breathing.
10. If no pulse: Start 5 additional cycles of 30 compressions and 2 breaths.	See step **8.**
11. If pulse: Reassess for adequate breathing	Reassess for adequate breathing; continue rescue breathing if necessary.
12. If there is a pulse, but inadequate breathing:	Continue rescue breathing.
13. If there is a pulse and adequate breathing:	Monitor until help arrives.

45

SOLO CHILD CPR Skill Sheet:
(1-Year-old to puberty)

What to Check for:	Skill to be demonstrated:

1. ASSESSES:
Check for Responsiveness.
Check for Breathing.

If you witnessed collapse: Follow steps for adult.
If you did not witness collapse: Give 2 minutes CPR, then get help and AED.

Shout "Are you OK?"
If no response, apply painful stimuli.
Check for no breathing or normal breathing.

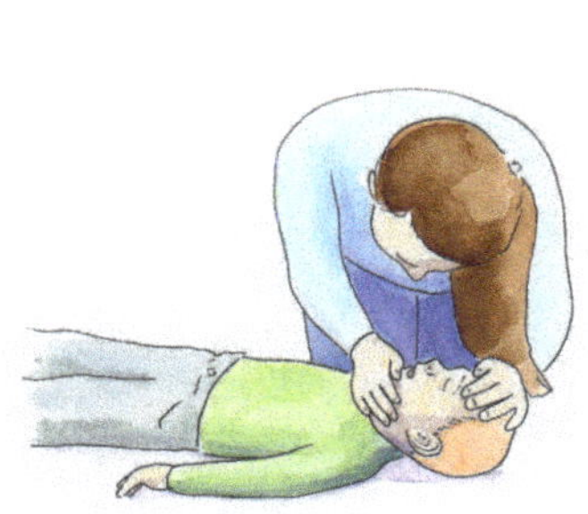
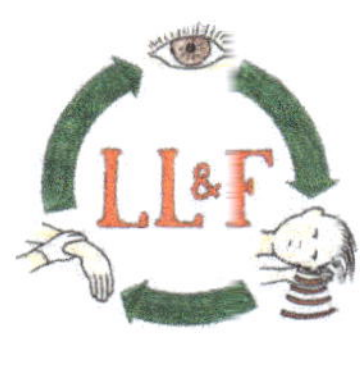

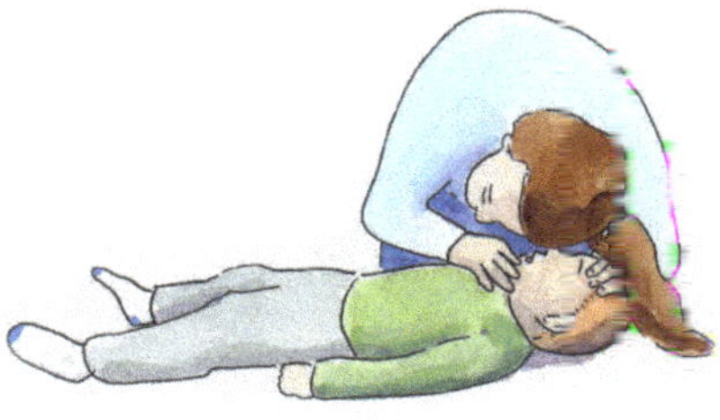

2. ACTIVATE:
Emergency response system if you have two rescuers or a second person on scene. If you are the only rescuer activate after 2 minutes CPR.

Shout for help; direct someone to call for help.
Activate Emergency Response System and get an AED/defibrillator if available.

3. PULSE:
Check for pulse

Check for carotid pulse
(less than 10 seconds).

4. If there is a pulse but no breath sounds:
Start rescue breathing.

Ventilate Patient once every 3-5 seconds, 12 breaths per minute.

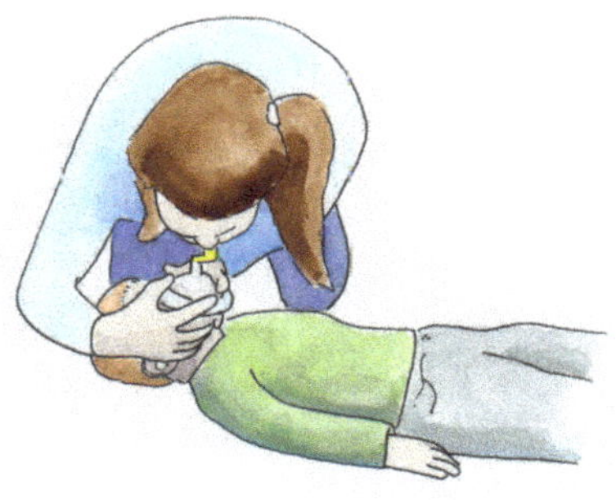

5. If there is no pulse:
Start CPR.
Check for Correct hand placement.
Check for adequate rate.
Check for adequate depth.
Allow for complete chest recoil.
Minimize interruptions.

Activate ERS if you have not already done so.

Begin compressions within 10 seconds of identifying cardiac arrest.
Place one or two hands on lower half of patient's sternum.
Compress the chest at least 2 inches (5cm, or 1/3 body depth) 30 times in 20 seconds, allowing chest to fully recoil.
Follow with 2 rescue breaths.
One rescuer: Continue 30 compressions followed by 2 breaths.
Two rescuers: Continue 15 compressions followed by 2 breaths.

What to Check for:	Skill to be demonstrated:
6. AED and CPR	Apply and use AED as soon as it arrives.
7. AED	Turn on AED. Place proper size pads in correct locations. Clear patient and allow AED to analyze rhythm. If advised by AED, clear patient and deliver a shock. Resume CPR immediately after shock delivery. Do not turn off AED during CPR. *If shock not advised*, check for pulse. If no pulse resume CPR five cycles of 30:2
8. After 5 cycles (approximately 2 minutes) of 30 compressions to 2 breaths, reassess for pulse	After approximately 2 minutes the AED will tell you to stop CPR so it can analyze the rhythm. Follow prompts from the AED. If 'Shock advised," repeat step **7,** re-shock and continue CPR. If "no shock advised," reassess patient for pulse and breathing.
9. If no pulse: **Start 5 additional cycles of 30 compressions and 2 breaths**	See step **7.**
10. If pulse: Reassess for adequate breathing	Reassess for adequate breathing; continue rescue breathing If necessary.
11. If there is a pulse, but inadequate breathing:	Continue rescue breathing once every 3-5 seconds.
12. If there is a pulse and adequate breathing:	Monitor until help arrives.

SOLO INFANT CPR Skill Sheet:
(0-12 months-old)

What to Check for:	Skill to be demonstrated:
1. ASSESSES: Check for Responsiveness Check for Breathing.	Tickle bottom of infant's foot to check for responsiveness. If unresponsive, check to see if infant is breathing.
2. ACTIVATE: Emergency response system if you have two rescuers or a second person on scene. If you are the only rescuer activate after 2 minutes CPR.	Shout for help; direct someone to call for help. Activate Emergency Response System.
3. PULSE: Check for pulse.	Check for a brachial pulse (not carotid). 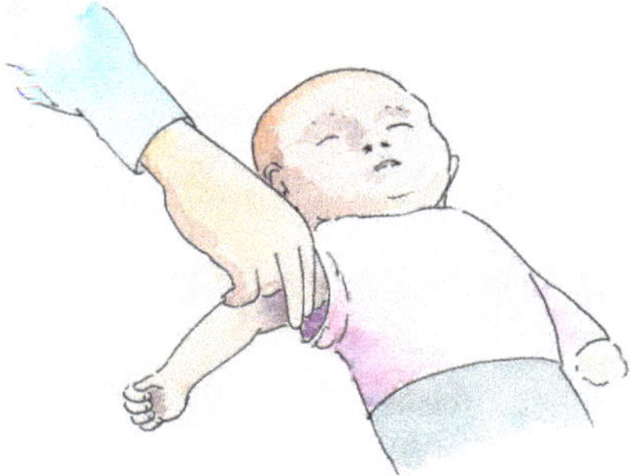
4. If there is a pulse but no breath sounds: Start rescue breathing.	Ventilate Patient once every 3-5 seconds, 12-20 breaths per minute.
5. If there is no pulse: **Start CPR.** Check for Correct hand placement. Check for adequate rate. Check for adequate depth. Allow for complete chest recoil. Minimize interruptions. **Compression to ventilation ratios: One Rescuer CPR** Activate EMS if you have not already done so.	Begin compressions within 10 seconds of identifying cardiac arrest. Place two fingers just below the nipple line. Compress the chest 1/3 depth of the chest (aprox 1 ½ inches, or 4cm) 30 times in 20 seconds, allowing chest to fully recoil. Follow with 2 rescue breaths. 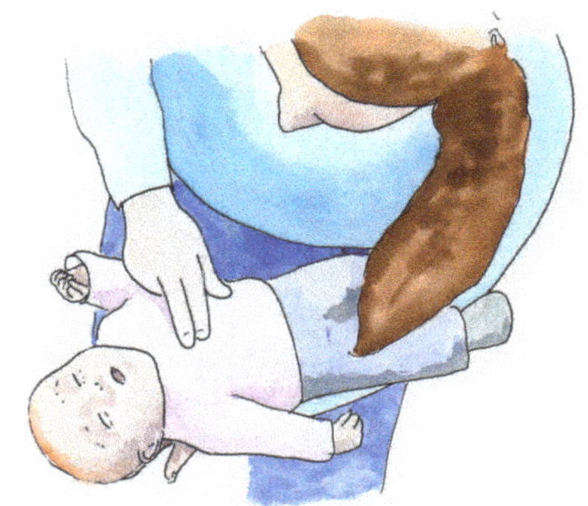 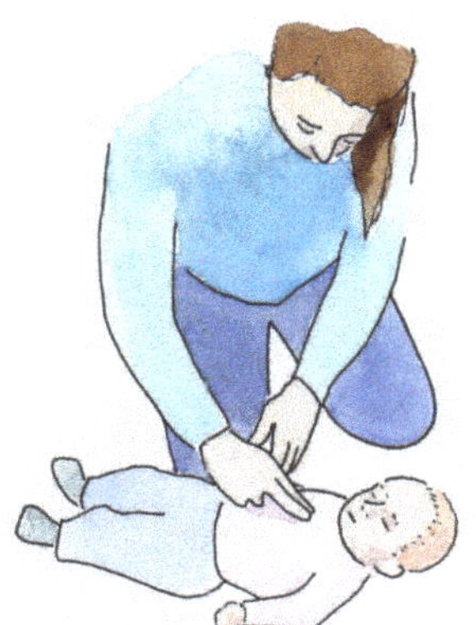 One Rescuer CPR: 30 compressions to 2 breaths, 2 fingers at the nipple line

SOLO INFANT CPR Skill Sheet:
(0-12 months-old)

What to Check for:	Skill to be demonstrated:
Compression to ventilation ratios: Two Rescuer CPR	Two Rescuer CPR: 15 compressions to 2 breaths, thumb encircling chest method at nipple line. 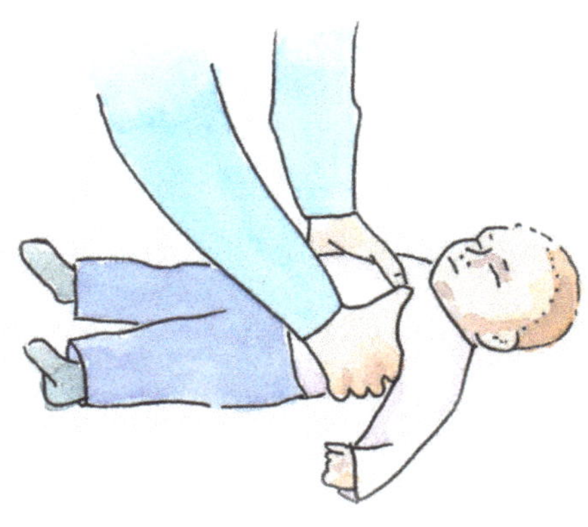
6. After 5 cycles (approximately 2 minutes) of 30 compressions to 2 breaths, or 15 compressions to 2 breaths, reassess for pulse.	Check for brachial pulse for at least 5 seconds, but not more than 10 seconds.
7. If no pulse, begin five additional cycles of 30:2 or 15:2 ratio of compressions to breaths.	See step **6**.
8. If pulse: Reassess for adequate breathing.	Look for chest rise, listen and feel for air movement.
9. If there is a pulse, but inadequate breathing:	Continue rescue breathing; ventilate once every 3-5 seconds.
10. If there is a pulse and adequate breathing:	Monitor until help arrives.

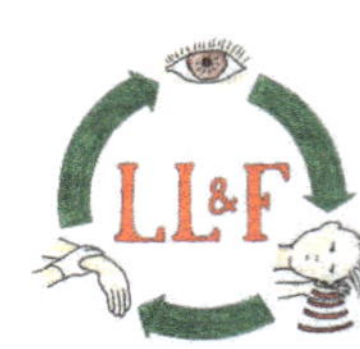

SOLO FOREIGN-BODY AIRWAY OBSTRUCTION
ADULT AND CHILD SKILL SHEET
(1 year of age and older)

What to Check for:	Skill to be demonstrated:
1. Assess for airway obstruction	Poor or no air exchange, increased respiratory difficulty, possible cyanosis of the lips and nail beds (bluish), universal choking sign. 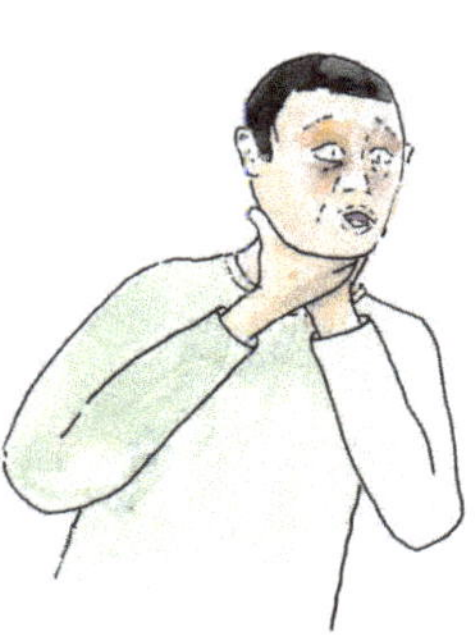
2. Position patient for abdominal thrusts	Stand behind the patient and wrap your arms around the patient's waist. Place the thumb side of your fist against the patient's abdomen, midline, above the navel and well below the sternum. 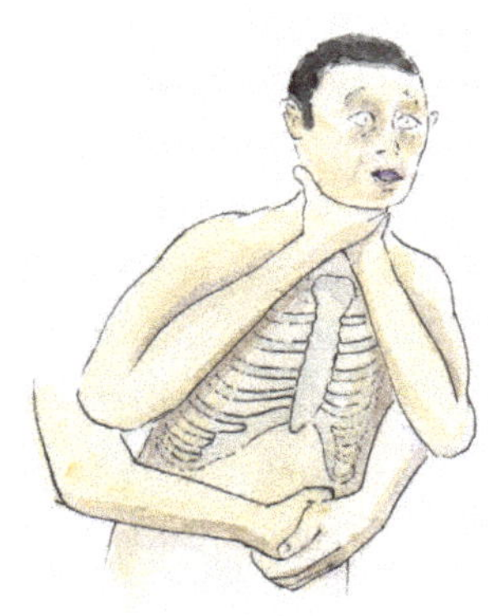 *Position for adult* 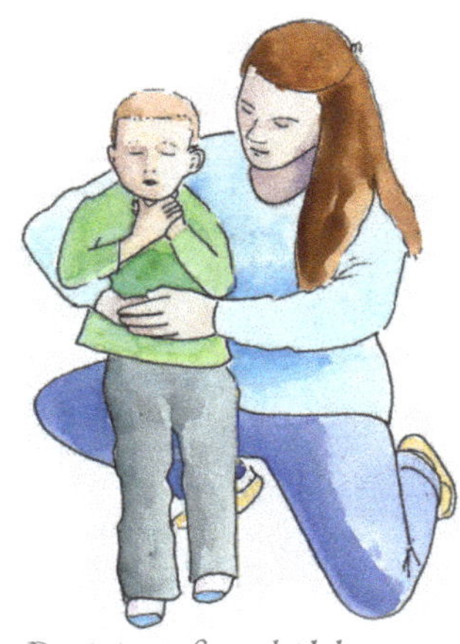 *Position for child*
3. Deliver abdominal thrusts	Grasp your fist with your other hand and force both hands together into the patient's abdomen with a quick, forceful upward thrust. 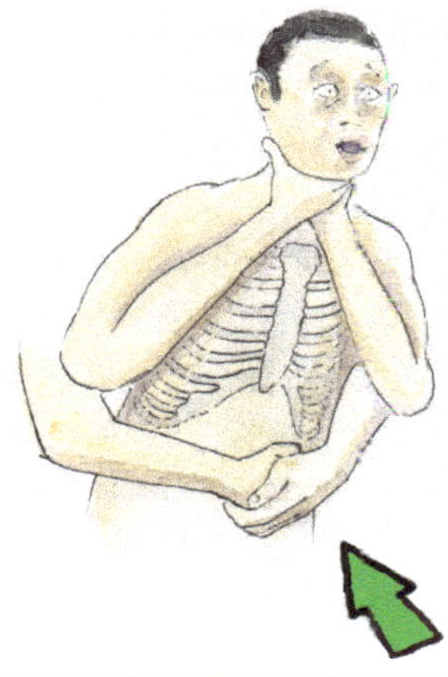

SOLO FOREIGN-BODY AIRWAY OBSTRUCTION
ADULT AND CHILD SKILL SHEET
(1 year of age and older)

What to Check for:	Skill to be demonstrated:
4. Repeat thrusts	Repeat thrusts until object is expelled from the airway or until patient becomes unconscious. Give each thrust as a separate and distinct movement to dislodge the obstruction.
5. Obese or pregnant	Perform chest thrusts instead of abdominal thrusts.

If the patient becomes unresponsive:

What to Check for:	Skill to be demonstrated:
1. Activate the Emergency Response system:	Send someone to call for help, but do not leave the patient alone.
2. Begin CPR: **30 compressions to 2 rescue breaths.**	Lower the patient to the ground and begin chest compressions. Each time you go to give ventilations, open the patient's mouth and look inside for the obstructing object. If the object is visible, remove if possible.
3. After 5 cycles of 30 compressions and 2 rescue breaths, check that the Emergency Response System has been activated.	Check that Emergency Medical help has been notified and continue CPR. Remember to look in the airway before giving rescue breaths.

SOLO FOREIGN-BODY AIRWAY OBSTRUCTION
INFANT SKILL SHEET
(0-12 months old)

What to Check for:	Skill to be demonstrated:
1. Assess for airway obstruction.	Poor or no air exchange, increased respiratory difficulty, possible cyanosis of the lips and nail beds (bluish), inability to cry.
2. Position patient for back slaps.	Kneel or sit with the infant in your lap. Hold the infant facedown resting on your forearm with the head slightly lower than the chest. Support the infant's head and jaw with your hand. Rest your arm on your leg or lap to support the infant. 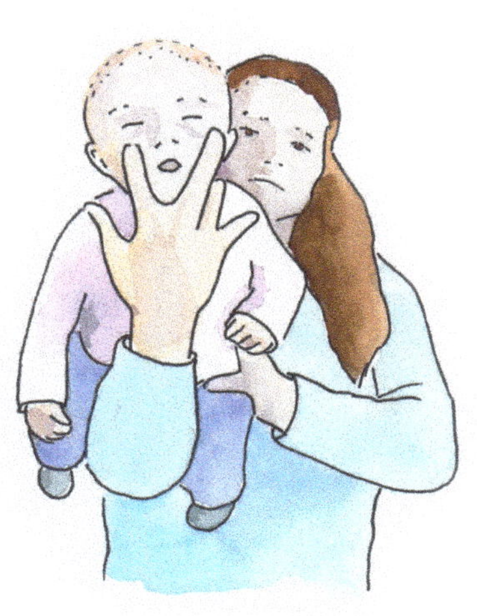 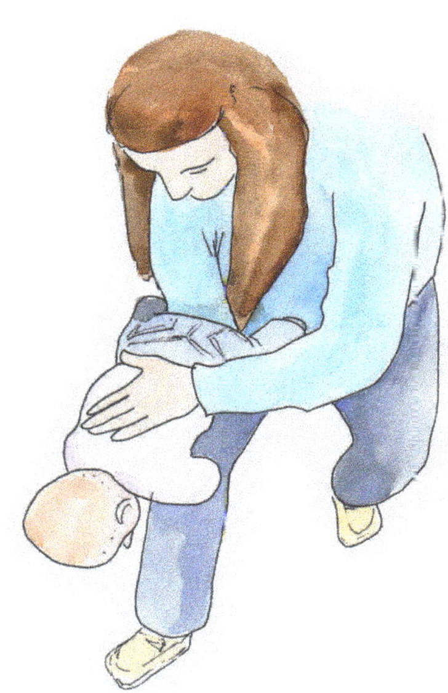
3. Deliver 5 back slaps.	Slap the infant forcefully in the middle of the back between the shoulder blades using the heel of your hand.
4. Position the infant for chest thrusts	Place your free hand on the infant's back supporting the back of the head with the palm of your hand. The infant should be cradled between your two forearms. Turn the infant as a unit while carefully supporting the head and neck. Hold the infant on its back with your forearm resting on your lap or thigh. 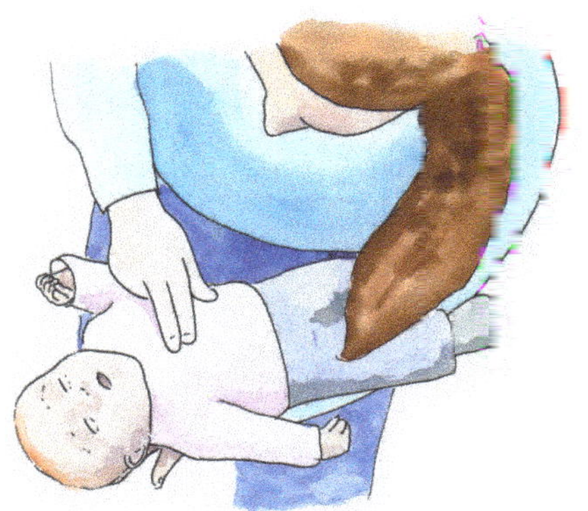

SOLO FOREIGN-BODY AIRWAY OBSTRUCTION
INFANT SKILL SHEET
(0-12 months old)

What to Check for:	Skill to be demonstrated:
5. Deliver up to 5 chest thrusts.	Provide up to 5 quick downward chest thrusts in the same place as chest compressions. Deliver chest thrusts at a rate of 1 per second.
6. Repeat until the object is removed or the infant becomes unresponsive.	Continue the sequence of 5 back slaps and up to 5 chest thrusts.

If the patient becomes unresponsive:

What to Check for:	Skill to be demonstrated:
1. Activate the Emergency Response system.	Send someone to call for help, but do not leave the patient alone.
2. Begin CPR with one extra step.	Each time you open the airway, look for the obstructing object in the back of the throat. If the object is visible, remove if possible.
3. After 5 cycles, check that the Emergency Response System has been activated.	Check that Emergency Medical help has been notified and continue CPR. Remember to look in the airway before giving rescue breaths.

SUMMARY OF BASIC LIFE SUPPORT

Action	Adult:	Child:	Infant:
AIRWAY	Head tilt chin lift		Neutral in-line position
BREATHING	2 breaths at 1 breath per second	2 effective breaths at 1 breath per second.	
Rescue breathing without compressions	1 breath every 5 seconds: 10-12 breaths per minute	1 every 3-5 seconds: 15-20 breaths per minute	
Rescue breaths for CPR with advanced airway	Adults 30 compressions to 2 breaths, approximately 10 breaths per minute	Children and infants, One Rescuer CPR: same rate as adult. Children and infants, Two rescuer CPR: 15 Compressions to 2 breaths.	
Foreign-body Airway obstruction (Conscious patient)	Abdominal thrusts Chest thrusts if obese or pregnant		Back slaps and chest thrusts
Foreign-body Airway obstruction (Unconscious patient)	If patient becomes unconscious from choking, activate the Emergency Response System and begin CPR. Each time you open the airway to ventilate, check throat and mouth for foreign objects.		
CIRCULATION Pulse check 10 seconds	Carotid		Brachial
Compression landmarks	Lower half of sternum		Just below nipple line
Compression method	With fist covered by other hand, thrust hard and fast. Allow complete recoil.		1 rescuer CPR: 2 or 3 fingers 2 rescuer CPR: 2 thumbs encircling chest technique
Compression depth	At least 2 inches	2 inches	1 ½ inches
Compression rate	Approximately 100/120 compressions per minute		
Compression to ventilation ratio	30:2 one or two rescuer	Children and infants—one rescuer 30:2 Children and infants—two rescuer 15:2	
Two-rescuer CPR	One rescuer ventilates; one rescuer does compressions. Switch every two minutes. Switch should take less than 5 seconds.		Same as for child or adult using thumbs—encircling chest method
DEFIBRILLATION AED	Use adult pads. Do not use child pads.	Use AED after 5 cycles of CPR. Use pediatric system if available.	No recommendation for infant less than one year of age

CPR CONSIDERATIONS IN THE REMOTE ENVIRONMENT

When to begin CPR:
Street and Wilderness: For any pulseless individuals.

EXCEPTION: Do NOT begin CPR if:
Street:
Scene is unsafe.
Rigor mortis is present.
Dependent lividity is present.
Injuries are incompatible with life.
DNR orders are present.
Putrefaction (rot) is evident.

Wilderness:
All the street protocols plus:
Frozen/uncompressible chest.
Hypothermic patient.
Putrefaction (rot) is evident.

When to stop CPR:
Street:
Scene becomes unsafe.
Patient returns to life.
Rescuer is relieved by equally or more highly
　　trained personnel.
Patient is declared dead by an MD, DO, or
　　Medical Examiner.
Rescuer is unable to continue efforts.

Wilderness:
All of street protocols plus:
May stop CPR after 30 continuous minutes
　　without patient exhibiting any signs of life.

EXCEPTION: DO NOT stop CPR if:
Patient was victim of:
A lightning strike: electrocution—may have to
　　provide prolonged ventilations.
A drowning: cold water drowning victims can
　　survive longer durations of submersion.

AUTOMATED EXTERNAL DEFIBRILLATION

Many heart attacks are the result of irregular heartbeats. When cardiac arrest is caused by disorganized ventricular rhythm (ventricular fibrillation), a machine known as a defibrillator can deliver an electrical shock that disrupts or stops this irregular, lethal rhythm, allowing the heart to spontaneously develop an effective rhythm of its own. The sooner a patient in cardiac arrest caused by ventricular fibrillation receives a shock, the greater the chances for survival.

Not all cardiac arrests can be helped by a defibrillator. Differing dysrhythmias require differing treatments. Ventricular tachycardia, which is characterized by a very fast lower chamber heart rate, and accounts for less than 10% of pre-hospital cardiac arrests, may also be helped by defibrillation. Neither electromechanical dissociation, which is a very slow heart rate caused by an extremely sick heart muscle, or asystole, where there is no electrical impulse to the heart, can be helped by defibrillation.

Time is of the essence! Six minutes from the moment a person collapses to the moment the defibrillation shock is delivered is considered optimal. Responses are categorized into four segments between the arrest and the first shock, their ideal time components are as follows:

1. EMS (or Emergency Response System) access—from collapse to alerting the EMS system—1 min.

2. Dispatch—from EMS receipt of the call to alerting the rescuer—3 min.

3. Response—from the alert to reaching the patient—3 min.

4. Shock—from reaching the patient to delivering the shock—1.5 min.

If these ideal time goals are met, the survival rate for witnessed cardiac arrest with ventricular fibrillation will improve by 25%.

Public Access Defibrillators (PAD): In an effort to increase survival rates, PAD programs are in place across the country. PADs can be found at airports, malls, sporting events, etc.

Warnings to be heeded when working with all automated defibrillators:

1. Follow the same precautions that you would for operating any electrical device.

2. Do not defibrillate a patient who is not in cardiac arrest.

3. Do not defibrillate a patient who is in contact with rescuers, bystanders, or others.

4. Do not assess or shock a patient who is being moved or when the defibrillator (or its leads) are being moved.

5. Do not defibrillate a patient who has an obstructed airway-- the patient who is in respiratory arrest, but not cardiac arrest, does not need defibrillation.

6. Do not defibrillate a patient who is in the water.

7. Do not defibrillate a patient who is lying on a metal surface that may transfer the electrical shock to others.

8. Do not defibrillate a child who is less than 12 years of age or weighs less than 80 pounds (30 kilograms) unless directed to do so by a physician.

9. All defibrillators are different, but public-access defibrillators are increasingly simple.

BLS, BLS, BLS...

1. Perform primary survey to confirm the patient is in cardiac arrest.

2. Begin CPR. If two or more rescuers are available, one performs CPR while the other prepares and attaches the defibrillator to the patient. If only one person responds, they should follow local protocols.

3. If possible, place the device on the left side of the patient close to the head and work from the left side.

4. Bare the patient's chest. If the chest is wet, quickly wipe it dry.

5. Remove the backing from the first pad and place it adhesive side down on the patient's upper right chest. Make sure the adhesive area makes full contact with the skin, and do not press on the mid-section of a pad with a sponge center. The top of the pad should touch the skin over the top of the clavicle while the medial edge is next to the sternum. The pad should not be placed on the sternum.

6. Remove the backing from the second pad and place it on the skin below and left of the left nipple.

7. Tightly connect the lead cables from the AED to the pad following the manufacture's instructions.

8. Follow the defibrillator's prompts:

A. "Stop CPR"—All rescue efforts cease while the AED analyzes.

B. "Stand back"—All persons must clear themselves of contact with the patient.

C. "Analyzing rhythm"

D. If "Shock advised," you may be instructed to push the shock button.

E. After the shock is delivered, immediately restart CPR.

F. Perform CPR 5 cycles of 30 compressions to 2 breaths.

G. After approximately 2 minutes the AED will tell you to stop CPR so it can analyze the rhythm. It will then either tell you "shock advised" or it will tell you "no shock advised".

H. If a shock is advised, deliver the shock and restart CPR for 5 cycles of 30:2.

I. If shock is not advised, check pulse. If no pulse, restart CPR.

J. Perform CPR 5 cycles of 30 compressions to 2 breaths.

K. Continue CPR stopping every 2 minutes to either analyze rhythm again or to check for pulse.

TROUBLESHOOTING

Most problems, correctable by the rescuer, involve the attachment of pads and/or cables.

Check to ensure pads are in full contact and cables are tightly connected.

If pads are not in full contact:

1.　Make sure that the patient's chest is dry and free of anything in contact with its surface.

2.　Remove all dressings and nitro patches on placement site.

3.　Wipe off any nitropaste.

4.　Shave the pad placement area if necessary.

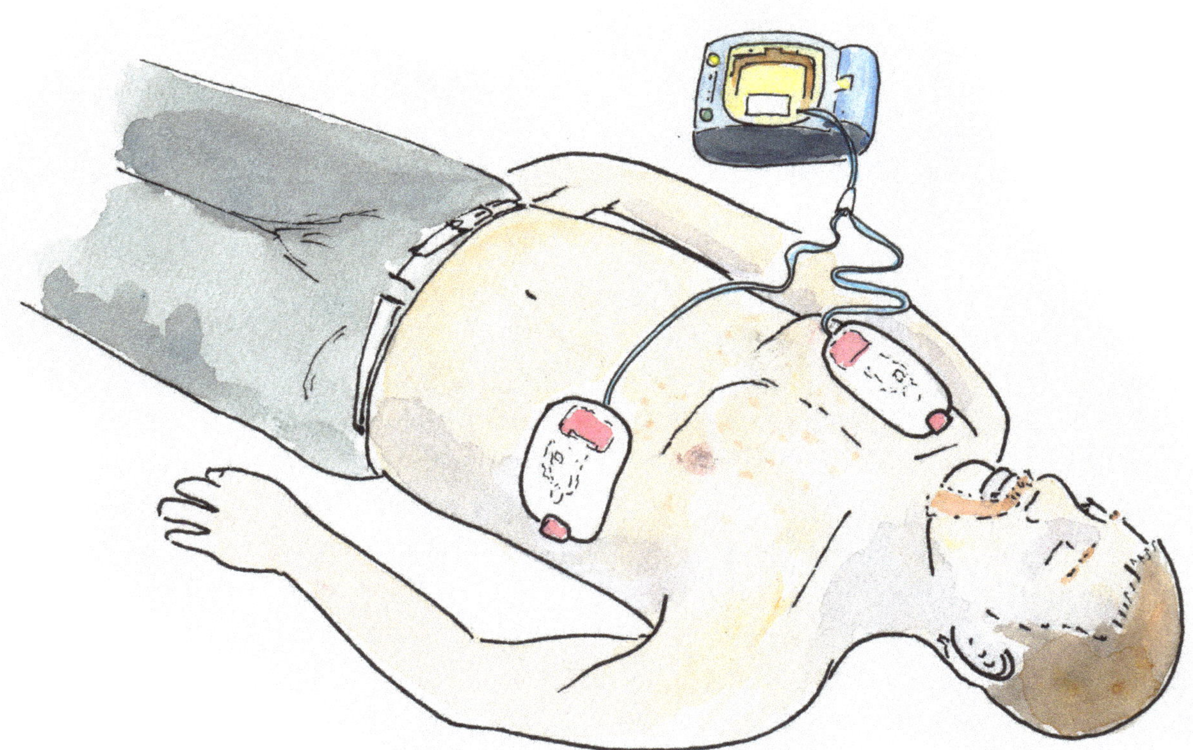

The curriculum for SOLO Basic CPR-AED and Advanced CPR-AED satisfies the requirements for CPR training according to the latest ECC/ILCOR and American Heart Association guidelines. No organization exists that provides a national endorsement or approval for CPR, so each CPR certification provider can develop their own curriculum and implement their own instructional strategies. The SOLO CPR curriculum meets the American Heart recommended guidelines.

Shock and Wound Care

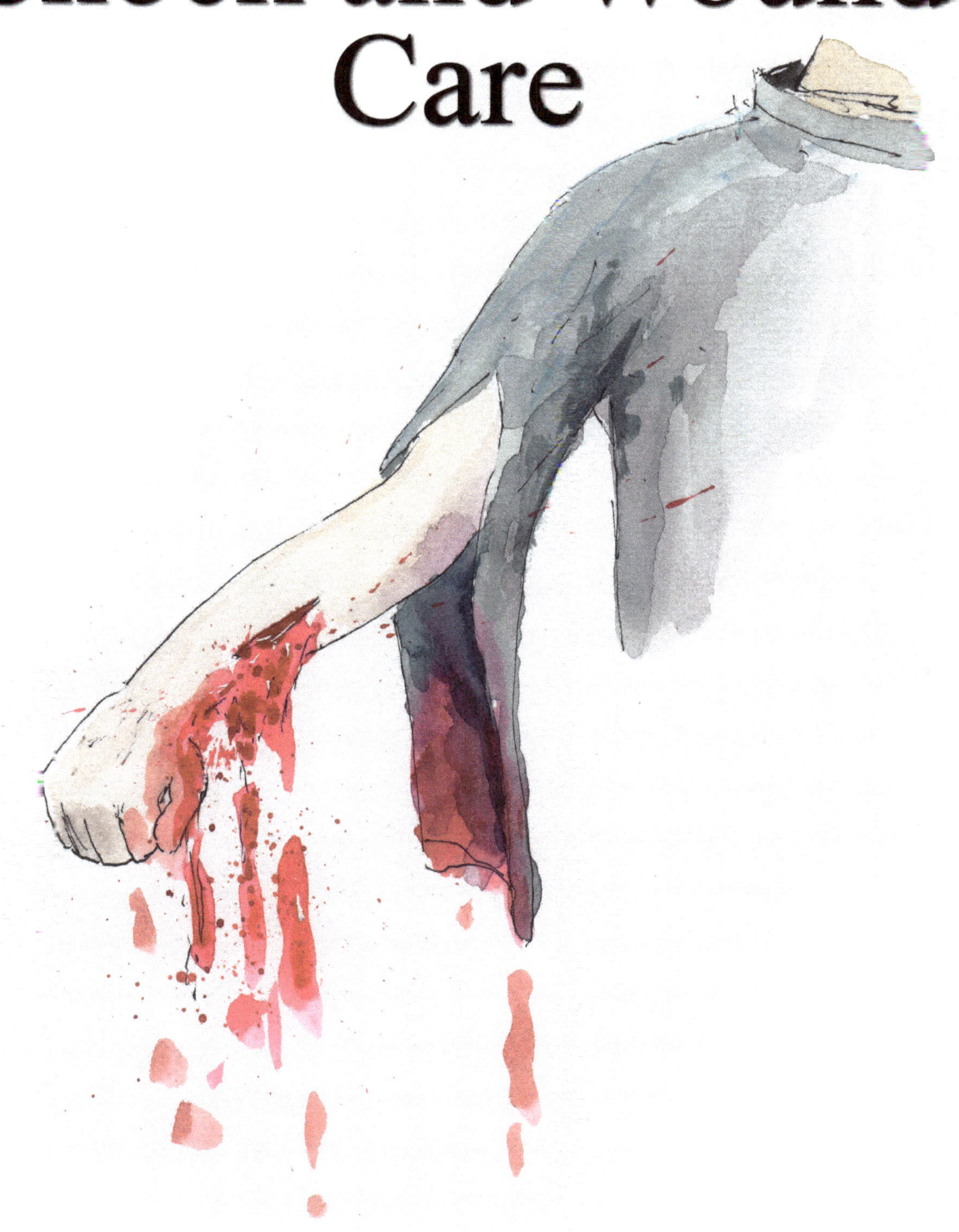

SHOCK

Shock is not a chief complaint

like the other problems described in this critical care section. No one has ever said, "My vasculature feels compromised." Instead, shock is a condition that you may discover as you monitor a patient's vital signs. Shock occurs when the cardiovascular system fails to provide sufficient circulation to every part of the body, causing tissues to eventually suffer from a lack of oxygen. If the cause goes untreated, and the shock is severe enough, it can kill.

The cardiovascular system consists of

Heart—pumps the blood
Blood vessels—carry and distribute the blood
Blood—carries O_2 and nutrients around the body

Shock is a compensatory mechanism designed to keep the brain well-oxygenated during times of cardio-vascular insufficiency by vasoconstricting the peripheral circulation, thus pulling blood into the body core. It also increases the heart rate, which sends more blood to the brain, and increases the respiratory rate to maximize the amount of oxygen in the blood. Initially shock is a life-saving condition that preserves blood flow to the brain, but shock kills if it continues for too long.

types of shock

Hypovolemic shock is caused by decreased blood volume due to blood loss, dehydration, sweating, diarrhea, vomiting, or a thermal burn.

Cardiogenic shock is caused by pump failure, a heart attack (an MI or cardiac arrest).

Neurogenic shock, also called **Distributive** shock, is caused by vasodilation, a loss of vascular tone. This vasodilation results in an increase in vascular space. The space in the vasculature for the blood volume becomes too large for the blood volume, creating the same effect as hypovolemic shock. This can be caused by a spinal cord injury, acute allergic reaction (anaphylaxis), or life-threatening infection (septic shock).

Shock is often an amorphous, misunderstood, and mis-attributed term. It is NOT feeling icky as a result of a flush of adrenalin in the moments and minutes after a traumatic event or accident. Shock is a specific medical condition, and it is ALWAYS the result of a major compromise to the circulatory system.

Decompensatory shock

Shock is a mechanism that compensates for a failing cardiovascular system. It is what keeps us alive until the underlying problem can be repaired. However, the shock condition cannot be maintained forever. If shock continues for too long it will begin to fail or decompensate.

Decompensatory shock means, that the effort to maintain vasoconstriction begins to fail and the blood vessels throughout the body begin to vasodilate and the compensatory mechanism that was keeping us alive is now failing and the patient is starting to die.

This change in status from compensatory shock to decompensatory shock is recognized by a fall in their blood pressure. As the blood vessels vasodilate, their blood pressure begins to fall.

THE CARDIOVASCULAR SYSTEM CONSISTS OF:

Heart – pumps the blood to every cell in the body.
Blood – the fluid that carries oxygen and nutrients to the cells and removes the carbon dioxide and other waste products from these cells.
Blood Vessels – the pipes that carry and distribute the blood to every cell in the body.

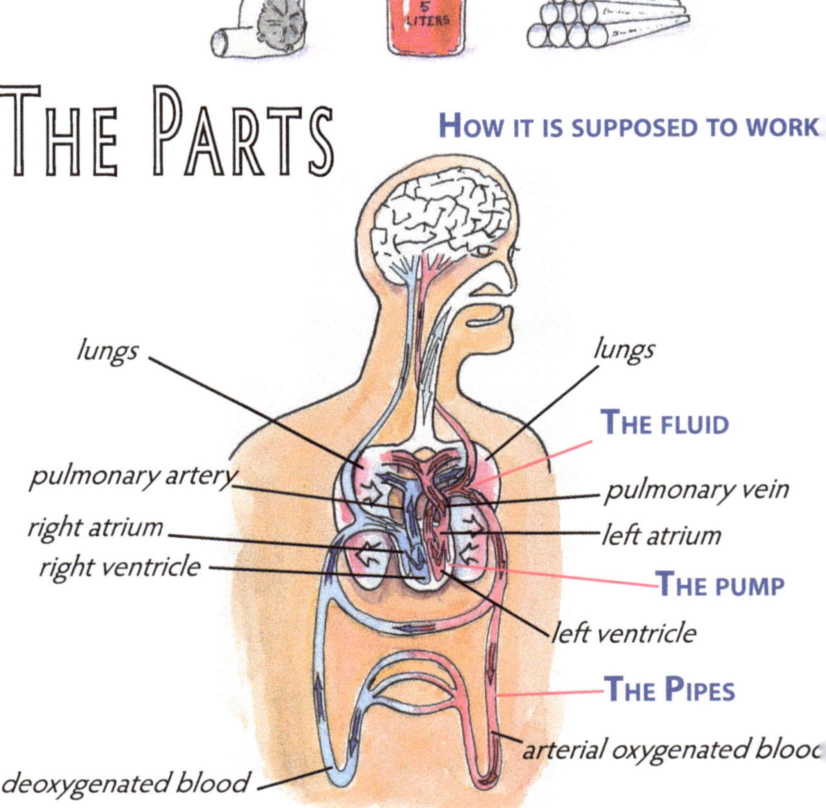

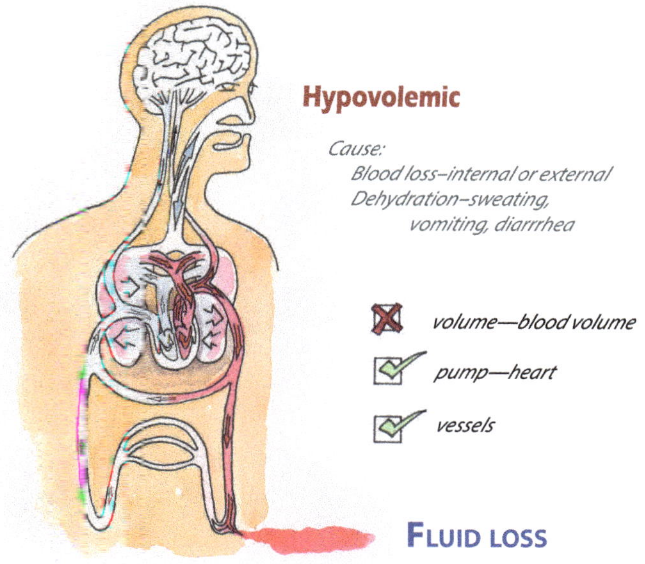

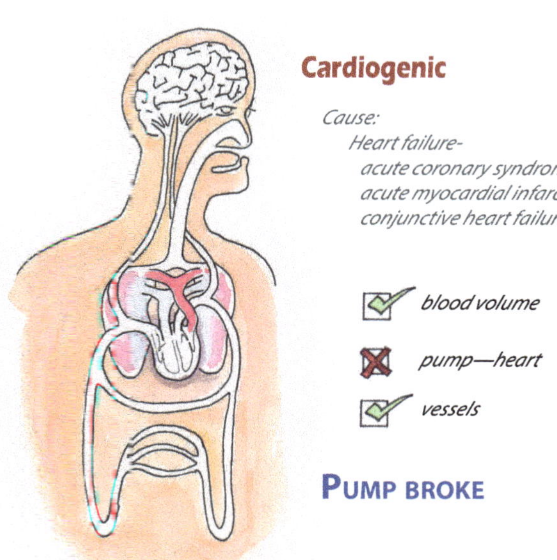

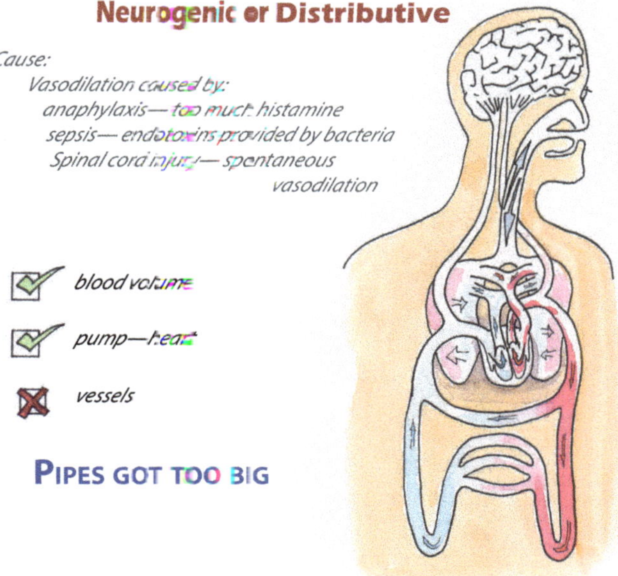

SIGNS AND SYMPTOMS of shock

→ Individuals in shock may be awake, but they seem distant, not in touch with reality.

→ They may stare off into space or be unconscious.

→ They may not know who you are or understand that you are there to help.

→ They may not feel pain or respond to pain

→ They may have an obvious wound or injury that they ignore. (They may try to walk on a broken leg or use a broken arm.)

→ They may not know how seriously injured they are.

→ They may have a sense of impending doom.

vital signs for shock

LOC restless, anxious, may be disoriented, or unconscious.

RR rapid and shallow (the respiratory rate increases because the brain wants more oxygen).

RR rapid, weak, and thready (the heart rate increases to deliver more blood to the brain).

Skin pale, cool, and clammy (PCC) due to vasoconstriction of the capillaries in the skin, which helps to shun blood away from the extremities.

BP begins to fall as the compensatory mechanism (shock) begins to fail.

The patient may **collapse** if they try to stand up.

They are typically **nauseated** and they may vomit

TREATMENT of shock

1 Check airway/breathing—no breath, no life.

2 Control bleeding to minimize blood loss.

3 Find and treat the underlying cause(s).

4 Treat all injuries to minimize pain.

5 Keep the patient lying flat in a position of comfort; you may elevate their legs.

6 Protect the patient from the environment and maintain body temperature.

7 Monitor vital signs, reassure the patient and get help.

8 Administer O_2 if available, 10 – 15lpm by non-rebreather mask.

SOFT TISSUE INJURIES

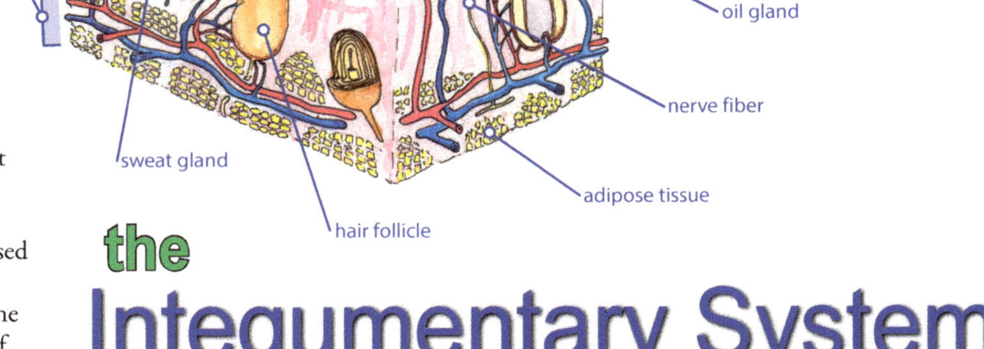

Anatomy and Physiology of the skin

EPIDERMIS

- This outer layer of the skin is composed of epithelial cells that create a protective shield.
- Most cells are made up of keratinocytes which are composed of tough, fibrous proteins.
  - These cells arise from the basal layer at the base of the epidermis and migrate toward the surface of the skin.
  - As they reach the surface and are worn away, new ones replace them.
- Other cells that make up the epidermis include melanocytes that produce the skin pigment melanin responsible for skin color.
  - When exposed to sun, the melanocytes cause the skin to tan by producing more melanin.
- There are also Langerhan's cells, (macrophages) that help activate our immune system and protect us from infectious disease, and Merkel cells that provide sensory receptors for touch.

DERMIS

- The dermis is a tough, flexible layer primarily made up of connective tissue.
- This semi-fluid matrix of collagen, elastin, and reticular fibers binds everything together.
- The dermis is supplied with nerves, blood vessels, lymphatic vessels, hair follicles, and oil and sweat glands.
- It is attached to the underlying hypodermis.

HYPODERMIS

- The hypodermis is not actually part of the skin, but it supports the skin, shares many of the same functions, and suffers the same insults.
- It is made up of adipose tissue (fat) and has a rich blood and nerve supply.
- The hypodermis gives the skin its insulation and thermoregulation capabilities.

61

Specific injuries

CONTUSIONS

- Rest, Ice, Compression, and Elevation (RICE), to limit swelling.
- Protect and watch injury closely in cold weather as it will freeze quicker than undamaged tissue

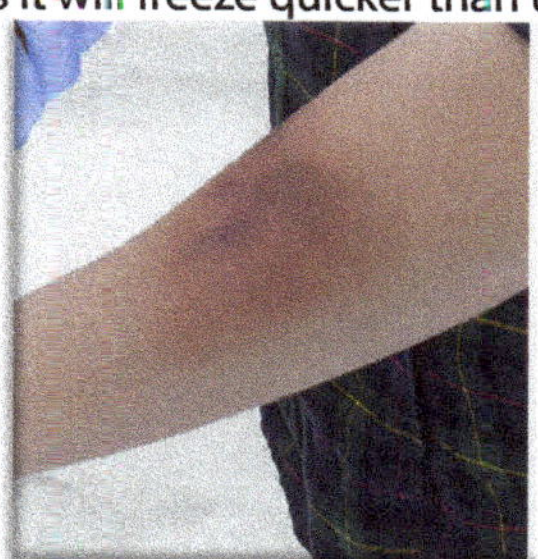

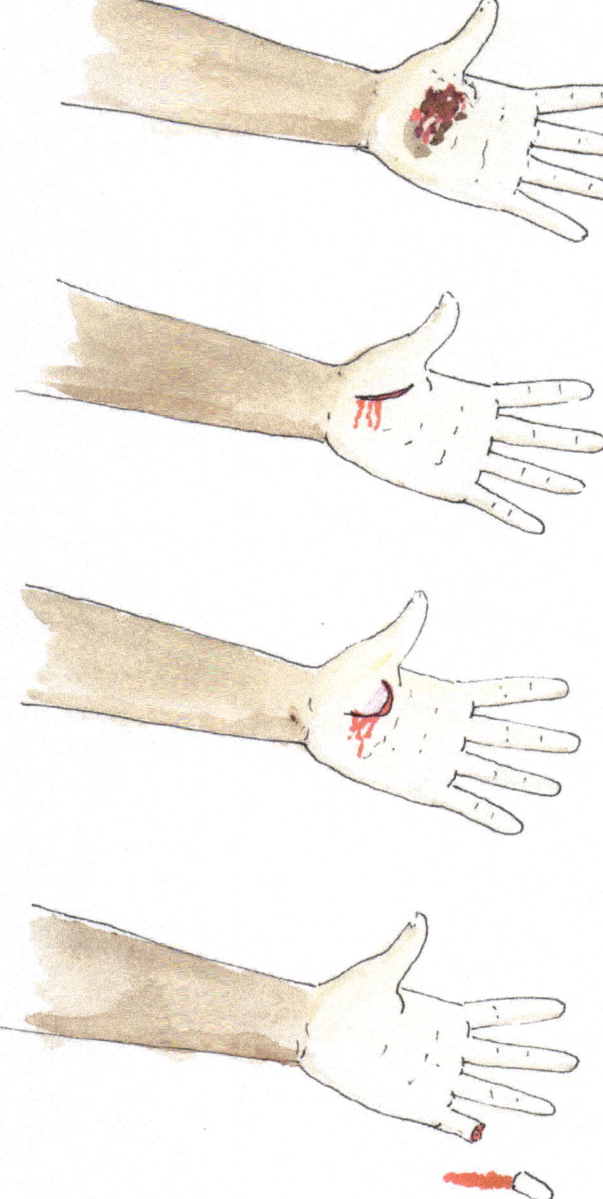

ABRASIONS

- Clean, debride, and wash thoroughly with soap and water.

LACERATIONS

- May bleed profusely or require pressure dressing
- Control bleeding and maintain hemostasis for 20 – 30 minutes.
- Cleanse well with copious irrigation.
- To treat a large gaping wound, control bleeding, cleanse with irrigation as usual, approximate the edges, but do not close tightly.

AVULSIONS

- Control bleeding.
- Rinse under flap with sterile water irrigation: place flap in proper anatomical position and bandage.

AMPUTATIONS

- Wrap the amputated part in a moist sterile dressing and seal in a plastic bag.
- Immerse the bag in ice water and evacuate both the patient and the part to the hospital.

PUNCTURES

- Gently irritate to cause some bleeding to flush out wound.
- Monitor for infection. This is the most likely wound to become infected.

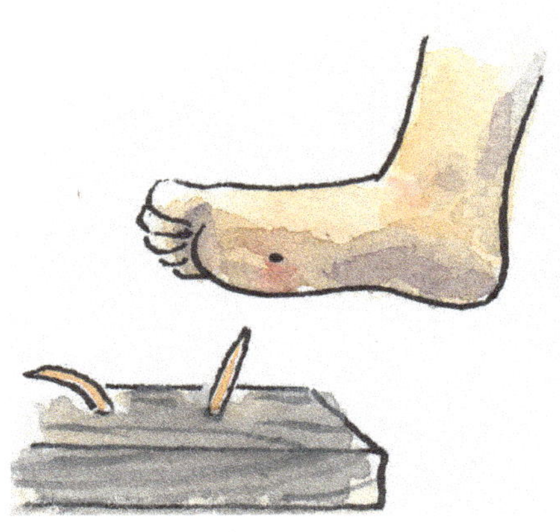

IMPALED OBJECTS

- Use common sense; if easily removed, remove it.
- Impaled objects **may be removed** if it is in an extremity, if it is metal in a cold environment, if it is too large or hard to cut off, or if it is in the cheek of the face (or the other one—buttocks) .
- An impaled object **should be bandaged in place** if it is in the skull, face, or neck, in the chest (possibly penetrating the lungs), in the abdomen (possibly penetrating the abdominal cavity and damaging organs).

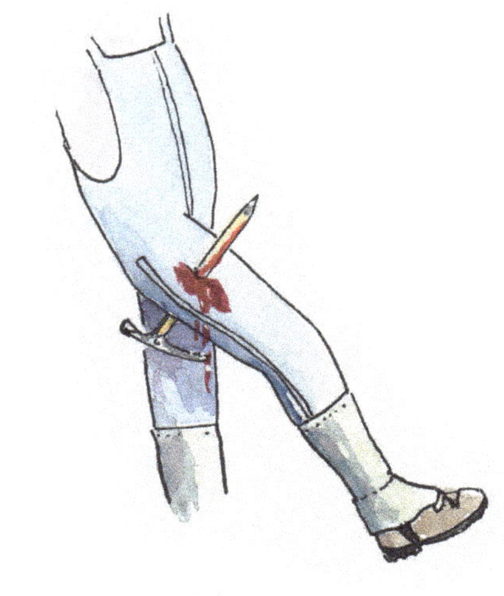

BURNS

Get the heat out

- Remove clothing over and around the burn site; cool with cold water for at least 15 minutes. (see pages 74-76)

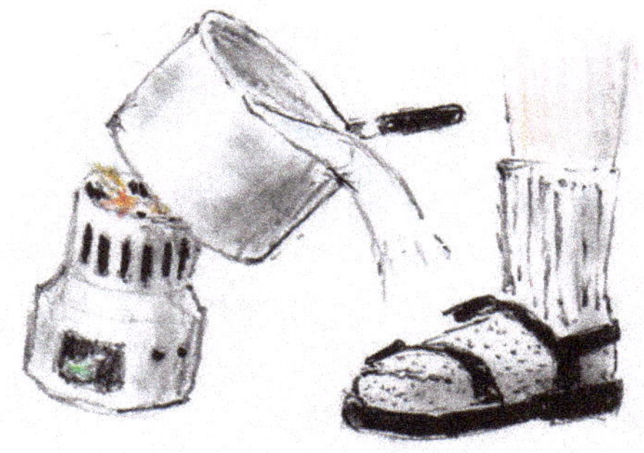

BLISTERS

- Use sterile techniques; deflate the blister; then protect with moleskin, antibiotic ointment, and tape. (see pages 80 and 81)

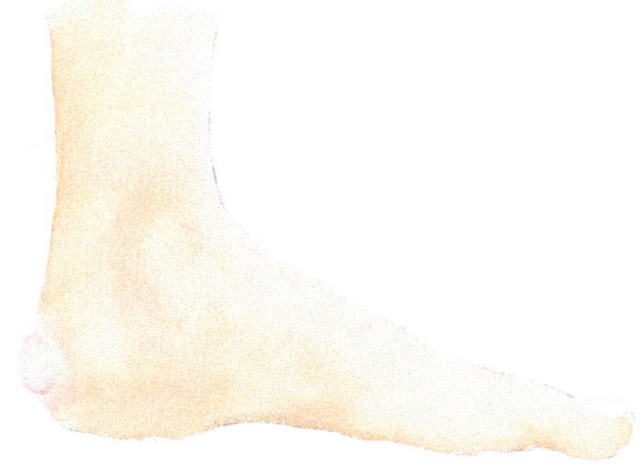

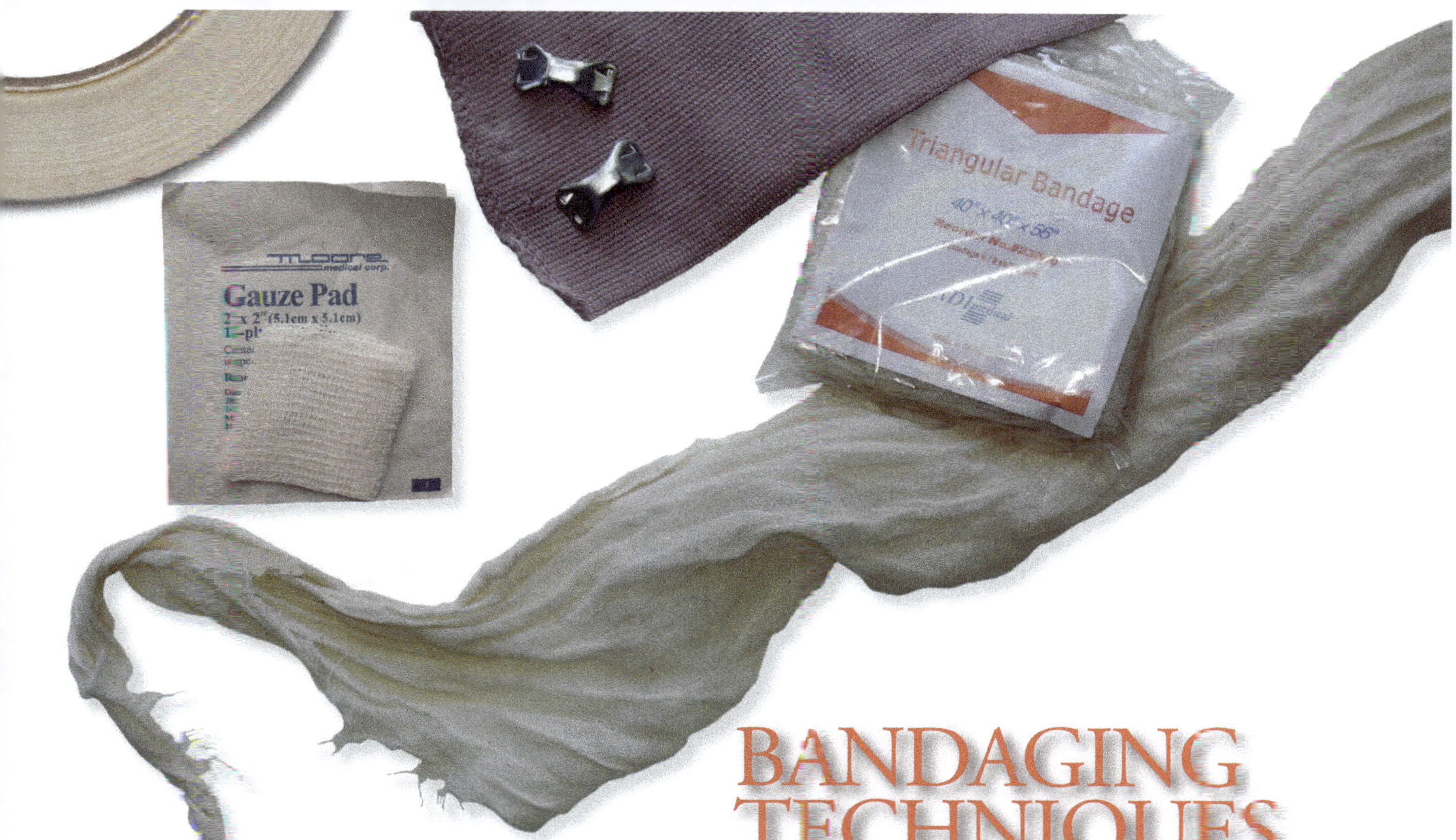

BANDAGING TECHNIQUES

BANDAGING MATERIALS

Dressings and bandages are soft items that are placed directly onto a wound to help protect the wounded tissues from further injury or insult. Common dressing and bandage materials include:

- **GAUZE PADS**—they come in a variety of shapes and sizes, from 12" x 9" trauma or abdominal dressings to smaller 4" x 4" or 2" x 2" square pads.
- **ROLLER GAUZE**—comes in a variety of widths and materials: 1" to 6" roller gauze is commonly used to hold gauze dressings and pressure bandages in place.
- **ELASTIC WRAPS**—available in widths from 2" to 6".
    - Very helpful to create pressure dressings
    - Perfect for stabilizing strains and sprains, and as the final wrap over splinting material to contain the entire splint
- **TRIANGULAR BANDAGES**
    - Tried and true, these large triangular pieces of cotton fabric are used to tie dressings and splints in place.
    - Cravat: a triangular bandage that has been folded in a 3" – 4" wide strips—"Cravat" is also the generic term used to describe any bandanna-sized triangular bandage—whether folded or not.

SPECIFIC BANDAGES

- **SCALP**
- **TOOTHACHE**
- **SHOULDER**
- **ARM SLING AND SWATHE**
- **HIP**
- **KNEE**
- **SPRAINED ANKLE**

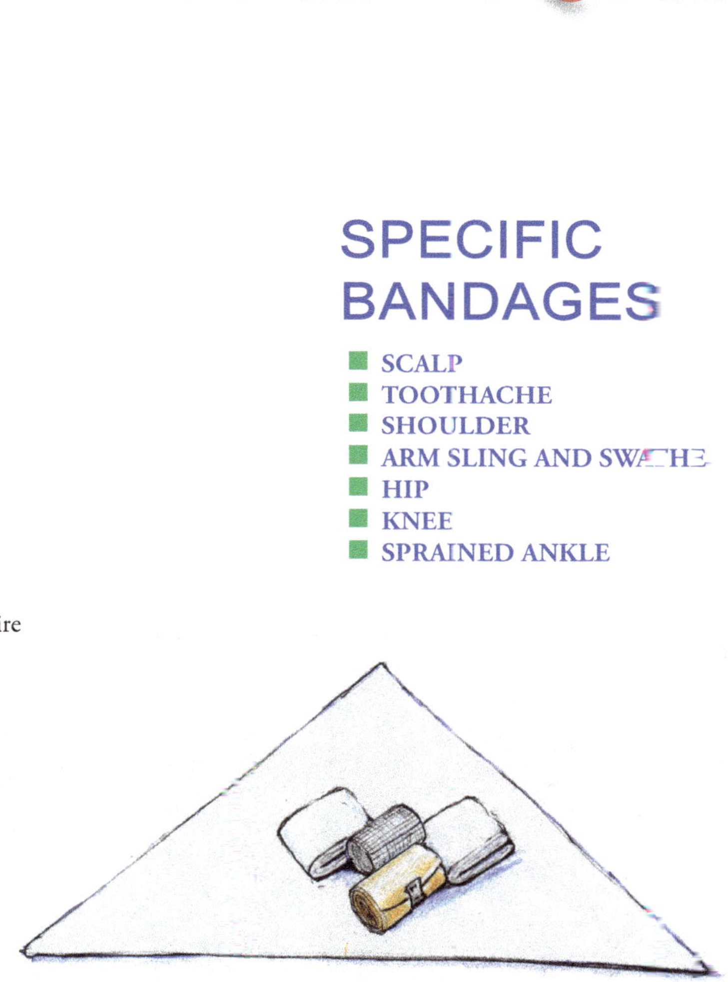

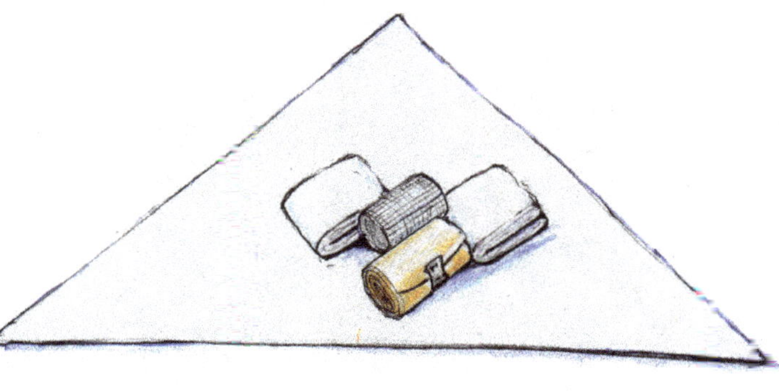

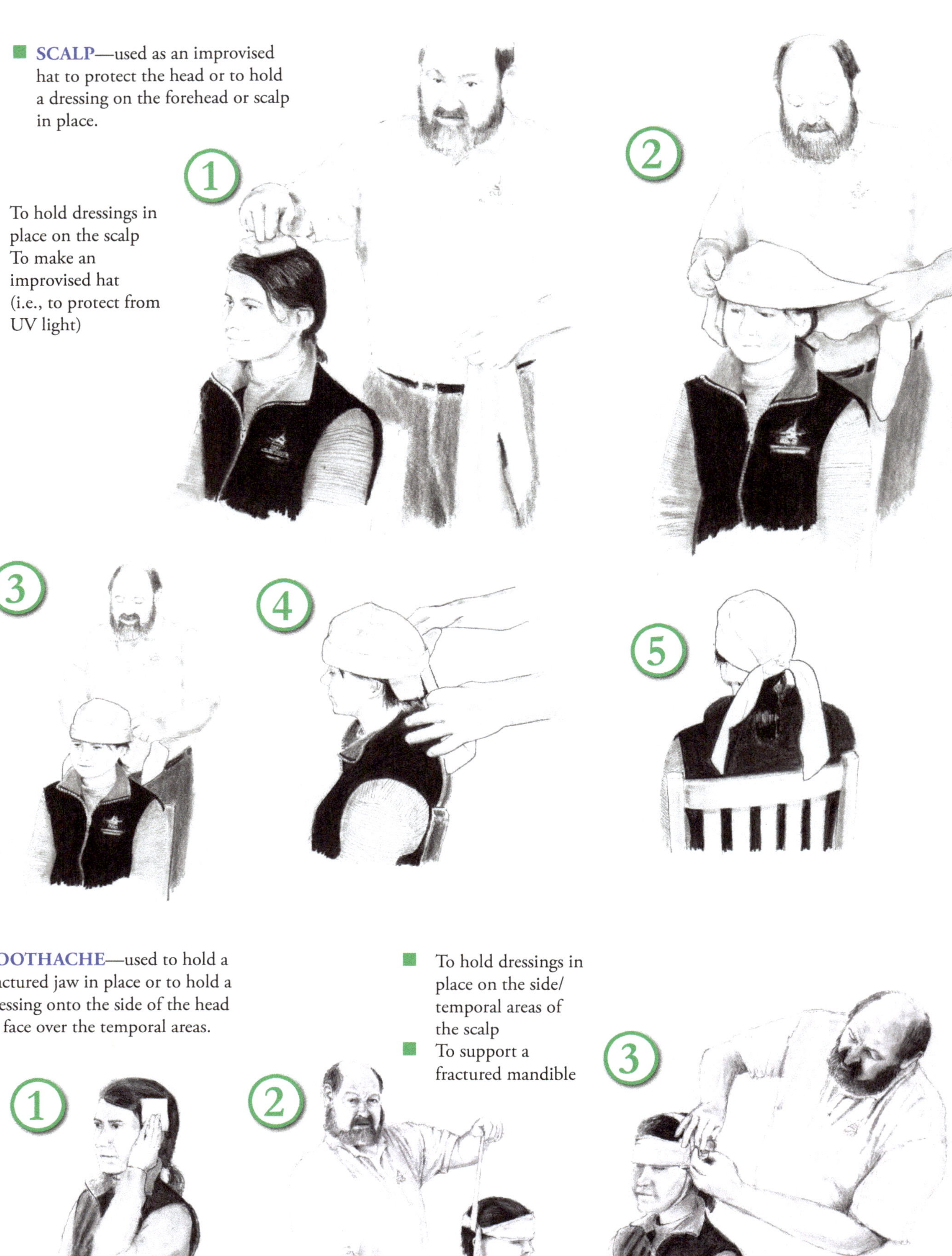

- **SCALP**—used as an improvised hat to protect the head or to hold a dressing on the forehead or scalp in place.

- To hold dressings in place on the scalp
- To make an improvised hat (i.e., to protect from UV light)

- **TOOTHACHE**—used to hold a fractured jaw in place or to hold a dressing onto the side of the head or face over the temporal areas.

- To hold dressings in place on the side/temporal areas of the scalp
- To support a fractured mandible

SHOULDER—used to support and
hold dressings onto the shoulder or
upper arm.

To hold dressings in
place on the shoulder
and upper arm

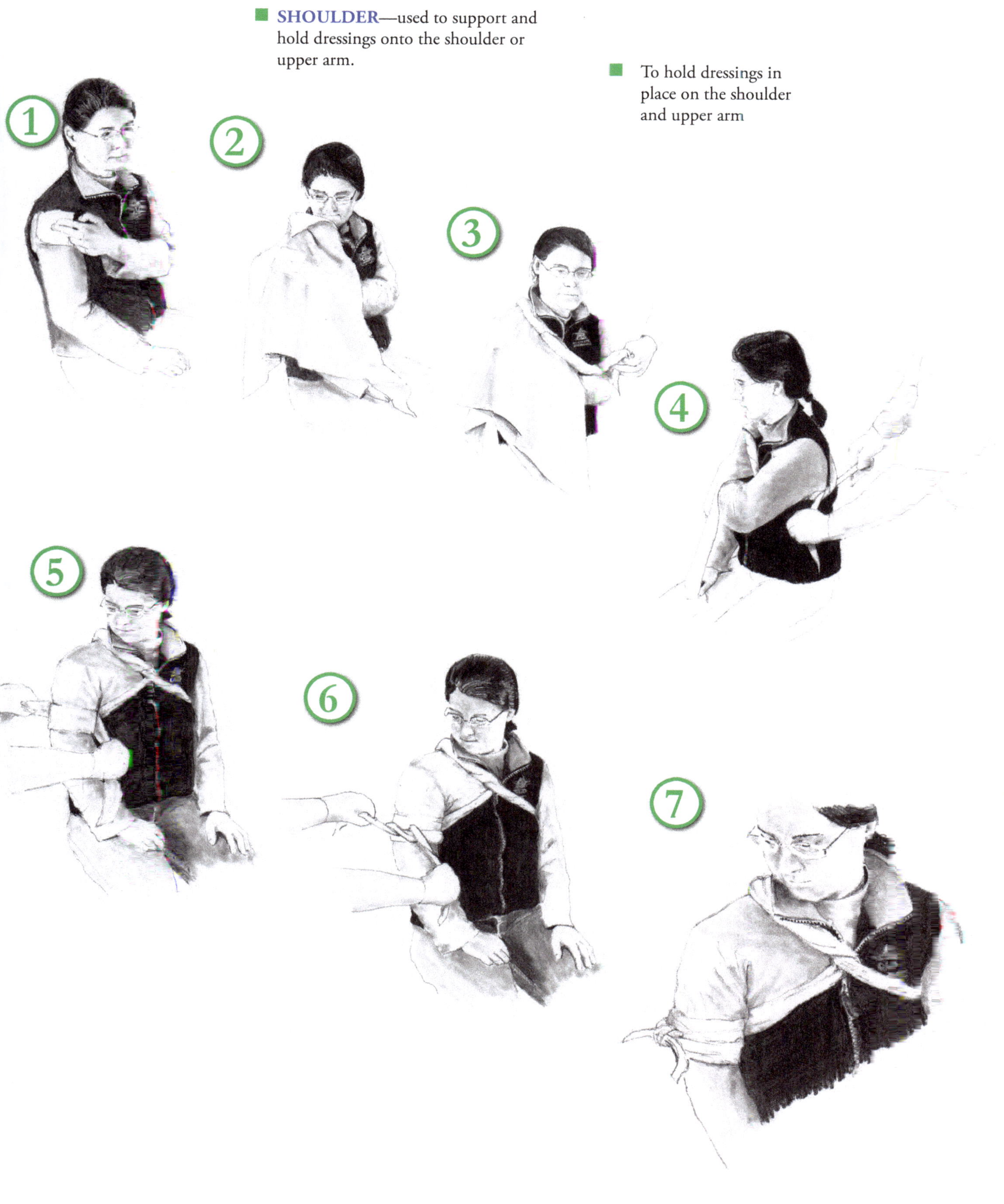

66

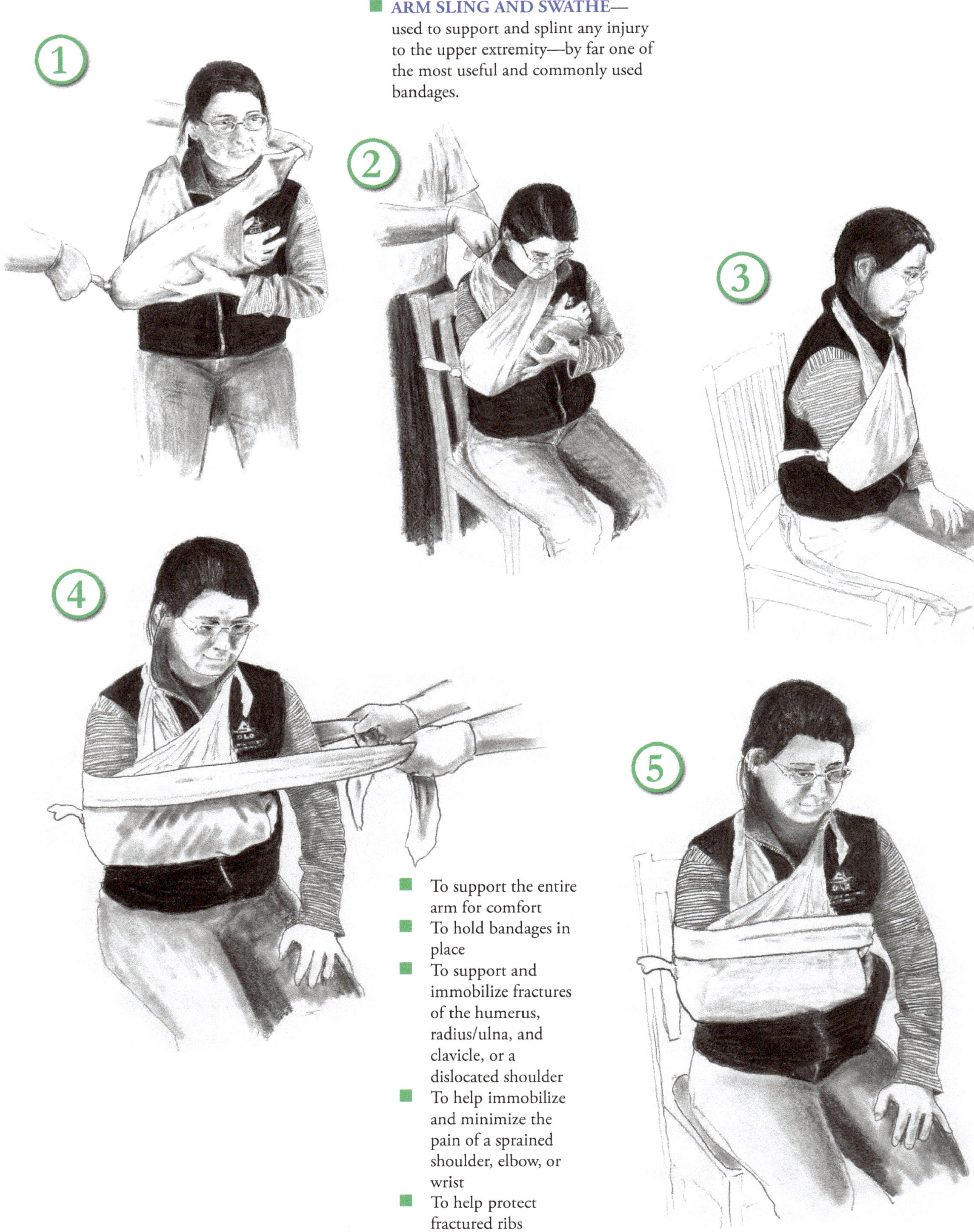

ARM SLING AND SWATHE—
used to support and splint any injury
to the upper extremity—by far one of
the most useful and commonly used
bandages.

- To support the entire
  arm for comfort
- To hold bandages in
  place
- To support and
  immobilize fractures
  of the humerus,
  radius/ulna, and
  clavicle, or a
  dislocated shoulder
- To help immobilize
  and minimize the
  pain of a sprained
  shoulder, elbow, or
  wrist
- To help protect
  fractured ribs

67

HIP—used to support and
hold dressings on to the hip,
buttocks, or upper leg.

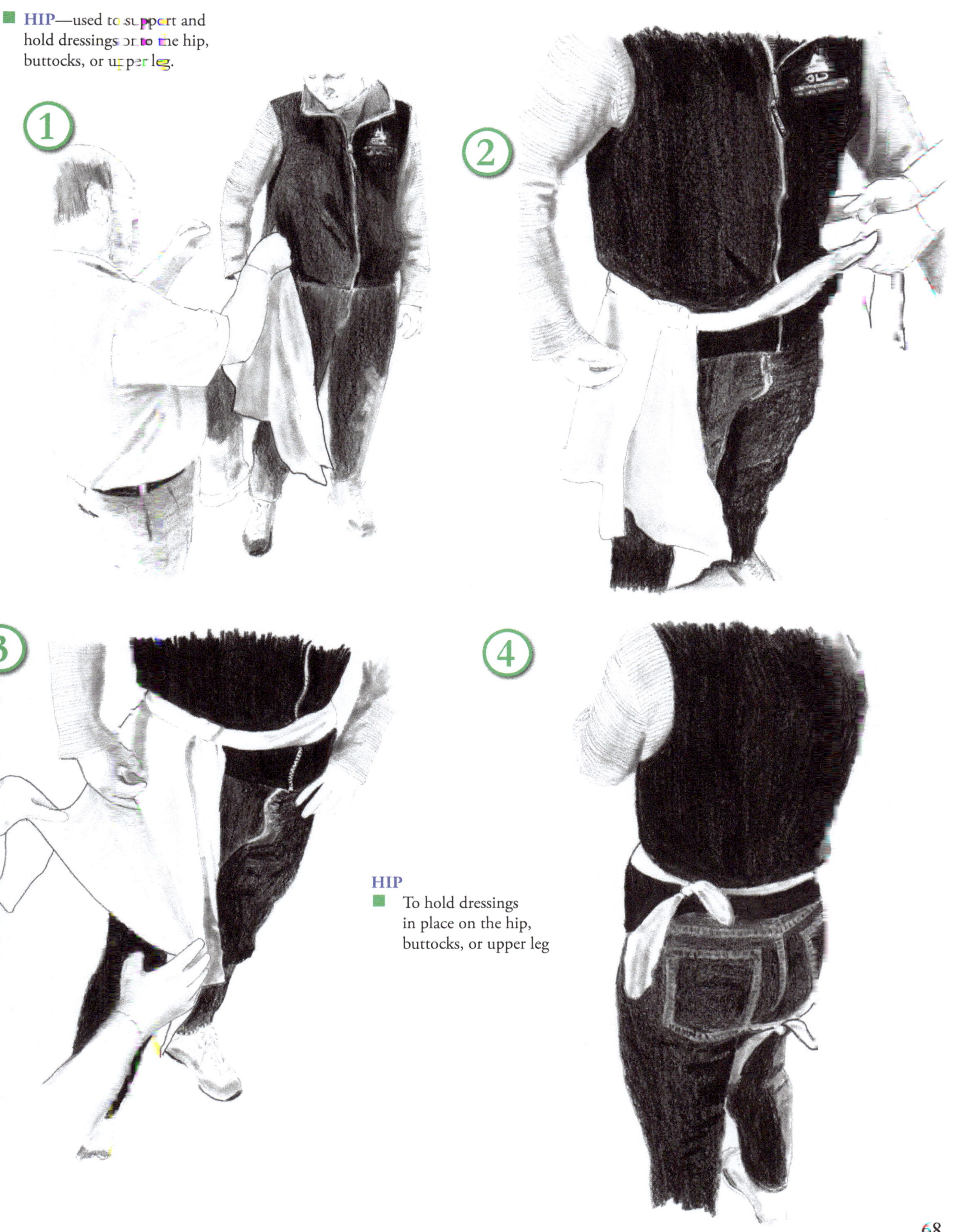

HIP
To hold dressings
in place on the hip,
buttocks, or upper leg

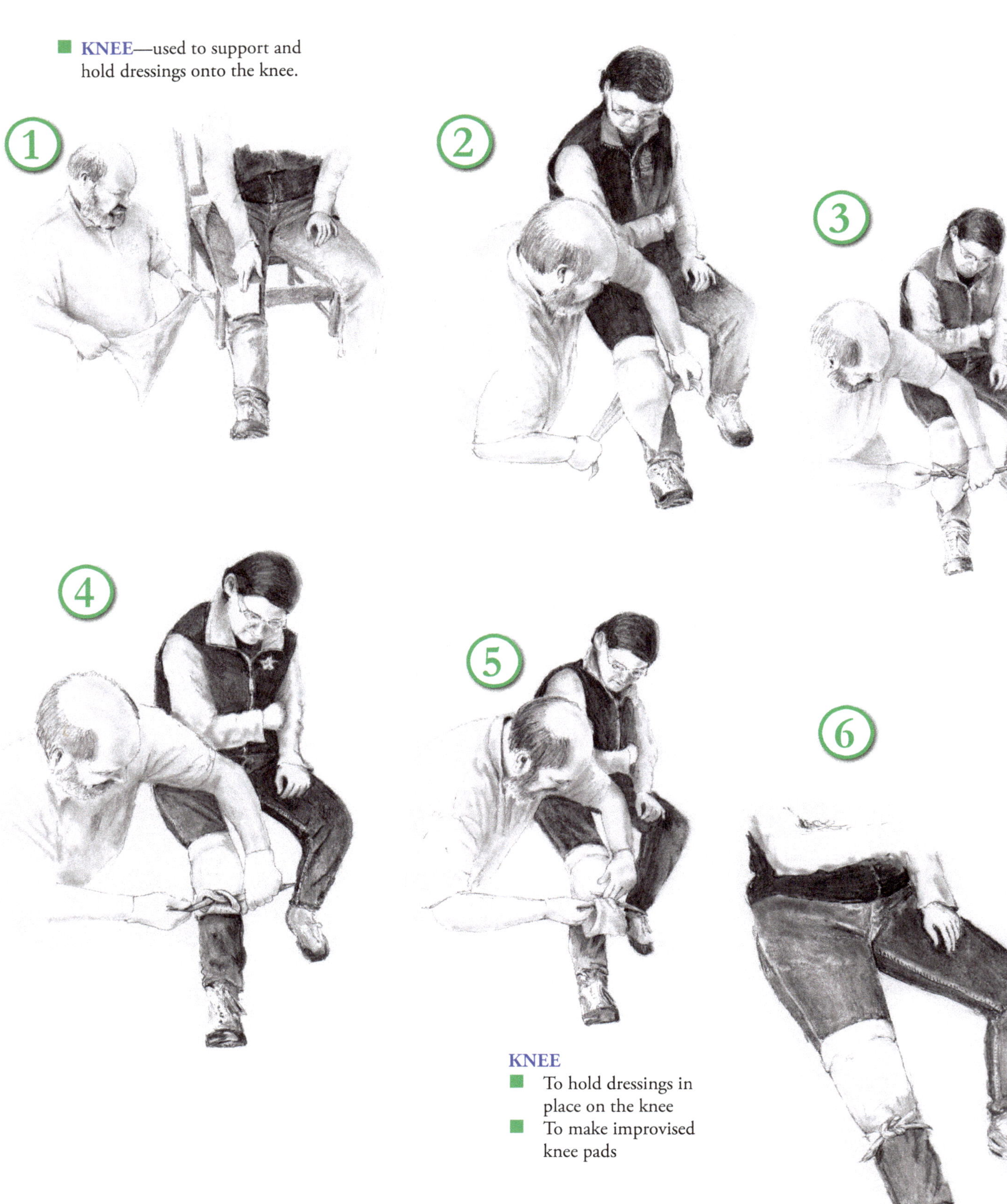

SOLO Wilderness First Responder

- **SPRAINED ANKLE**—or "S" hitch, used to support and stabilize a sprained ankle. Can also be used as the ankle hitch for an improvised traction splint. Here shown using a cravat.

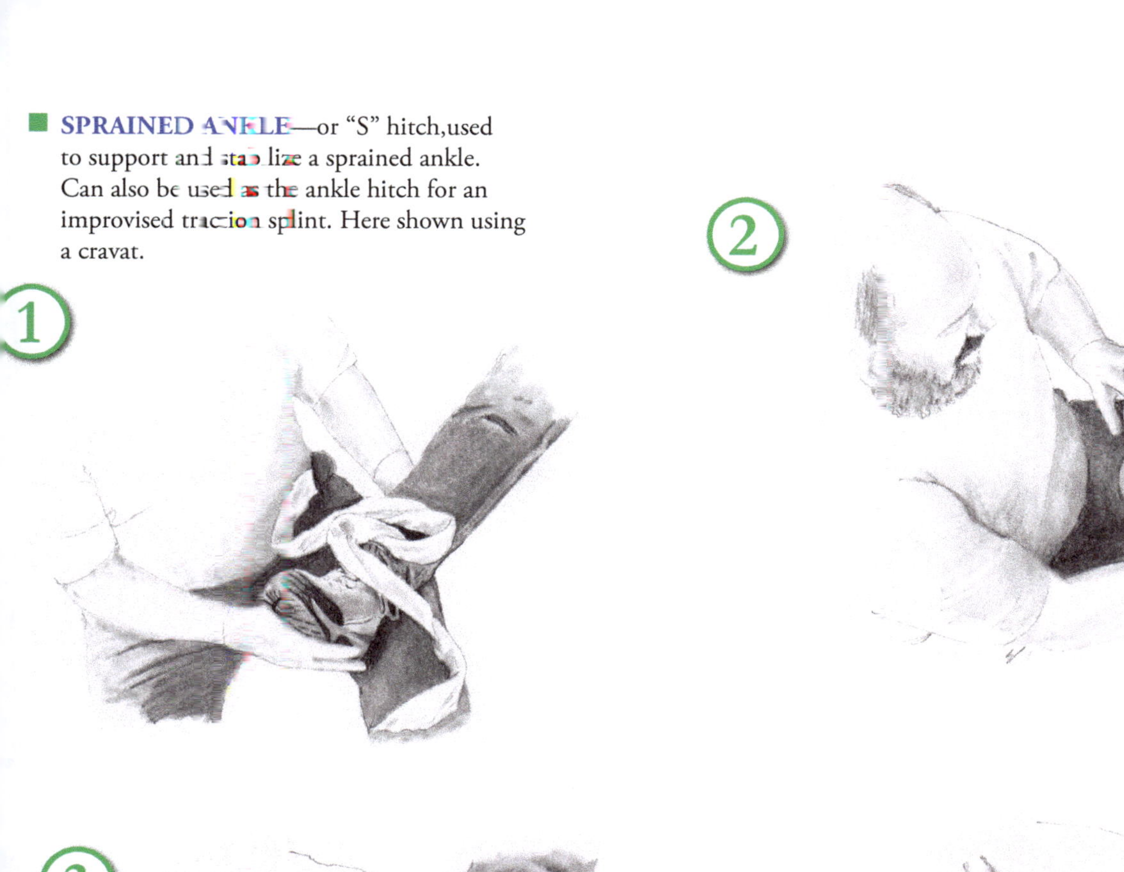

- **SPRAINED ANKLE**—used to support and stabilize a sprained ankle. Here shown using a cravat. Here shown using an elastic bandage.

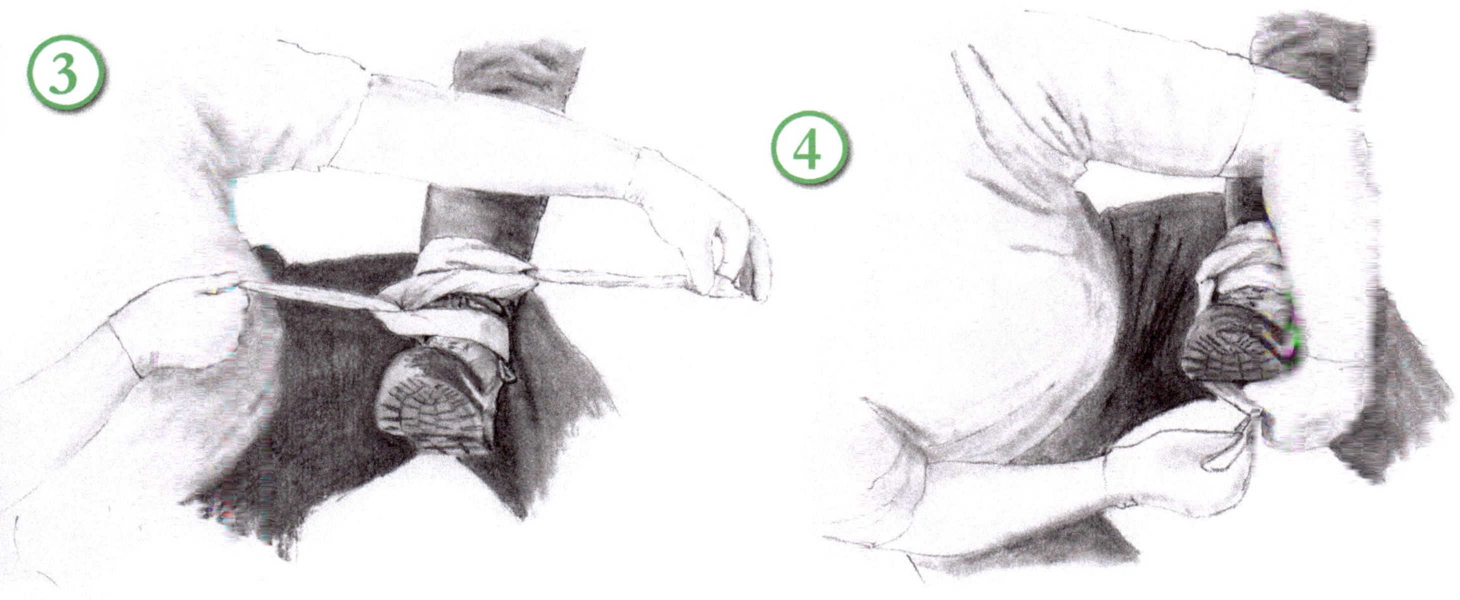

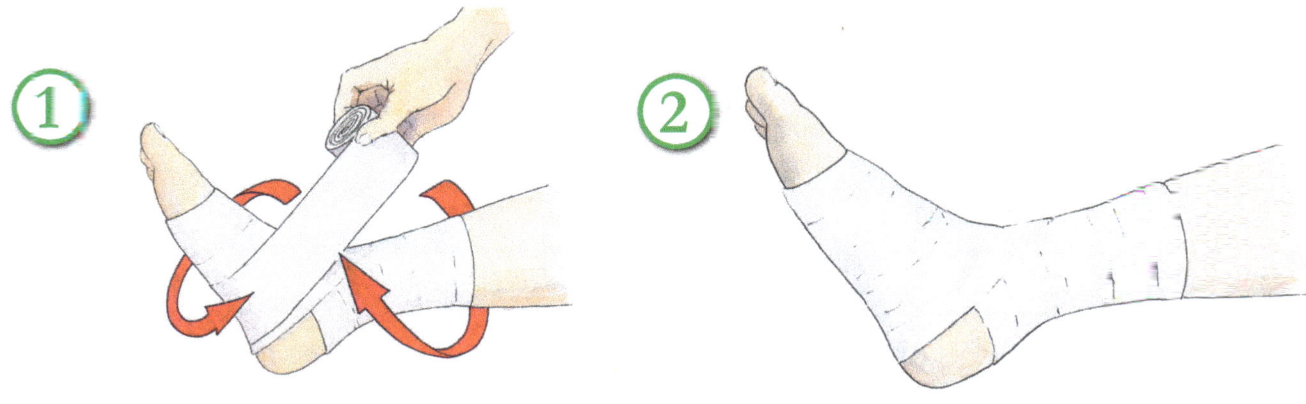

Since almost all soft tissue injuries involve open wounds, it is vital to protect your patient from infection and do everything possible to encourage fast healing. For the most part, this is simple and straightforward—but do not take it lightly. Even a minor wound can become life-threatening (due to infection) if it is not treated properly.

1. EXPOSE AND EXAMINE THE WOUND

- Is there evidence of **nerve damage** (demonstrated by loss of sensation)?
- Is there evidence of **muscle or tendon damage** (demonstrated by loss of function)?
- Is there evidence of a **severed artery** (demonstrated by the inability to control bleeding)?
  - If there is **evidence** of nerve, muscle, tendon, or artery damage, care for the wound properly, and plan to evacuate the patient as soon as possible—surgical repair will likely be needed.

2. CLEAN AND DRESS THE WOUND

- **Prepare** a dilute solution of iodine in water.
  - The amount you will need depends on the size of the wound—up to 4 liters may be needed.
  - The iodine will continue to kill bacteria that gets into the wound during the healing and evacuation process.
- **Examine** the wound closely and remove any gross debris (e.g., grass, sticks, dirt, rocks, glass, etc.). Forceps or tweezers will aid the process.
- **Clean** the wound with soap and clean water. Then rinse the wound several times with the dilute iodine solution 1) by pouring directly from a container, 2) by using a syringe, or 3) by improvising a device that will squirt the solution.
- **Dry** off the wound and cover with a sterile dressing or with a wet dressing containing the dilute iodine solution (the latter if the wound is still dirty).

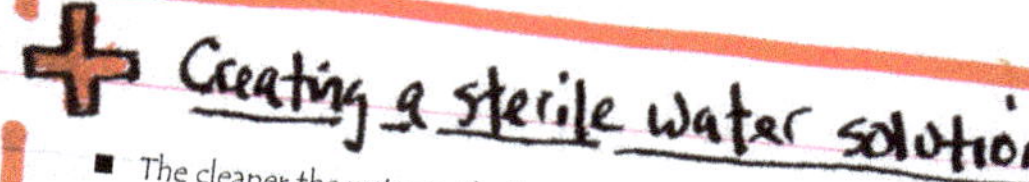

Creating a sterile water solution

- The cleaner the water is, the better, but don't hesitate to use stream or pond water—as long as you sterilize it first.
- You can sterilize water by making a dilute iodine solution (e.g., 20 milliliters iodine to 1 liter of water—a 2% solution).
- Do not exceed a 2% concentration—iodine in too high a concentration can cause damage or even death to tissues.
- The water/iodine solution should stand for 30 minutes prior to using.
- Iodine is available without prescription under the generic name povidone-iodine or the brand name Betadine.
- Sterile water can also be made by bringing it to a boil—just be sure it is cool before using it. (Don't put ice in it to cool it; the ice may not be sterile—but you can use ice to cool the container from the outside, e.g., one way is to double-bag the ice in zip-lock bags).

3. LONG-TERM WOUND CARE

- **Protect** the patient and the injured area from further injuries.
- **Monitor** for signs of infection: **tumor** (swelling), **rubor** (redness), **calor** (heat), **dolor** (aching), **purulence** (pus formation: a collection of white blood cells).
- Signs of a **worsening** infection: **lymphangina** (red streaks traveling up the lymphatic ducts), **lymphadenopathy** (swollen lymph nodes when the infection reaches them), **fever and chills** as the infection begins to spread systemically, **septic shock** (a dangerous medical emergency caused by decreased tissue perfusion and oxygen delivery as a result of severe infection; can lead to organ failure and death; the mortality rate is approximately 25% – 50%)
- Treatment if infection occurs:
  - **Apply** non-scalding hot water with Epsom Salts to the infection every 6 hours.
  - **Consider** starting an oral antibiotic, such as Keflex (500mg) every 6 hours.
  - If an abscess forms, **drain** it (see specific directions in the section on cellulitis).
- **Inspect** the wound and change the dressings every 12 hours (more often if dirty).
- If the wound is on an extremity, **check regularly** for circulation, sensation, and movement distal to the wound site.
- **Find out** when the patient last had a tetanus booster (if it's been more than 10 years, another booster will be needed quickly, within 48 hours, if possible).

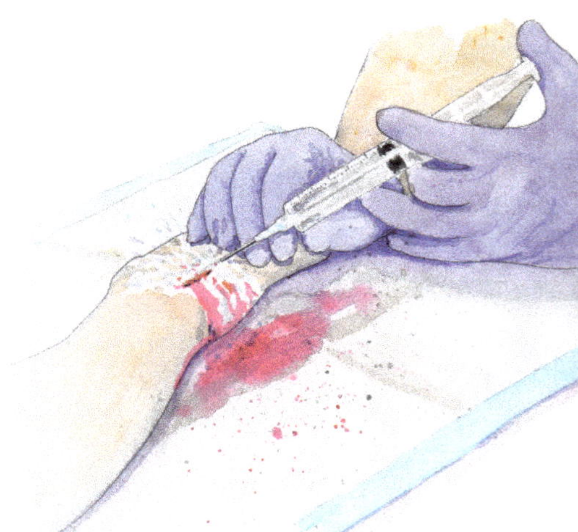

Thorough cleaning is one of the most important aspects of wound treatment—a few minutes of concentrated effort can eliminate days of painful infection.

Special considerations

IMPALED OBJECTS

GENERAL TREATMENT PRINCIPLES

◆ **It is usually best to remove an impaled object, if it comes out easily.**
  - However, sometimes removing an impaled object (such as one that has damaged a major artery or is in a dense vascular area, like the abdomen) will put the patient at risk of severe bleeding—in cases like this the impaled object provides perfect direct/digital pressure (see sidebar).

◆ **Examine the object.**
  - *How big is it?*
    - Is the object too big, too heavy, or too long?
    - Can the patient be moved and transported without the object shifting and causing more damage?
  - *What is it made of?*
    - Can it conduct heat or cold? A metal object can increase the risk of hypothermia and frostbite—a good reason to consider removing it.
  - *How is it shaped?*
    - Is it smooth, serrated, barbed, or some shape that would be difficult to remove?
  - *Where is it embedded?*
    - If in an arm or leg, treatment is typically straightforward.
    - Has it damaged a major artery or vein? These injuries may bleed profusely when the object is removed.
    - In the chest or abdomen? Organ damage may have occurred, or major blood vessels may be damaged.
    - If the object appears to have penetrated the chest or abdominal cavity and is firmly stuck in place, since there is no way to determine what vital organs may have been injured, pad and immobilize the object.
    - If the object is loose and ready to fall out, gently remove it to eliminate its potential for causing more damage by moving around. If you remove the object, take it with the patient to definitive care to aid in evaluating the injury.
    - Head, face, or neck? If the object appears to have penetrated more than 1cm (1/2") and is firmly in place, leave it and package it to maintain its position.
      - Evacuate.
      - For impaled objects in the eye, see the eye injury section.

◆ **Infection is a major concern.**
  - Microbes have likely been driven deep into the body.
  - Clean the wound and surrounding tissue thoroughly.
  - Gently irritate the wound to promote bleeding and to aid in flushing out the wound.
  - If the wound is open, leave it open.
  - Monitor for signs of infection.
  - If more than 10 years have lapsed, the patient needs a tetanus booster.

IMPALED FISH HOOKS

- ◆ **Method 1 (for a barbless hook)**
    - ◆ If you're dealing with a barbless hook, just back it out the same way it went in—simple catch and release.
- ◆ **Method 2 (for a barbed hook)**
    - ◆ Force the hook to continue through the skin until it re-emerges.
    - ◆ Cut the barbed portion of the hook with pliers or wire cutters.
    - ◆ Back the original part of the hook out the way it came in.
    - ◆ This is a painful technique that requires a cutting device, but it is effective.
- ◆ **Method 3 (for a barbed hook)**
    - ◆ Grab the shank and push the hook down and back, and it should pop out.
    - ◆ This is a less barbaric—and less traumatic—method than the previous method and is the same method you use to remove a hook from a fish (although the fish isn't usually as big a baby about it).
- ◆ **Method 4 (for a barbed hook)**
    - ◆ This "push-me-pull-you maneuver" is kinder, gentler, a little less painful, and causes less tissue damage than the previous methods for a barbed hook.
    - ◆ Gently pull on the hook to feel how well it is seated.
    - ◆ Attach a loop of fishing line to the bend in the hook close to the skin—this will aid you in pulling the hook out.
    - ◆ Now, perform the maneuver (you will have to do two things at once—having a helper will make it a lot easier).
    - ◆ Push the hook shank toward the surface of the skin.
        - ◆ Pliers or a hemostat will make this easier.
        - ◆ This will force the back of the bend of the hook to push the tissues deeper, helping to free the barb.
    - ◆ At the same time, gently pull on the fishing line attached to the bend of the hook—parallel to the skin
    - ◆ As the barb becomes free, the fishhook will come out.
    - ◆ Do not yank during the maneuver—the hook may pop out and embed itself elsewhere.
    - ◆ Note: even with your best efforts, tissue damage may occur.

The problem with most hooks is that they are barbed, which greatly increases their holding power (whether in a carp or the guy next to you)—especially when you are trying get them out. And, despite your best efforts, it's really hard to remove them without doing damage. Note: each of the techniques described also works with multiple hooks (e.g., treble hooks), although things will be more complicated.

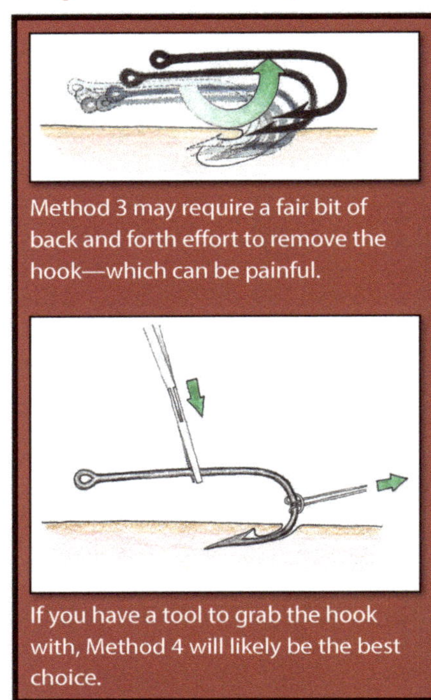

Method 3 may require a fair bit of back and forth effort to remove the hook—which can be painful.

If you have a tool to grab the hook with, Method 4 will likely be the best choice.

Once the hook is out, treat the injury as a puncture wound.

WORK WITH WHAT YOU HAVE GOT!

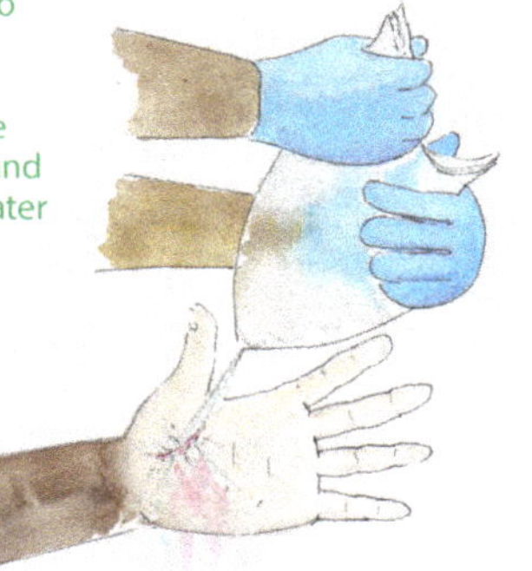

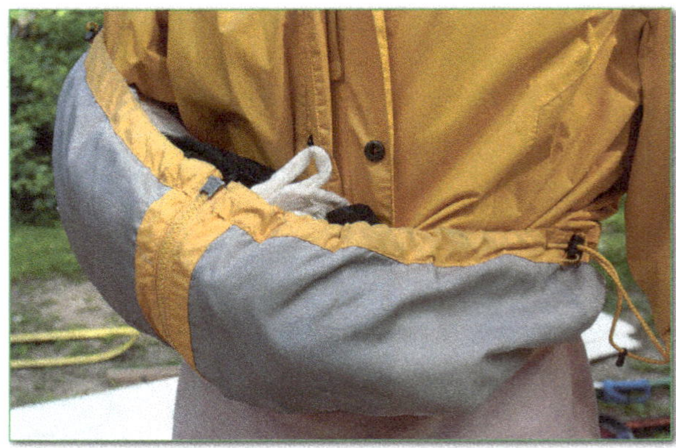

By its very nature, wilderness medicine often takes imagination and creativity—and improvisation is at the heart of it. You find a person who needs a sling/swathe but you don't have a backpack full of cravats? No problem! Just roll up their jacket and the rummage around for something to make a swathe with (e.g., a long-sleeved shirt), and you're good to go!

BURNS

TYPES OF BURNS

THERMAL BURNS

al burns are caused by an external heat source: fire, a hot stove, hot water, hot food.

- What you see is the extent of the burn.
- It is usually easy to estimate the depth and extent of the burn.

ELECTRICAL BURNS

Electrical burns are caused by resistance to electrical current flowing through tissue: lightning, contact with a man-made electrical source (e.g., household wiring). In addition to tissue damage at the contact point (the skin), electrical burns can cause additional problems.

- Respiratory arrest
- Seizures
- Fractures
- Extensive muscle damage—the current can extend well below the skin surface, so what may appear to be a relatively minor injury may actually be quite extensive beneath
- Can also have associated entry and exit wounds

CHEMICAL BURNS

Chemical burns are caused by both the heat produced by some chemical reactions, as well as direct chemical interaction with the skin. Examples of strong corrosives (either strong acids or bases) that can cause chemical burns:

- Bleach
- Concrete mix
- Drain cleaner (lye)
- Metal cleaners
- Pool chlorinators
- Battery acid

RADIATION BURNS

Radiation burns are caused by exposure to alpha, beta, gamma, or X-ray radiation, typically in an industrial or medical setting. This ionizing radiation can cause damage to cells and their DNA—this is very rare, as the victim would have to be exposed to a radioactive source (e.g., the Fujita nuclear power plant accident, following the 2011 tsunami in Japan, caused ionizing radiation damage to some rescue workers).

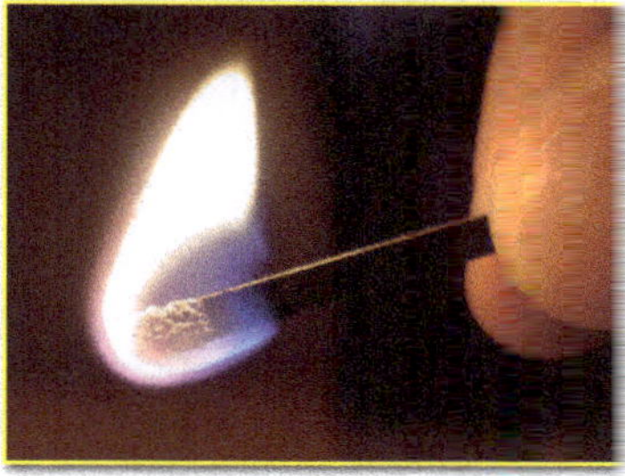

THERMAL

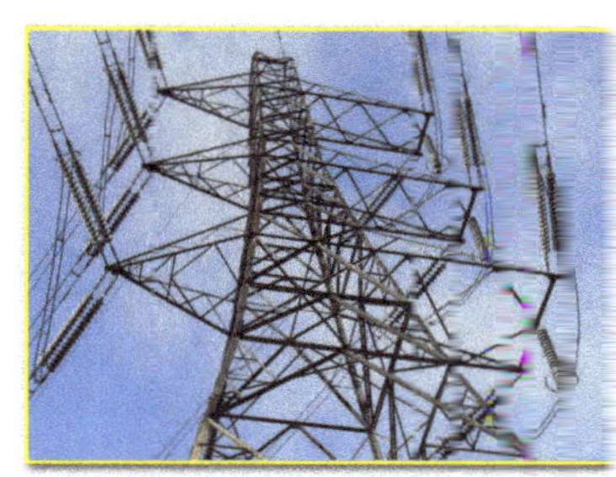

ELECTRICAL

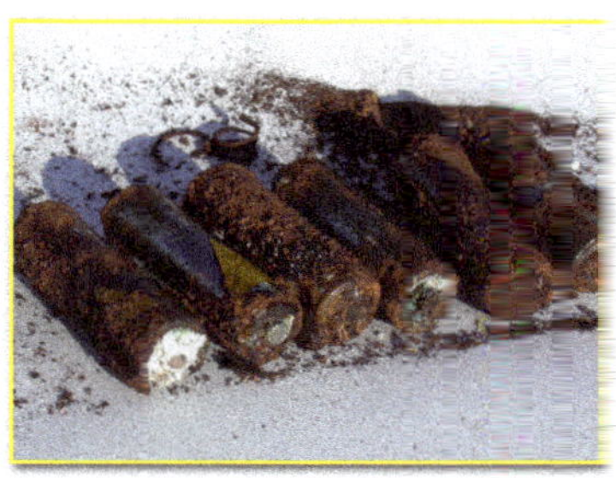

CHEMICAL

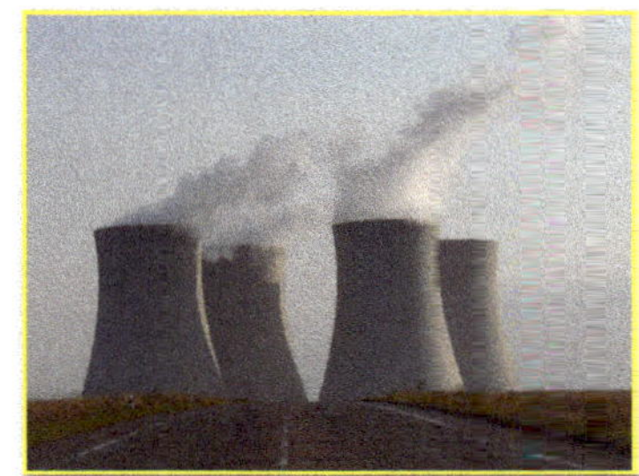

RADIATION

DETERMINING THE SEVERITY AND EXTENT OF THERMAL BURNS

Thermal burns are like many injuries—both the things that you do (and the pace that you do them) depend to a great extent on how bad the injury is. With burns, there are two things to determine:

1. The severity of the burn (how deep it goes into the tissue).
2. The extent of the burn (the surface area affected as a percentage of total body surface area).

In general, the deeper the burn and greater surface area it covers, the more severe the burn is. But it can be more complicated than that: a small full-thickness burn (that goes all the way through the hypodermis) may not be as severe (and thus, not require as fast and furious an evacuation) as a surface burn over a large area.

In addition to determining the depth and measuring the extent of a burn (below), there are other factors that you should consider when determining the overall seriousness of the injury—keep the following things in mind.

- Burn damage to the face, genitals, and airway make things more serious.
  - Genital burns can be very painful.
  - Even a minor burn to the airway can produce swelling significant enough to threaten the airway (this may take time to develop—pay attention).
  - Burns rarely cause immediate death, except when the airway is involved.
- Circumferential burns (burns that encircle a limb) can impair circulation distal to the burn site (over hours to days), requiring surgical escharotomy (cutting through the dead tissue of a full-thickness burn to relieve pressure and re-establish circulation distally).

SEVERITY

- SUPERFICIAL (1st degree)
  - Damage is limited to the top layer of the skin, the epidermis.
  - The area is red (erythema).
  - It is mildly painful.
  - It is tender to the touch.
  - There is an increase in warmth.
  - It can be itchy.
  - Sunburn is a good example of a superficial burn.
- PARTIAL THICKNESS (2nd degree)
  - Damage extends through the epidermis into the upper layers of the dermis.
  - The area is red because of vasodilation.
  - It can be very tender.
  - It is quite warm to the touch.
  - Painful blisters form (in minutes to hours).
  - Contact with boiling water is an example of a partial thickness burn.
- FULL THICKNESS (3rd degree)
  - The burn extends through the epidermis and dermis and into the hypodermis.
  - The area can be red, black, pale, or charred.
  - There is no pain because the nerves have been destroyed.
  - There is little or no bleeding because the vasculature has been destroyed.
  - Surrounding the burn area there will typically be additional areas of painful partial-thickness damage.

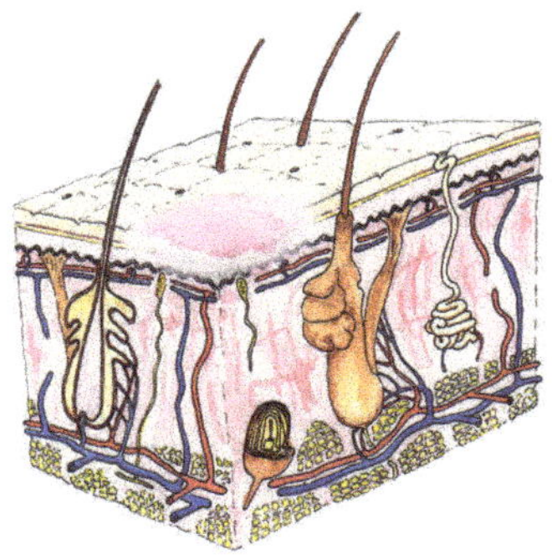

Superficial: damage just to the epidermis

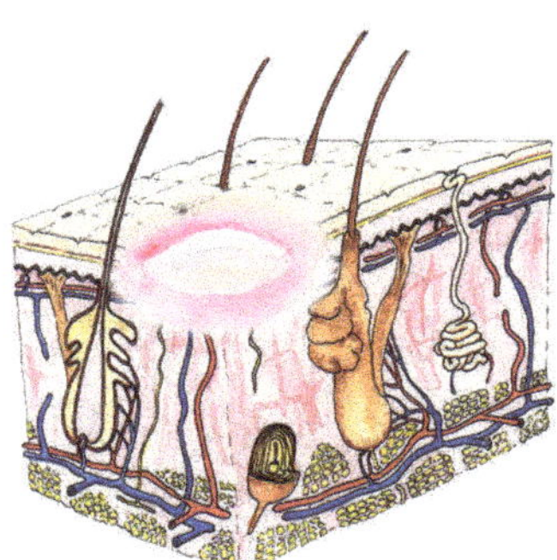

Partial Thickness: damage extends into the dermis; blisters may form

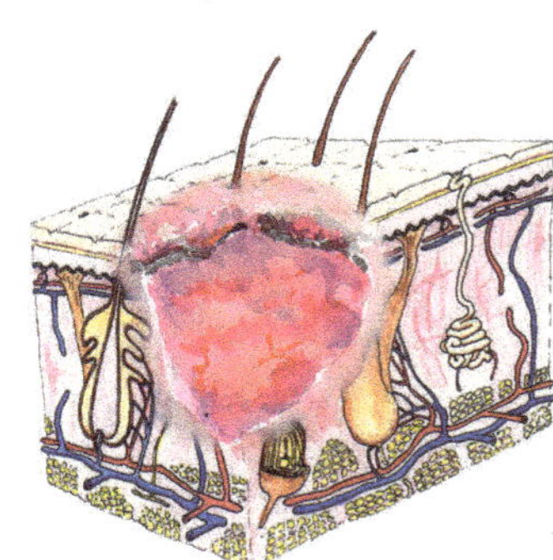

Full Thickness: damage extends into the hypodermis; subcutaneous tissue, nerves, and vasculature is destroyed

75

EXTENT

There are two common methods for estimating the percentage of total body surface area (TBSA) covered by a burn: the Rule of Nines and the Rule of Palm.

- The Rule of Nines
    - This method divides the body of a typical adult into 12 areas, and assigns either 4.5%, 9%, or 18% to each area, with the genitals taking up the final 1%, for a total of 100%.
    - Because it uses relatively large increments, this method is most useful for burns that cover an extensive area.
    - With modifications (see chart below) it can also be used for the obese, children, and infants (their proportions are different so the numbers are not divisors or multipliers of 9).
    - In the chart below, if you do the math, only the column for adults adds up to 100% (the others are close, but not perfect)—the Rule of Nines is not meant to be precise; it is an *estimating* tool.
    - Also, bear in mind that burns may cover more than one body part or may not fully cover a particular body part—for complicated or fragmented burn patterns, consider using the Rule of Palm.

- The Rule of Palm
    - This is not the preferred technique because anatomical proportions are inconsistent with age groups and populations.
    - This method assumes that the area of an adult palm (not including the fingers) equals approximately 1% on a typical adult.
    - Because it measures in smaller increments, this method is *only* useful for burns covering a relatively small area.
    - *It should not be used* for children and infants because their proportionally smaller body sizes would give deflated values and underestimation of the total burn area—use the Rule of Nines for children and infants.

- Rule of nines Babies and small children:
    - Head 18%
    - Front of torso 18%
    - Back 18%
    - Each arm 9%
    - Each leg 14%

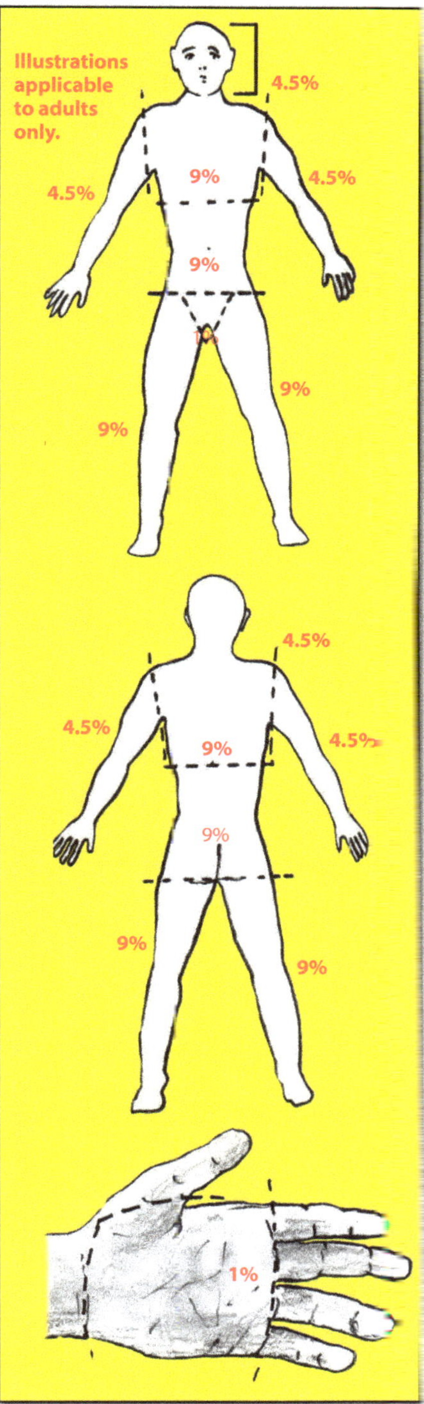

GENERAL TREATMENT PRINCIPLES

COOL IT FAST!

IMMEDIATE CARE FOCUSES ON FOUR AREAS

- Getting the heat out to minimize the extent of the burn
- Controlling all life-threatening problems
- Remove all jewlery
- Minimizing fluid loss from evaporation
- Pain control

LONG-TERM MANAGEMENT OF THE BURN PATIENT

- Fluid and electrolyte replacement
- Pain control
- Additional calories to aid in healing
- Thermal regulation

BURNS CAUSE SIGNIFICANT PAIN

and damage, plus long-lasting physical and emotional scars. Annually in the US there are about 1 million burn cases seen in emergency rooms, over 45,000 hospitalizations, and about 4,000 deaths. (The number of annual deaths has dropped significantly over the last 20 years due to increased use of smoke detectors and fire suppressant systems.) When a burn occurs, there is a risk of significant fluid loss both from the intense heat of the burn and from the loss of the protective waterproof barrier (skin). In severe burns, the skin and associated tissues are destroyed and fluid loss will continue to occur (along with electrolyte loss) for hours, and in some cases days and weeks. Burn injuries do not resolve quickly.

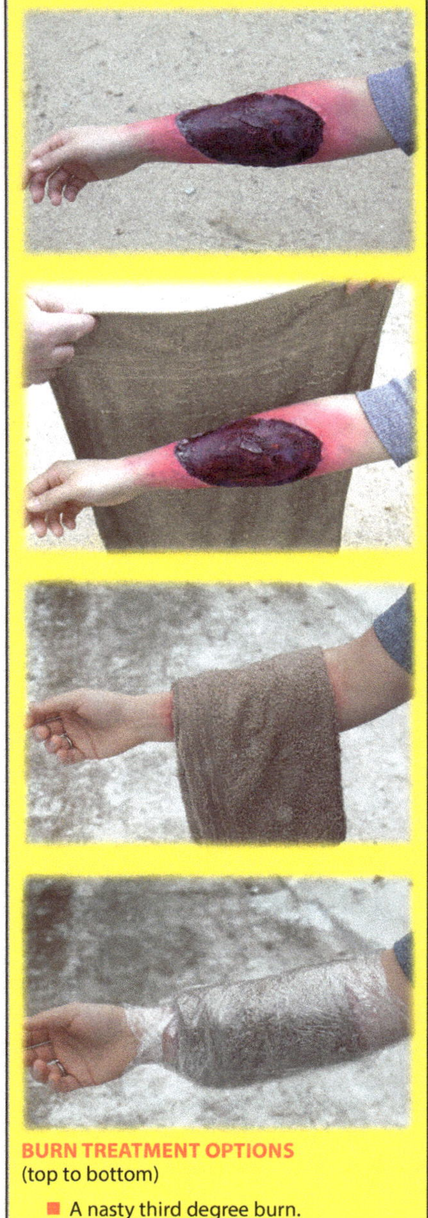

BURN TREATMENT OPTIONS
(top to bottom)

- A nasty third degree burn.
- A moist, sterile dressing (a towel, boiled and then cooled and soaked in a dilute Betadine solution).
- An occlusive dressing (minimized fluid loss through evaporation).
- Depending on the burn, an additional wet dressing can be applied over the occlusive dressing.
- Wrap the entire dressing packaged with an ACE wrap (not shown).

- **Minimize fluid loss, maintain fluid and electrolyte levels.**
  - When you re-dress the wound, help minimize the amount of fluid loss via evaporation by covering full-thickness burns with an occlusive dressing (e.g., plastic food wrap—this is airtight and waterproof and helps maintain core temperature and prevent hypothermia). Start with an under-dressing, moistened with a 1% dilute Betadine (see treatment section for formula) or 2% iodine solution, and finish with an occlusive dressing, and a final wrap.
  - You must replace electrolytes, too—use oral rehydration salts or rice water—cook rice with salt and continue to add water until the cooked rice dissolves into a milky-colored liquid (rice water is rich in electrolytes and carbohydrates).
  - Use vital signs and urine output to estimate fluid replacement—vital signs should stay in the normal range and adequate fluid volume should produce light amber urine. Minimal fluid output in an adult is at least 0.5cc/kg/hr, or at least 500cc per day (20⁺cc per hour). This minimal output cannot be sustained for long—urine output of 1000cc – 1500cc per 24 hours (50⁺cc per hour) is needed to maintain normal homeostasis.

- **Monitor vital signs.**
  - For severe burns, especially for extensive partial- or full-thickness burns, initially check vital signs every 10 – 15 minutes for the first two hours, then every 30 minutes after that.
  - If the vital signs deteriorate and indicate shock, treat the shock and evacuate the patient to definitive care immediately.

- **Control pain.**
  - Use a moist dressing as the outer layer—evaporation will provide cooling and comfort.
  - Administer Tylenol (acetaminophen or paracetamol) up to 3000mg total per 24 hours.
  - NSAID (aspirin, ibuprofen, naproxen): dosages vary depending on the med.
  - Note: Tylenol and an NSAID can be used together for very effective pain control.
  - Narcotics can be used and are extremely effective (codeine, hydrocodone, oxycodone).

- **Minimize the risk of infection.**
  - A burn is sterile for the first 24 hours—after that, the risk of infection increases.
  - It is easier to prevent an infection than treat one.
  - Re-dress the wound twice a day, if possible—or as often as necessary to prevent seepage through the dressing.
  - Use sterile dressings each time.

- **Keep the burn site clean**—reassess and debride the burn 2 - 3 times per a day.

- **Monitor blisters.**
  - Blisters form with partial thickness (2nd degree) burns.
  - If possible, leave them intact—they are sterile and leaving them intact helps minimize the risk of infection.
  - If a blister ruptures, gently debride the site by removing dead skin.

- **Provide proper nutrition.**
  - Cellular repair with any injury requires significant calories from carbohydrates and protein.
  - Burn patients have a very high calorie demand

- **Use ointments**—most over-the-counter ointments and antibiotic creams do little or nothing to aid in the healing process of a burn.

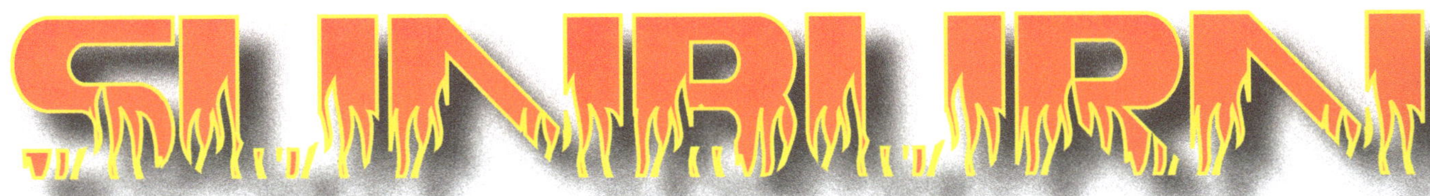

Sunburn is a unique and very common form of radiation burn caused by the direct effects of intense sunlight on exposed skin—the ultraviolet wavelengths A and B (UVA and UVB) account for the damage.

- These wavelengths cause chemical changes in the skin cells.
    - These changes, in turn, cause the blood vessels to dilate and stimulate the melanocytes (melanin-producing cells in the bottom layer of the epidermis) to crank out melanin.
    - This increase in melanin is our body's way of protecting us from future exposure to the sun—and it manifests itself by tanning. When we are over-exposed, we burn.
- The damage from UV exposure stimulates pain receptors, and the vasodilation produces increased erythema (redness) of the skin, which, in severe cases, produces blisters.
- Duration of sun exposure, altitude, and exposure to reflective surfaces (snow, sand, ice, water) increases the risk of severe sunburn.
- The damage is permanent and cumulative.
- There is very significant long-term increased risk of skin cancer from severe sunburns.
- Repeated sunburns or chronic tanning increases aging effects with wrinkles, areas of pigmentation, thickening, and precancerous lesions.
- With time these can turn into cancers: basal cell or squamous-cell cancer or malignant melanoma.

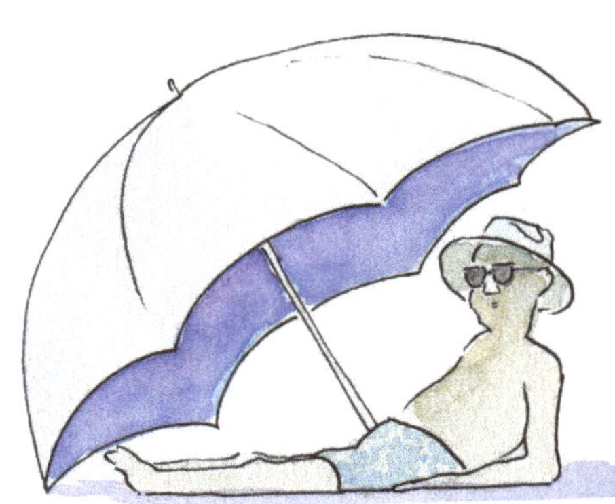

PREVENTION

- Wear proper clothing, use hats, umbrellas and sun block, avoid the sun, and don't go to tanning salons.

TREATMENT

- Eliminate further exposure—find shade, put on clothing.
- Assess for signs of heat exhaustion or heat stroke.
- Hydrate with water and salt replacement.
- Use non-steroidal anti-inflammatory drugs (NSAIDs) such as aspirin, ibuprofen (Advil, Motrin) or Naprosyn (Aleve)
- Acetaminophen (Tylenol), although not an NSAID, helps relieve pain and can be taken along with an NSAID.
- Moisturize the skin with an aloe-based skin cream.
- If blisters occur, leave them intact.
- Certain medications do cause increased photosensitivity to UV light, thus increasing the likelihood and severity of sunburn—if you are taking one of these drugs, take all measures to prevent sun exposure (sidebar).

(SOME) PHOTOSENSITIVE AGENTS

ANTIDEPRESSANTS
ANTIHISTAMINES
ANTIBIOTICS:
ANTIPSYCHOTIC DRUGS
DIURETICS
HYPOGLYCEMICS
NON-STEROIDAL ANTI-INFLAMMATORY DRUGS
OTHER DRUGS

BLISTERS

(FROM FRICTION)

DESCRIPTION

Blisters are caused by something rubbing against the skin (e.g., a wet sock)—friction forces the layers of the skin to shear and separate. As the connective tissues between these layers fail and pull apart (in effect, delaminating), the body secretes fluid into the area in an attempt to protect it. Wet macerated skin is much more likely to develop blisters than dry skin (that explains why wet socks in wet hiking boots are so often the culprit). A blister starts out as a "hot spot" which, if left unattended, will grow into a fluid-filled blister. Common causes of blisters are loose-fitting boots or shoes that rub against the heel, or a tool handle or oar loom that rubs against the palms of the hands.

PREVENTION

Easily prevented, blisters can be crippling if the early warning signs are ignored—literally stopping hikers in their tracks.

- Choose the correct sock combination—a thin synthetic sock next to the skin covered with a thicker sock is typical for most hiking boots.
- Fit boots properly; break them in.
  - This was much more important back in the old leather boot days.
  - Modern, composite hiking boots do not require nearly the same amount of break-in time.
- Wear gloves with hand tools.
- Keep feet dry. Change socks often. Use foot powder liberally.

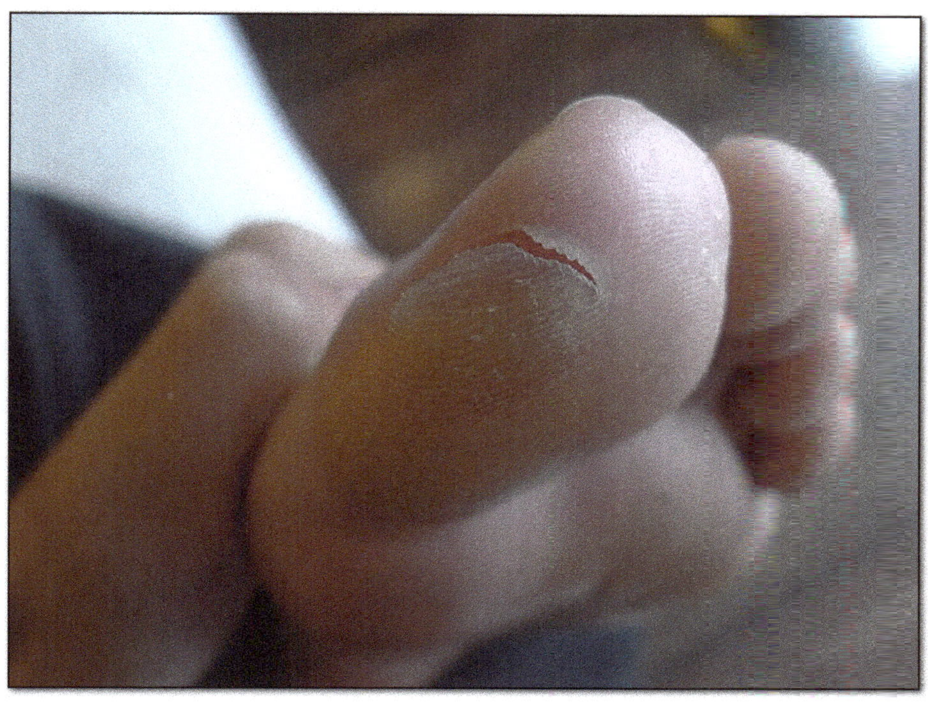

TREATMENT

- React early to hot spots that form on the hands or feet—don't wait!
- Make sure the area is dry and then protect it with athletic tape. (Be careful removing tape; you can easily pull off layers of skin.)
- If a fluid-filled blister forms:

  1. BSI—wash your hands and put on your gloves.
  2. Wash the blister gently and the surrounding tissue with soap and water, or swab the area with a Betadine/iodine solution or alcohol and allow to dry.
  3. Sterilize a needle or safety pin with a flame.
  4. Use the sterile needle to stab the base of the blister in several places.
  5. Gently press the blister with a gloved finger to deflate it.
  6. Leave the skin on the roof of the blister in place—do not debride the blister.
  7. Make a doughnut by cutting a hole in the center of a circle of Moleskin, Molefoam, Spenco 2nd

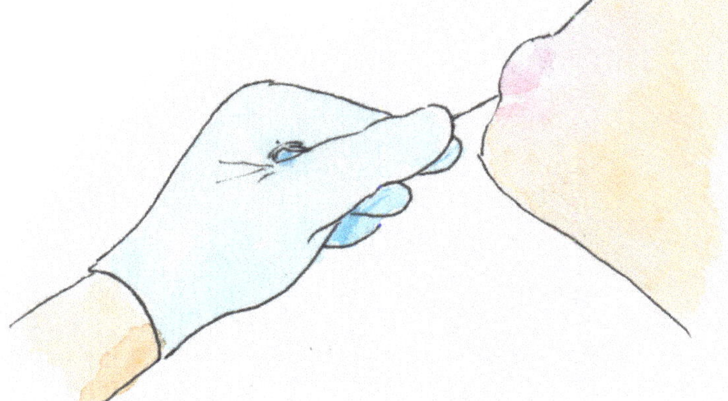

See next page for #8-12

Skin, etc.

8. Place this moleskin doughnut over the blister site to produce a protective well with the blister in the center.

9. Fill the well with Spenco 2nd Skin or antibiotic ointment.

10. Cover the area with tape.

11. Clean, inspect, and change the blister dressing twice daily.

12. Do not attempt to remove the moleskin doughnut, as this will most likely tear off more skin.

- If on the foot, re-dress, paying particular attention to sock and boot fit (use fresh, dry socks, making sure the boot is snug, with no slippage).
- Monitor the blister site for signs of infection: redness, swelling, tenderness, warmth, or red streaks extending from the wound.

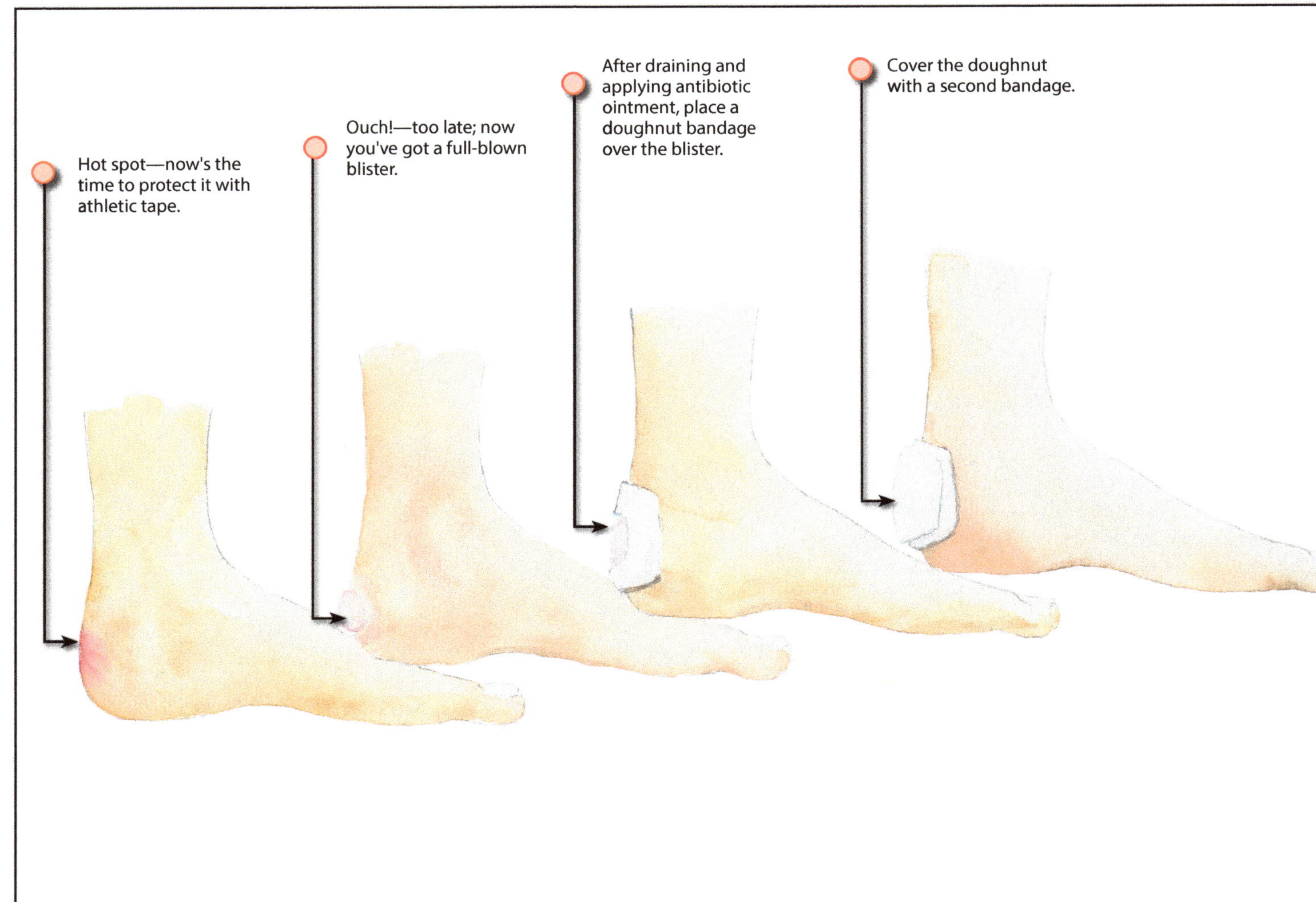

The Musculoskeletal system

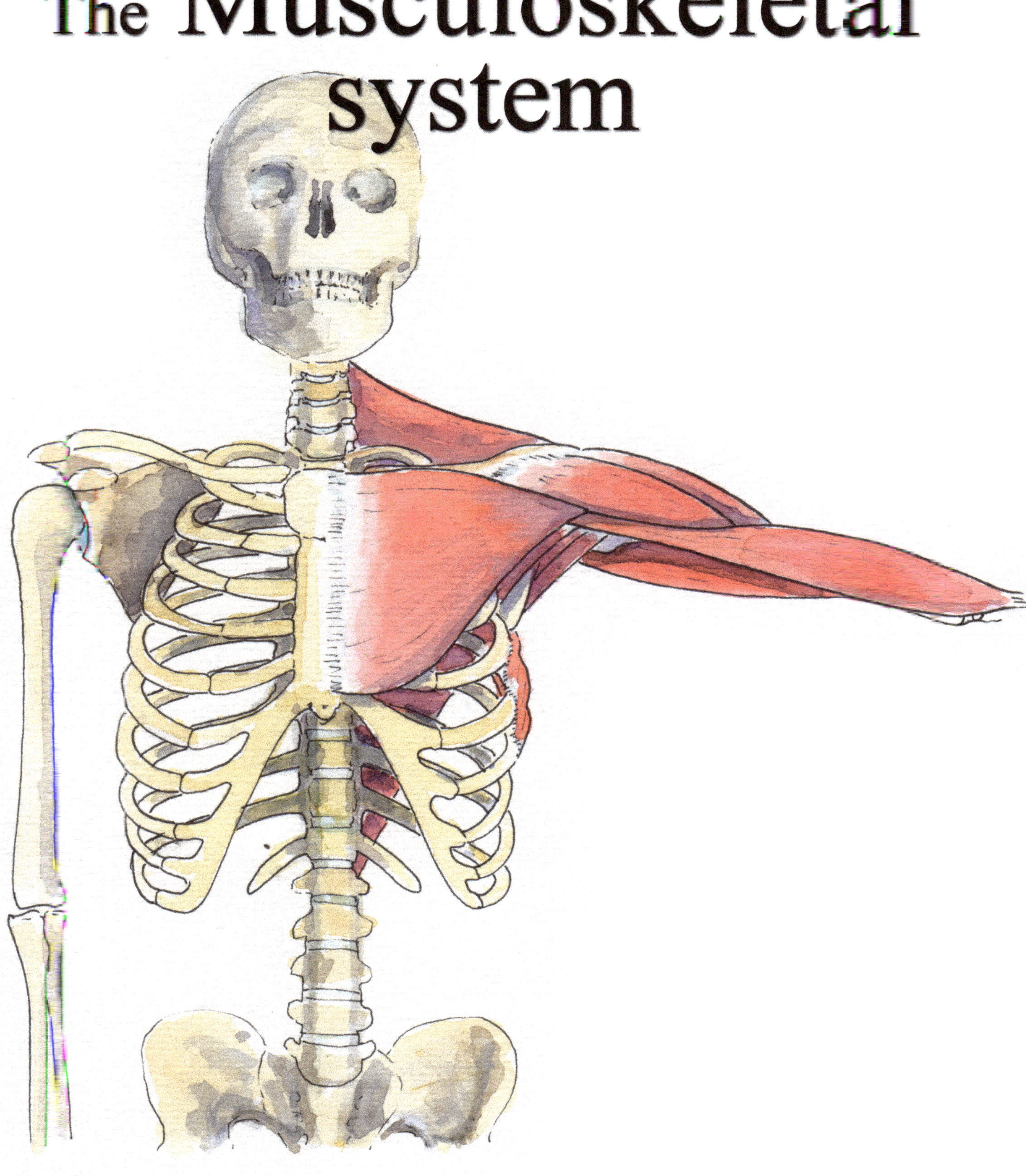

THE MUSCULOSKELETAL SYSTEM

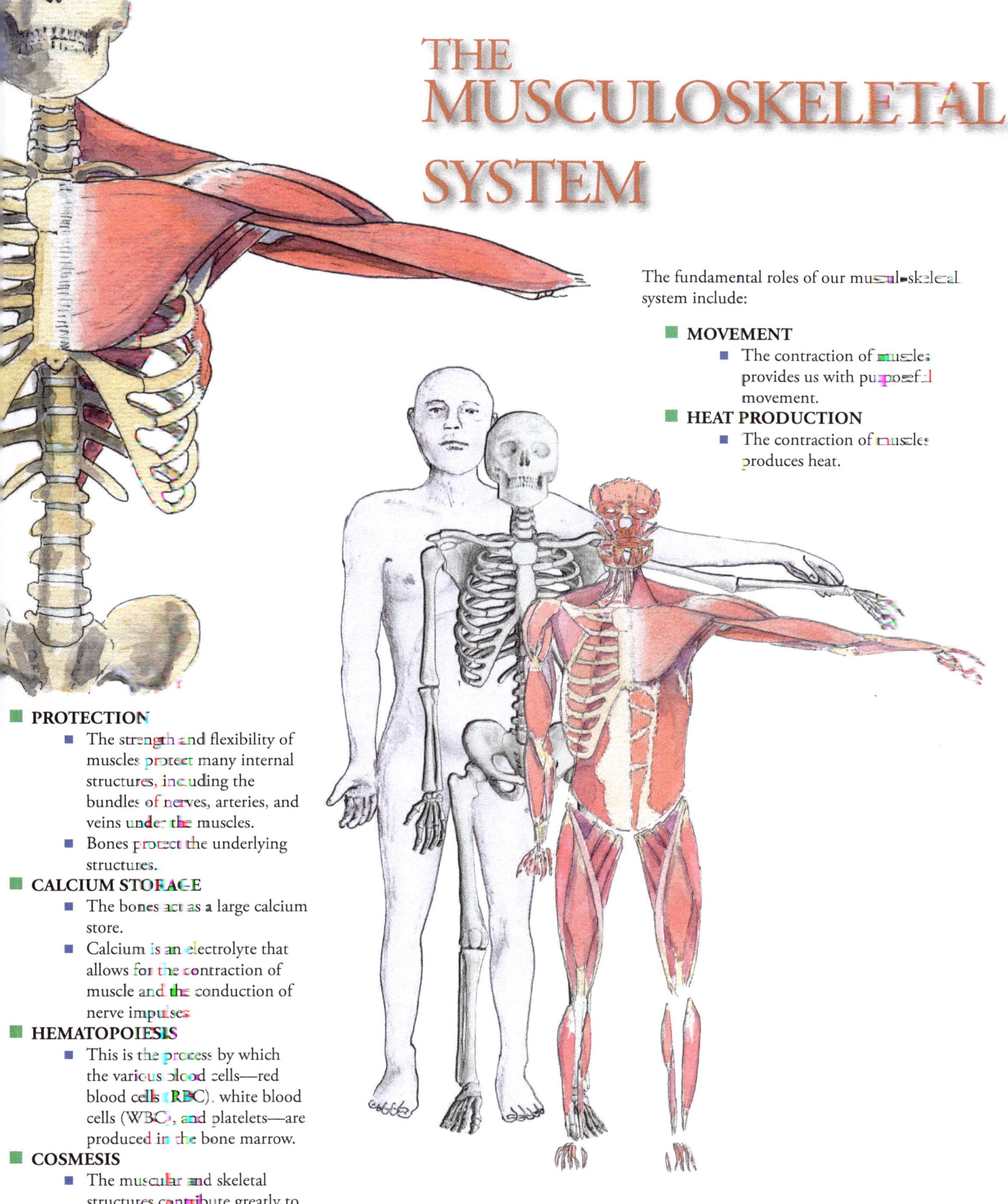

The fundamental roles of our musculoskeletal system include:

- **MOVEMENT**
  - The contraction of muscles provides us with purposeful movement.
- **HEAT PRODUCTION**
  - The contraction of muscles produces heat.

- **PROTECTION**
  - The strength and flexibility of muscles protect many internal structures, including the bundles of nerves, arteries, and veins under the muscles.
  - Bones protect the underlying structures.
- **CALCIUM STORAGE**
  - The bones act as a large calcium store.
  - Calcium is an electrolyte that allows for the contraction of muscle and the conduction of nerve impulses.
- **HEMATOPOIESIS**
  - This is the process by which the various blood cells—red blood cells (RBC), white blood cells (WBC), and platelets—are produced in the bone marrow.
- **COSMESIS**
  - The muscular and skeletal structures contribute greatly to how we look.

Bones
Provide structure, protection, motion, calcium storage, and red blood cell production.

Muscles
Provide the power for movement by contracting. Give our body form (cosmesis).

Functionality

Tendons
Attach muscle to bone or muscle to muscle. They span the joints to help facilitate movement. They operate in conjunction with ligaments, bones, and nerves to do work.

Ligaments
Tough, fibrous bands that span the joints and attach bone to bone. They help hold the joints together and control range of motion.

Cartilage
Provides cushioning between bones at the joints. Acts as a lubricated, durable cap on the ends of bones so that the joint can flex and rotate smoothly with little friction. Provides durable support for muscle in areas where more flexibility than what bone offers is needed.

Joint detail

Muscle

Bursa

Bone

Cartilage

Synovial cavity (synovial fluid)
The lubricant in the joint space, produced by the synovial lining of the joint capsule: reduces friction, provides shock absorption, facilitates nutrient and waste transportation.

Joint capsule and synovial lining

Ligament

Tendon

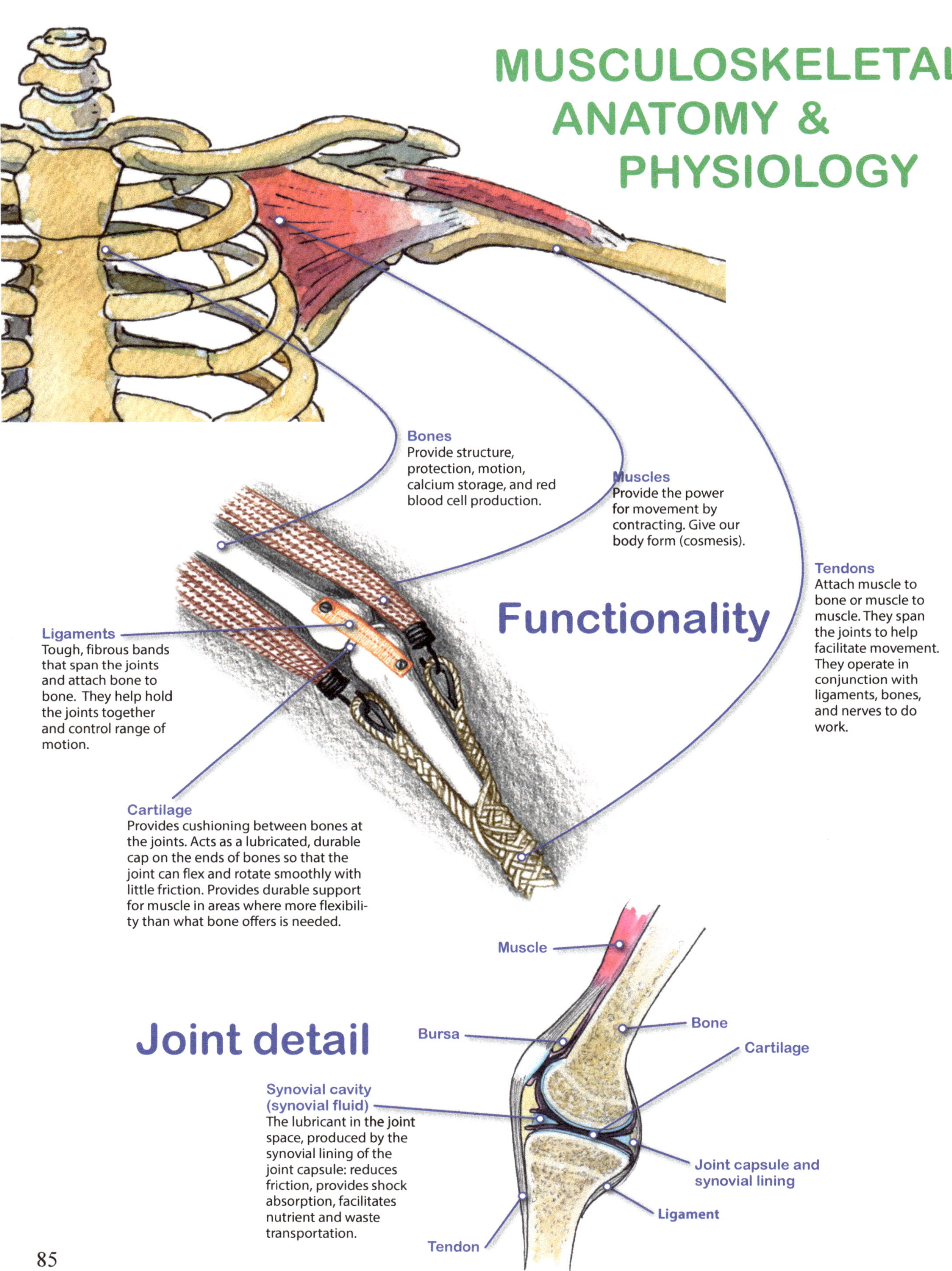

85

Types of musculoskeletal injuries

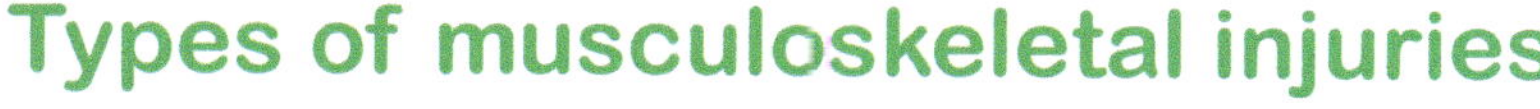

STRAINS AND SPRAINS

- Strains are overuse and/or over-stretching injuries, primarily involving muscles and tendons.
- Sprains involve the over-stretching of a joint (moving it beyond its range of motion) and typically cause damage to ligaments.

FRACTURES

- Sometimes abbreviated as Fx, a fracture is the break in the continuity of a bone.
- Fractures can result from high-force impact or stress, or from a seemingly trivial incident that occurs in people with bones weakened by disease (e.g. osteoporosis, bone cancer).
- There are two basic types:
    - Closed—fractures where the skin is not breached.
    - Open (compound)—where there is an accompanying wound that may expose the bone to contamination, risking infection.

DISLOCATIONS

- An injury where the bones in a joint become displaced or misaligned.
- Often caused by forceful impact or twisting action.
- There is always some accompanying soft tissue damage to the surrounding muscles, tendons, ligaments, and/or cartilage.
- Dislocations can be associated with a fracture.

Evaluating a musculoskeletal injury

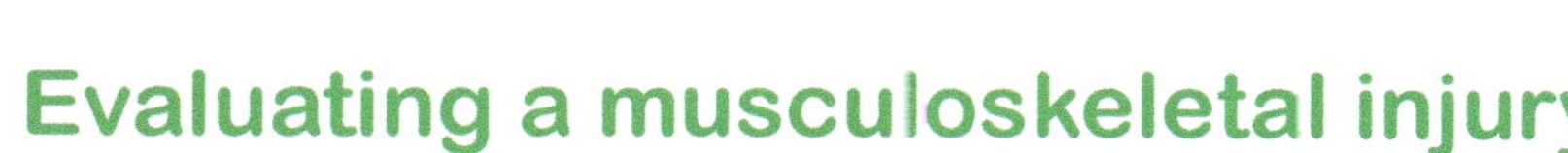

LOOK

- Is there normal movement and function?
- Is there any deformity or angulation?
- Is there any discoloration or swelling?
- Is there any guarding? They are trying to protect the injury—don't touch them.

LISTEN

- What happened—what was the mechanism of injury (MOI)?
- Where does it hurt—what is the patient's chief complaint (C/C)?
- Did the patient hear anything snap, crack, or pop?
- If the patient is unconscious, you will have to look for clues.

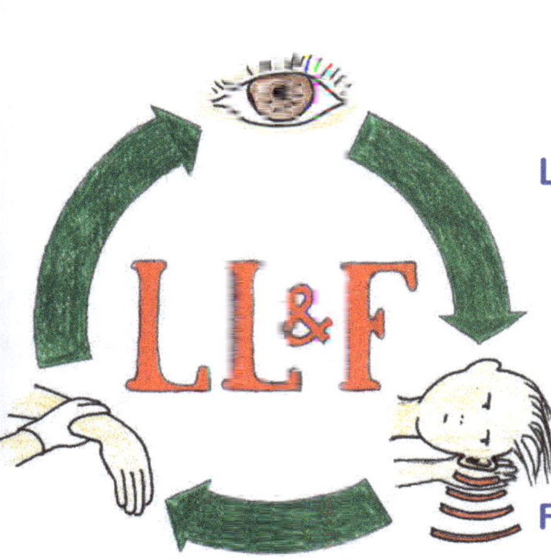

FEEL

- Is there point tenderness (pain felt when pressure is applied to a specific place—some injuries don't hurt unless palpated)?
- Is there crepitation (the crunching feeling or sound of broken bones grating against each other)?
- Is there any compromise in circulation, sensation, and movement (CSM), especially distal to the injury site?

STRAINS & SPRAINS

STRAINS AND SPRAINS are the most common musculoskeletal injuries (particularly involving the ankle). They will be considered together because the mechanisms of injury are similar; they typically occur together; they are hard to differentiate in the field; and they share the same treatment.

STRAINS

- Pulls or tears of the **muscles** and/or **tendons**—the injury occurs when the muscle and/or tendon is stretched to the point of tearing, causing slight (micro) internal bleeding.
- Strains occur when muscles are forced beyond their capacity because they are over-worked, stressed, or tired (because of recent activity).
- Strains can also be caused when the muscle is stressed before being properly warmed up (starting a long trail run by sprinting 200 yards is a bad idea).
- Strains most often occur in the lower back and hamstring.
- Most strains can be treated effectively in the field.

SPRAINS

- Overstretching of joints beyond their normal range of motion that causes injury to the associated **ligaments**.
- Sprains most often occur in the wrist and ankle.
- Muscle strains usually accompany sprains.
- Sprains can be very painful, and ankle or knee sprains may require litter evacuation.

SIGNS AND SYMPTOMS OF BOTH STRAINS AND SPRAINS

- Pain at the site can be mild to severe, depending on the injury, but is generally not debilitating.
- There is typically diffuse tenderness in the injured tissues.
- Pain is exacerbated by movement of the injured joint.
- Swelling and discoloration vary from minor to significant, depending on the severity of the injury and the speed of treatment. Swelling tends to increase with time. The faster the treatment, the less soft-tissue damage will occur.
- There is often decreased range of motion (ROM) secondary to the pain. Although ROM may not be compromised, the patient may say that they cannot move the injured area because it's too painful.
- Localized internal bleeding from the injured tissue may cause ecchymosis (the spread of blood under the skin—a minor bruise) and hematoma (localized collection of blood outside the blood vessels—larger and more serious than ecchymosis).

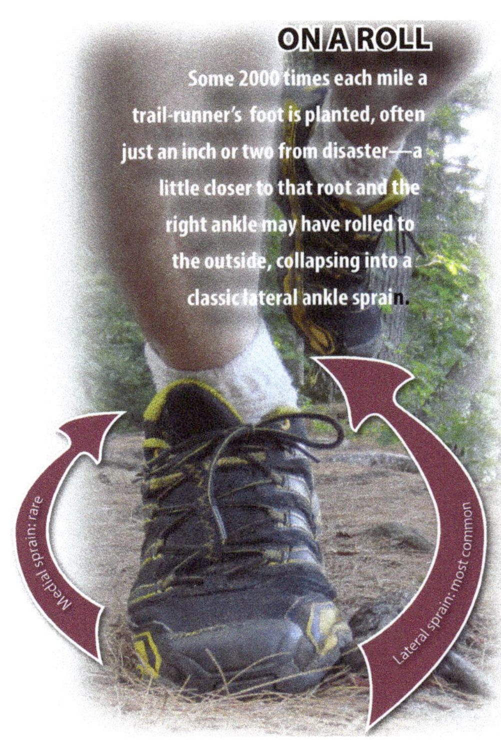

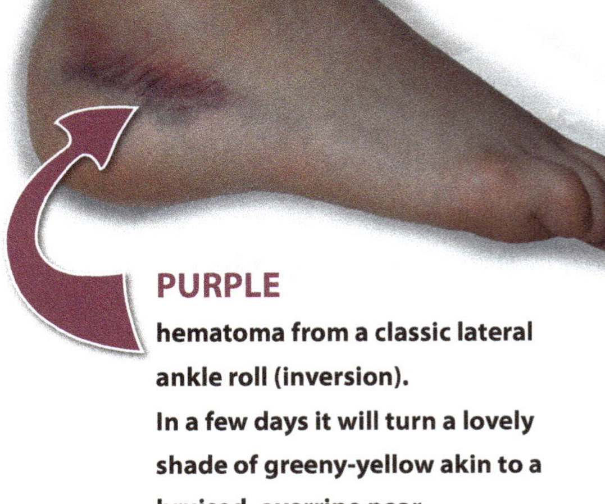

PURPLE hematoma from a classic lateral ankle roll (inversion).

In a few days it will turn a lovely shade of greeny-yellow akin to a bruised, overripe pear.

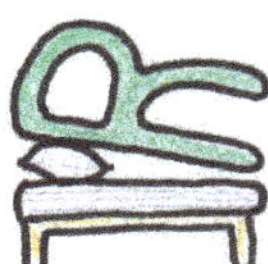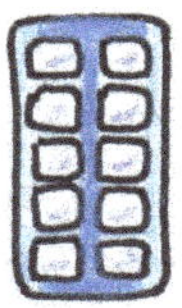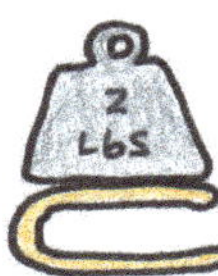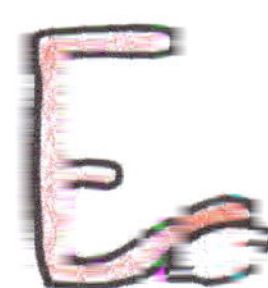

TREATMENT

1. **EXPOSE** the injury. If an ankle sprain, carefully and gently remove the boots and socks and examine.

2. **RICE: Rest, Ice, Compression, Elevation**
   Rest—Do not use the joint, get the patient off their feet.
   Ice—Apply ice or a cold compress to the injured area. Do not apply ice directly to the skin—wrap it in cloth or plastic first. A cold mountain stream is a good option if ice is not available.
   Compression—wrap the injured area with an elastic bandage to reduce swelling—but do not compromise circulation.
   Elevation—elevate the injured area above the level of the heart (this helps reduce swelling).

3. **RICE** for one hour, then re-evaluate:
   Can the ankle bear weight?
   - If it can't, then the patient must be evacuated.

   For possible fracture
   - The same MOI can cause a fracture or a strain/sprain, and each injury can present with a rapid onset of significant swelling, bruising, and pain.
   - With a sprain, the pain is usually more generalized and on one side of the ankle (lateral most often)—a fracture will be more severe and localized, with point tenderness and guarding.
   - Palpate the injury site, checking for misalignment, deformity, or crepitus.
   - If you suspect a fracture, splint the joint and start evacuation—a litter-carry may be inevitable.

   For functional ability
   - If a patient with a sprained ankle is ambulatory after an hour of RICE treatment, allow them to walk (a litter evacuation is a long and tedious affair).

4. **EVACUATE**
   - Go slowly and take frequent rests. You may have to assist them over rough spots.
   - Consider improvising a crutch or cane to help them minimize additional stress on the joint.
   - Have others carry the patient's gear.

5. **SPLINT**
   - The strain/sprain may benefit from splinting, which helps protect it from further injury and helps alleviate and control pain.
   - When in doubt, treat as a fracture and splint.

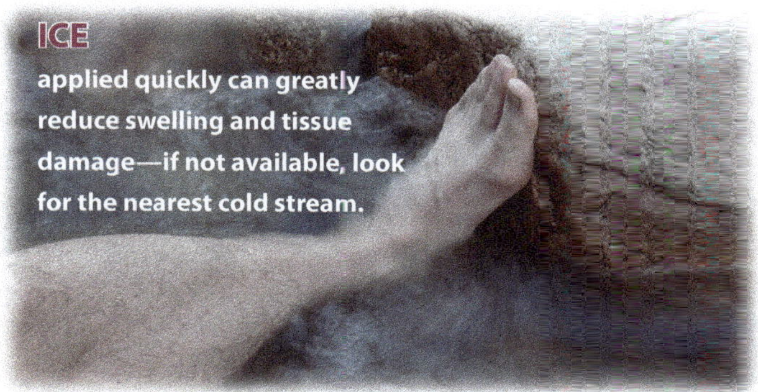

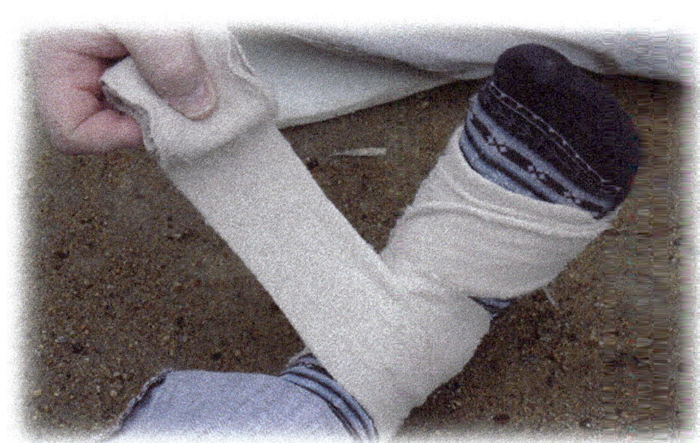

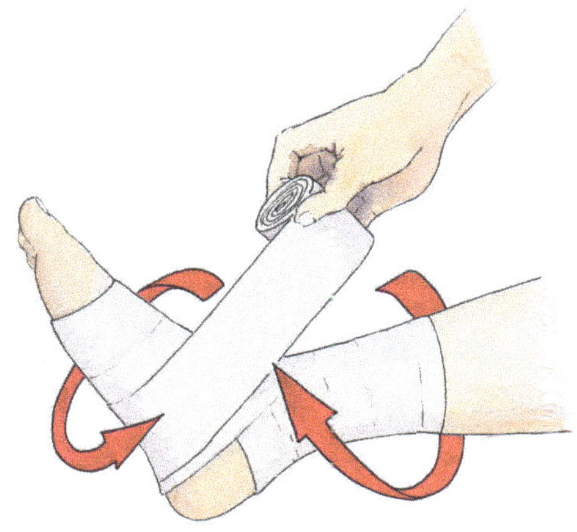

The hitch shown on page 96 can be used over a boot as an improvised ankle splint.

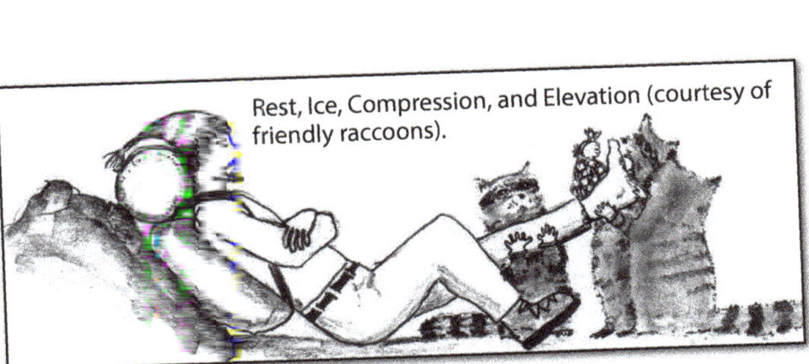
Rest, Ice, Compression, and Elevation (courtesy of friendly raccoons).

F_x is medical shorthand for "fracture."

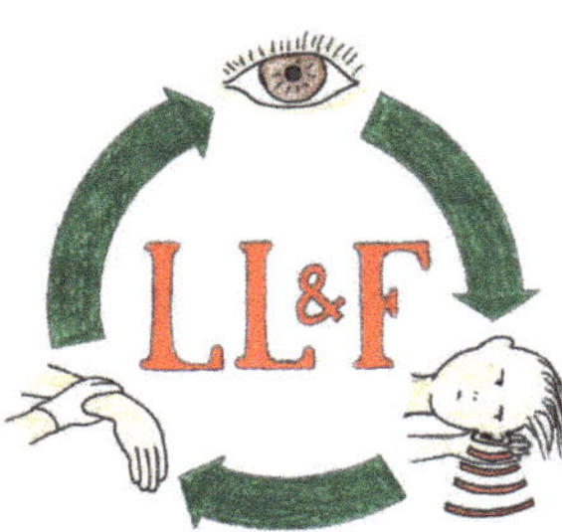

Fractures

A fracture occurs when enough force is applied to effect a break in the bone, causing pain and disruption of normal function. The pain results from the tear that occurs in the tissue surrounding the bone (the bone itself has no pain receptors).

Types of fractures

Although physicians differentiate between many kinds of fractures, because our treatment options in the backcountry are limited, the nuances are not that important. We're basically interested in answering two questions: **1)** Are the broken bones still in anatomical position? **2)** Is there an associated wound? And we keep the descriptions basic.

CLOSED (SIMPLE), IN-LINE FRACTURE
- There is a break in the bone's cortex, but the skin over the injury site is intact; the bones are in proper anatomical alignment; and there is no open wound.

CLOSED ANGULATED FRACTURE
- There is a break in the cortex, and the bone ends are angulated and not in anatomical alignment.
- Angulated fractures can be closed or open.

OPEN (COMPOUND) FRACTURE
- A fracture with an associated open wound—a break in the skin at the fracture site—with or without bone ends showing through the skin.

Diagnosing a fracture

Often, the mechanism of injury combined with the signs and symptoms will lead you to suspect a fracture.

1. **LISTEN TO THE PATIENT**—they will frequently say that they heard or felt a snap (a clear indication).

2. **LOOK**—expose the skin and examine the site.
   - Fractures may bleed internally, so there may be swelling and/or discoloration (ecchymosis).
   - There may be a wound associated with the fracture site: A) unrelated to the fracture, B) as a result of a compound fracture, C) from an impaled object.

3. **FEEL**—the injured limb
   - Check for CSMs distal to the injury site.
   - Check for proper anatomical alignment (when not associated with a joint, deformity indicates an angulated fracture).
   - Check for bilateral symmetry (i.e., compare the injured limb to the uninjured limb—asymmetry indicates a dislocation, a fracture, or both). See photo.
   - Palpate for point tenderness (can indicate a fracture).
   - Palpate for crepitation—the feeling of bones grating together (confirms a fracture).

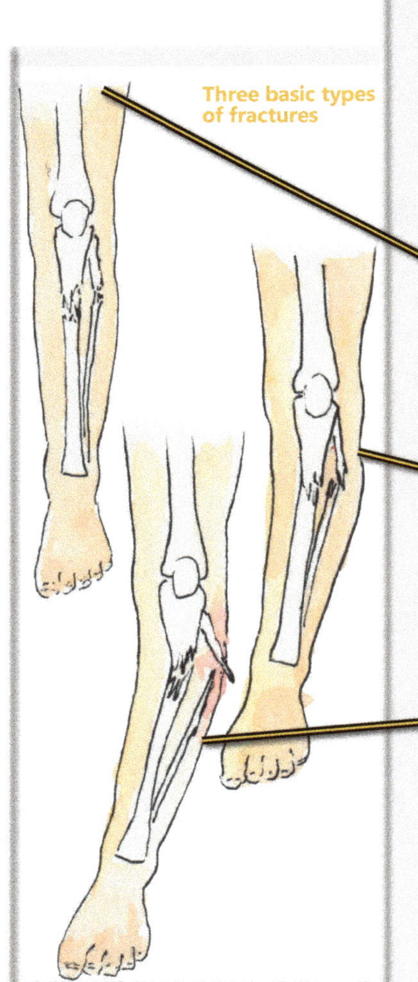

Three basic types of fractures

Basic goals for managing a fracture

All fractures will ultimately need to be seen by a physician—all will require treatment that cannot be done in the field, and some will require surgery. In the wilderness setting the goals are really simple.

1. **IF NECESSARY, USE TRACTION-IN-LINE (TIL)** to restore the fractured part to its anatomical position.

    - If this is not possible (e.g., because of shattered limbs or severely angulated fractures), immobilize in the position of greatest comfort and evacuate immediately.
    - With a closed, in-line fracture, TIL won't be necessary from an anatomical standpoint, but gentle TIL can help relax spasms and reduce pain until a splint is applied.

2. **CLEAN AND DRESS ANY ASSOCIATED WOUND,** minimize contamination, and dress the wound to protect it from infection.

3. **IMMOBILIZE THE FRACTURE** with a splint, making sure to preserve circulation.

4. **EVACUATE** to definitive care.

    - The rate of evacuation will depend, in part, on the severity of the fracture—for instance, a simple forearm fracture does not require as rapid an evacuation as a femur fracture would.
    - Check vital signs regularly, especially circulation distal to the injury.

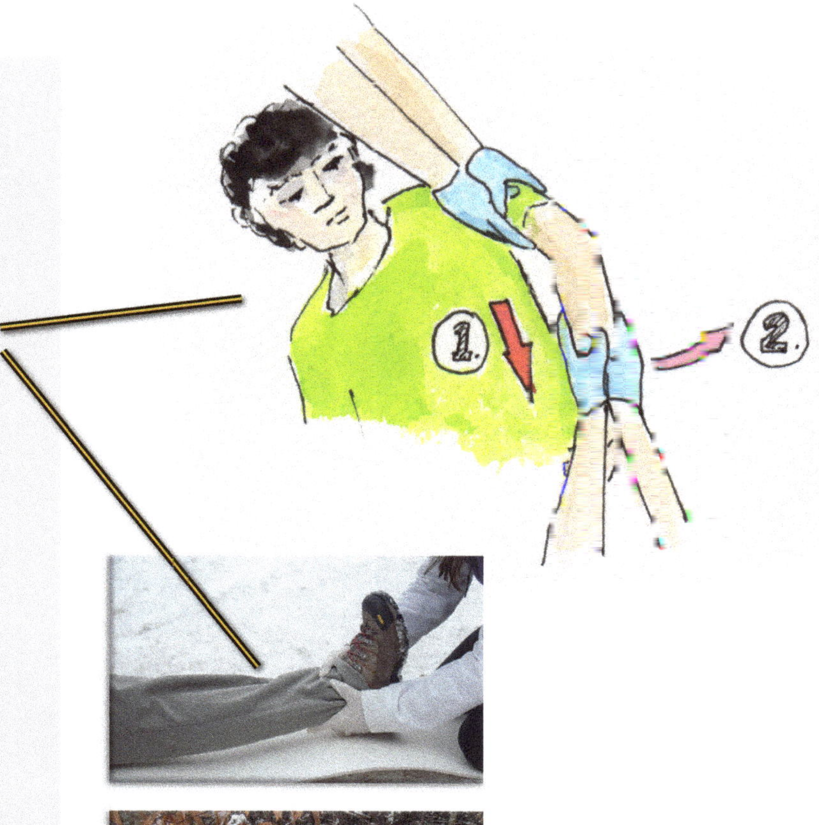

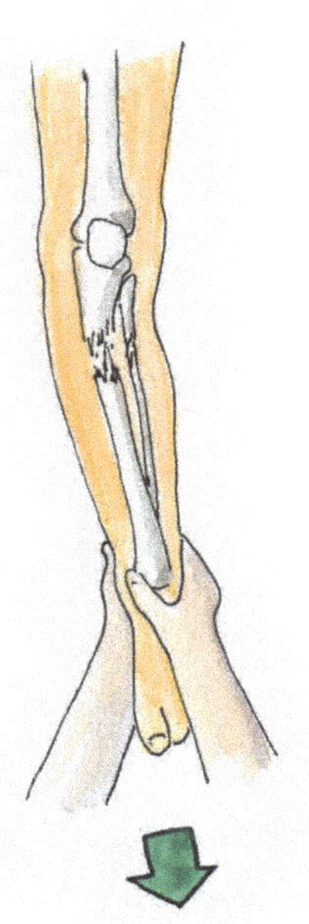

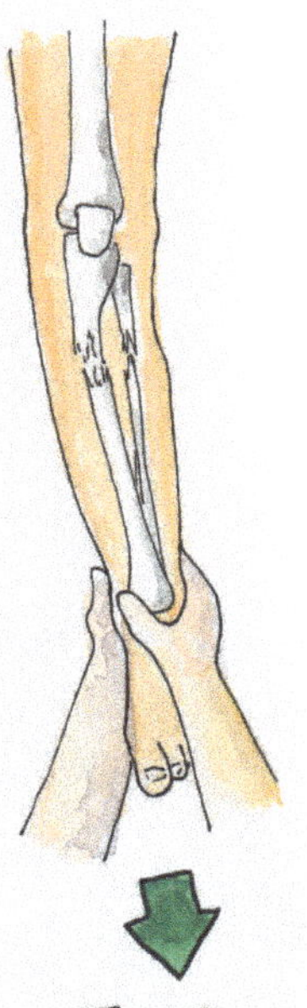

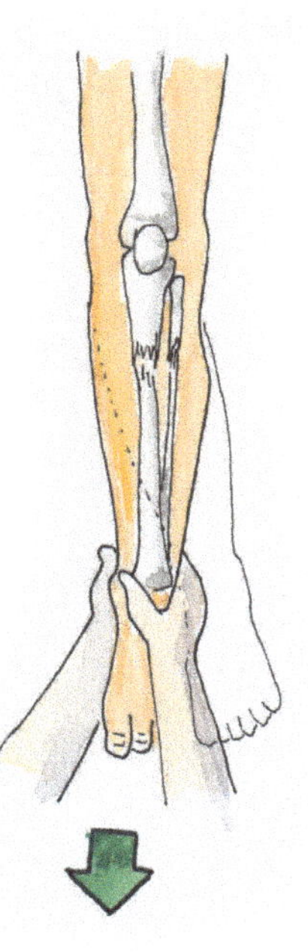

Simple Traction In Line

SPLINTING TECHNIQUES

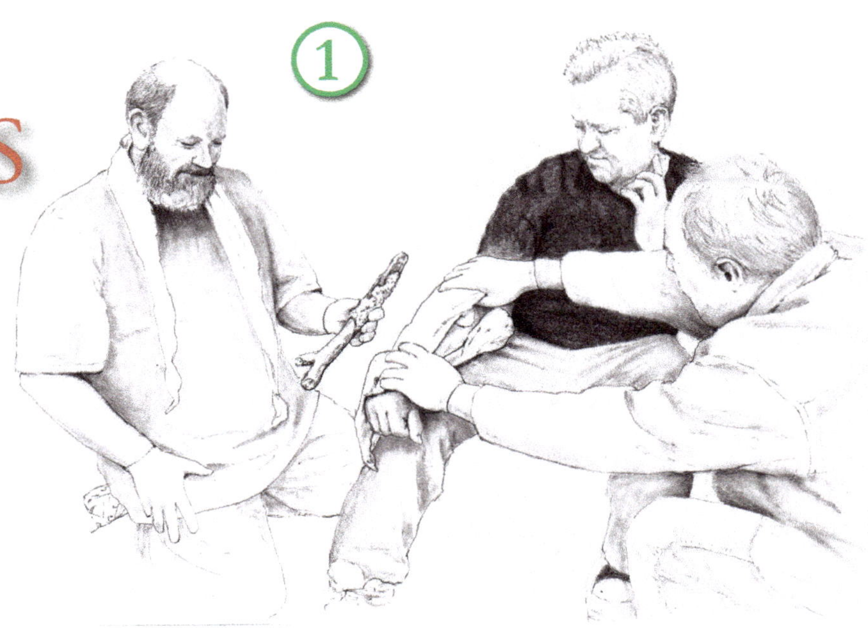

■ **LOWER ARM SPLINT USING STICKS AND CRAVATS**—used to support and stabilize alower arm.

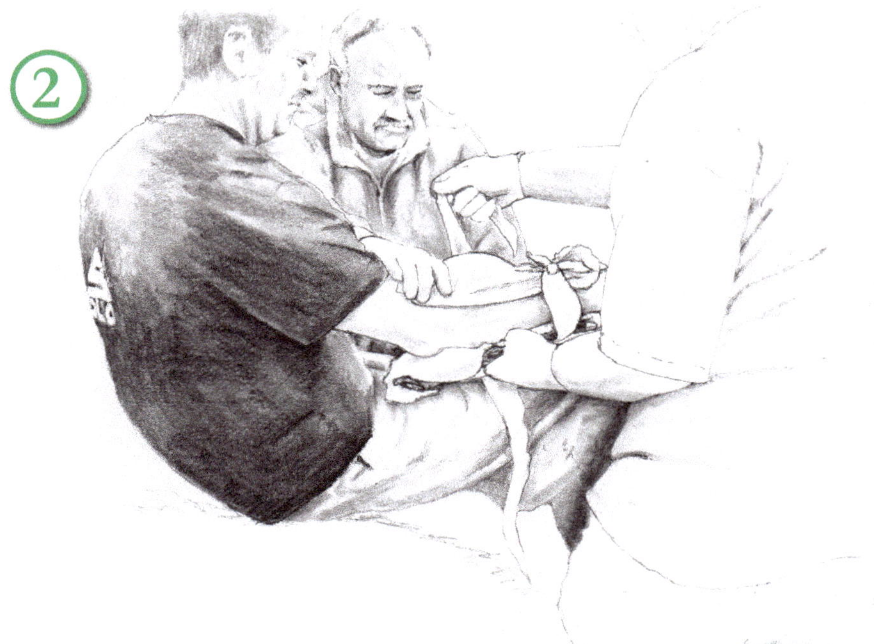

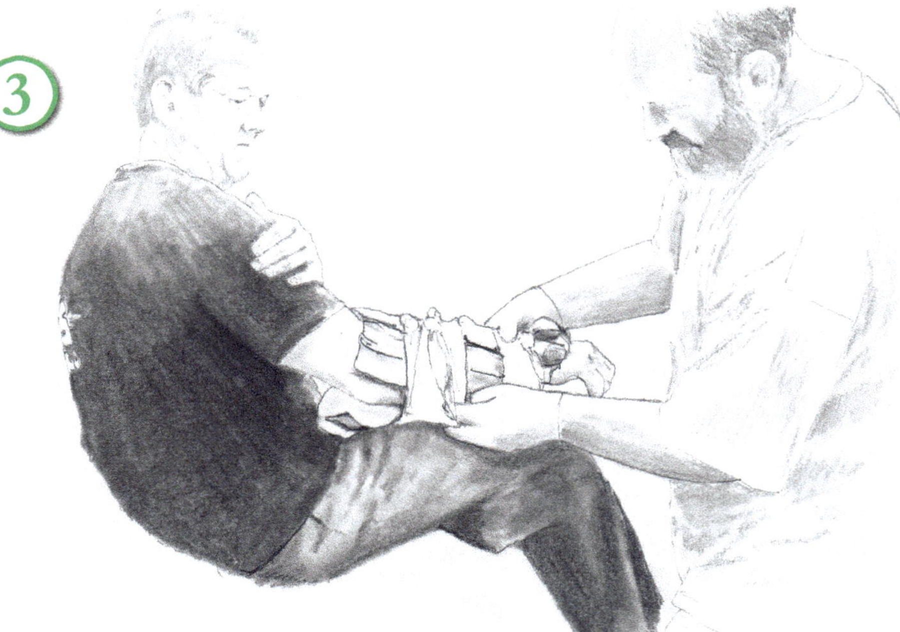

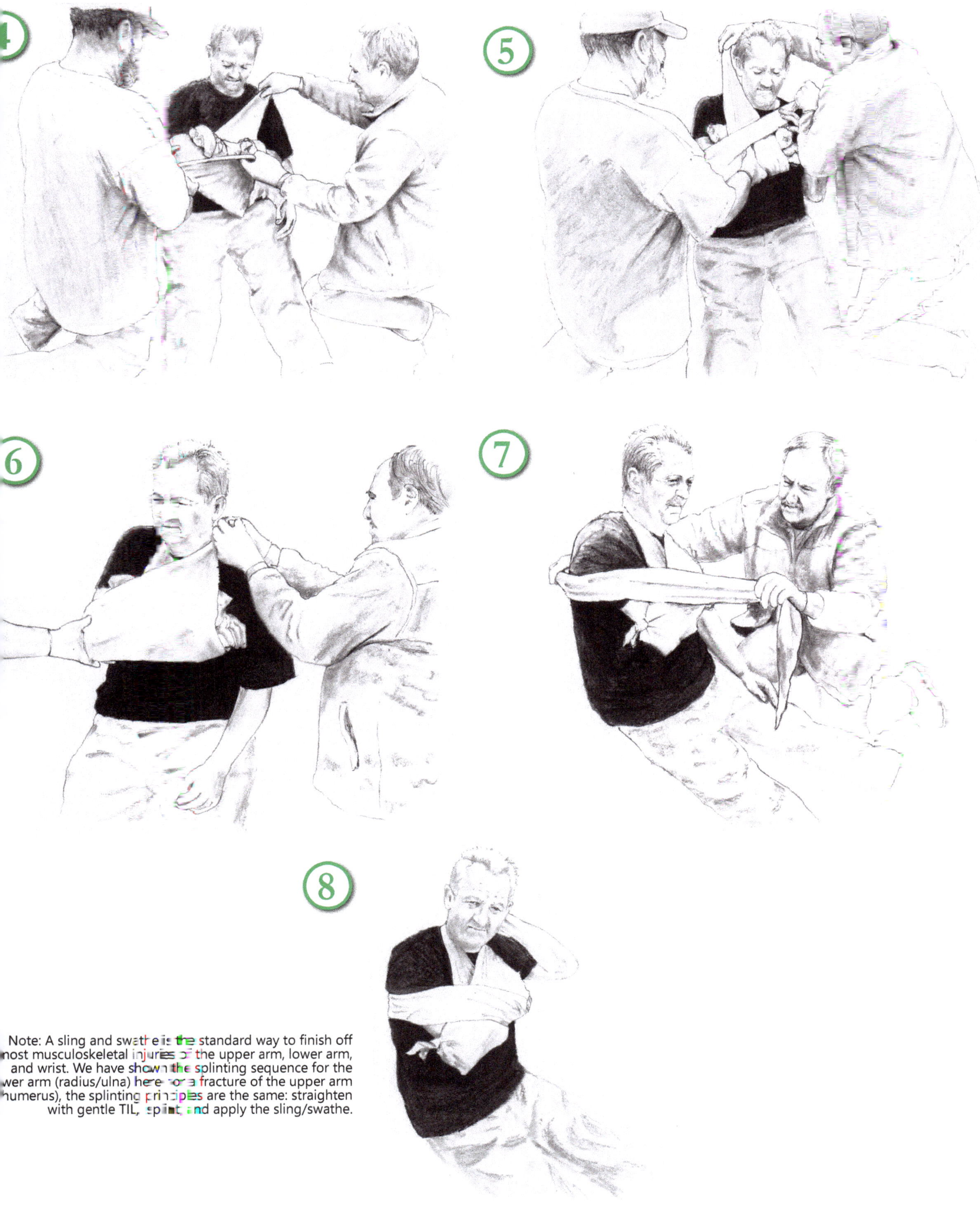

Note: A sling and swathe is the standard way to finish off most musculoskeletal injuries of the upper arm, lower arm, and wrist. We have shown the splinting sequence for the lower arm (radius/ulna) here. For a fracture of the upper arm (humerus), the splinting principles are the same: straighten with gentle TIL, splint and apply the sling/swathe.

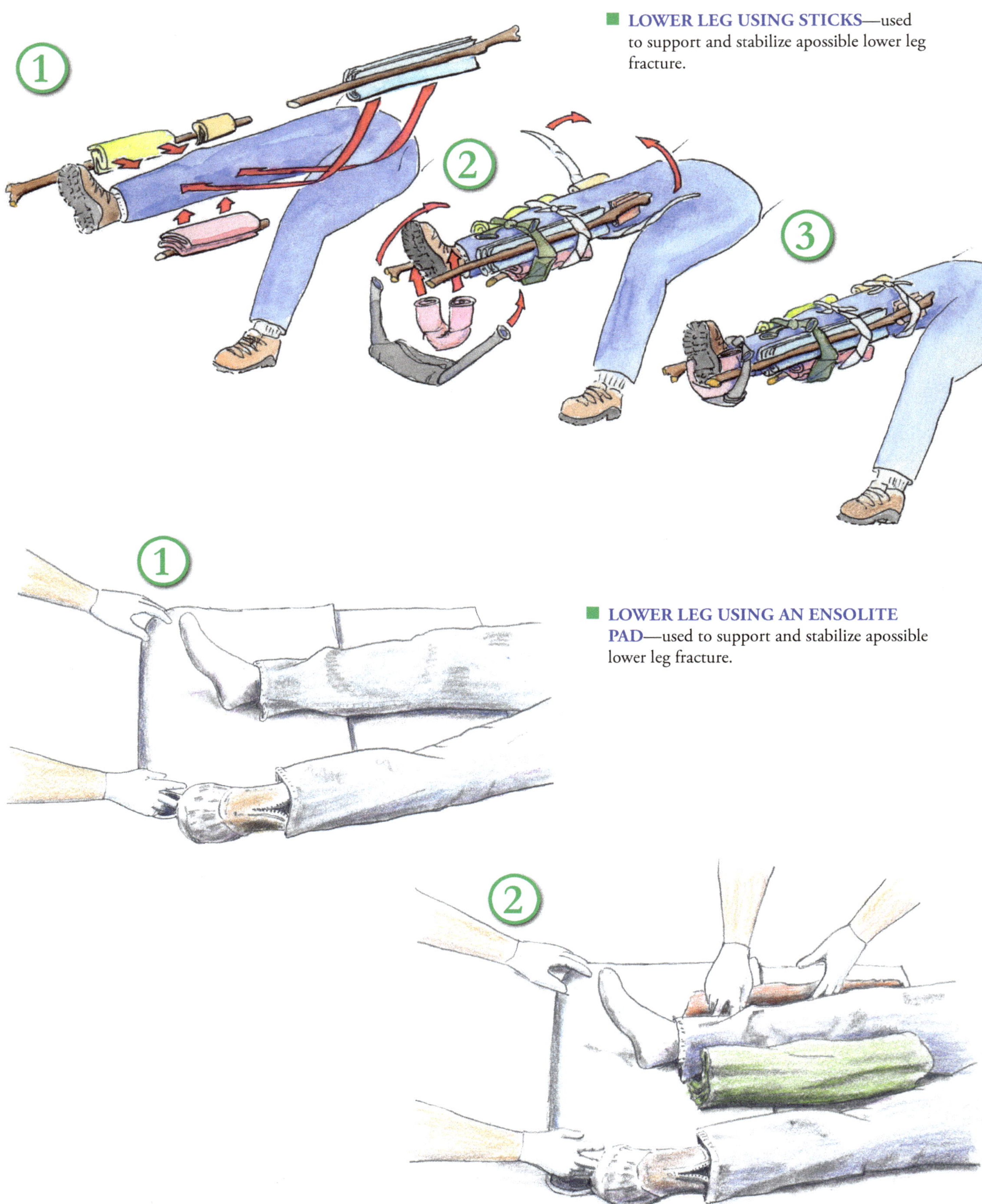

■ LOWER LEG USING STICKS—used to support and stabilize apossible lower leg fracture.

■ LOWER LEG USING AN ENSOLITE PAD—used to support and stabilize apossible lower leg fracture.

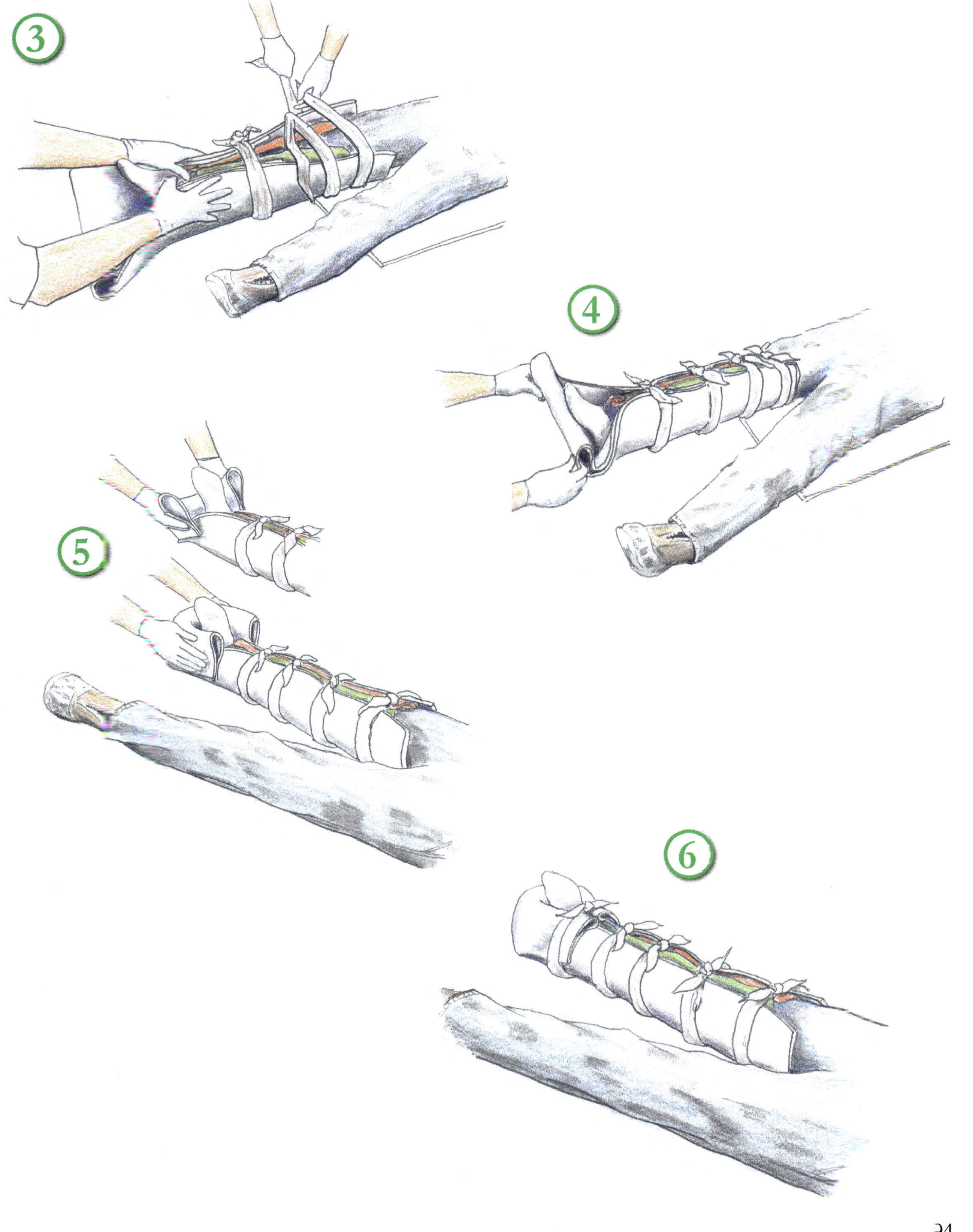

FRACTURED FEMUR

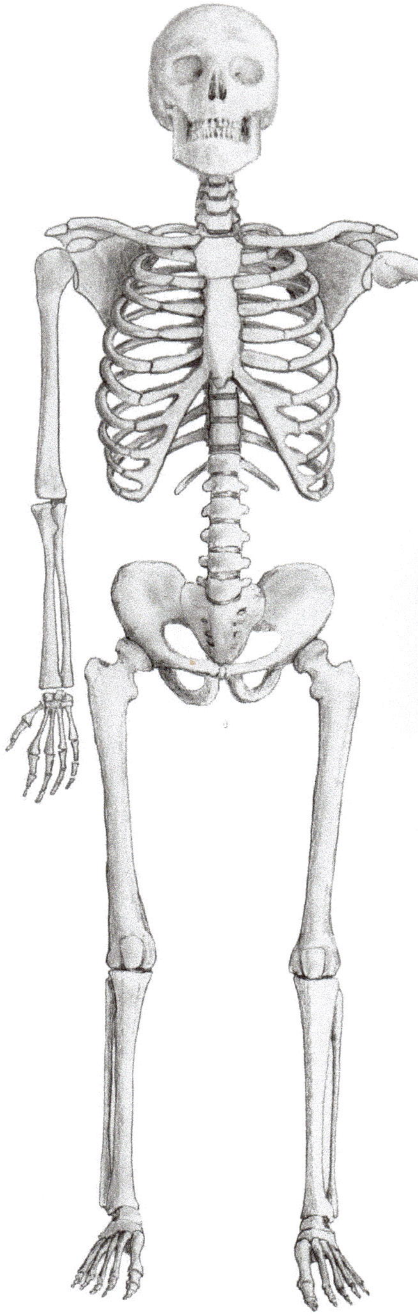

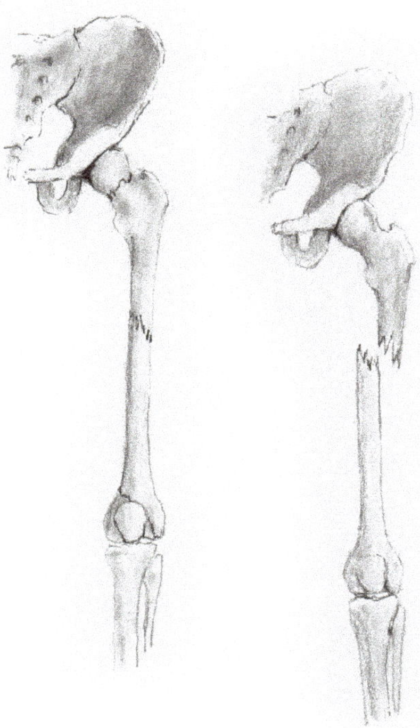

■ **THOUGH RARE, THIS INJURY IS POTENTIALLY LIFE THREATENING** — It takes a great deal of force to fracture a femur and the result is both very painful and a life threat. The treatment is the same for all other fractures, traction in line and splint. However, once to apply traction you cannot release that traction, you will need to apply a traction splint to maintain it.

■ Here is an improvised traction splint:

Apply steady, consistent, traction to the injured leg.
The waist hitch is a simple loop around the injured leg at the groin. Use a wde cravat or belt to spread the load.

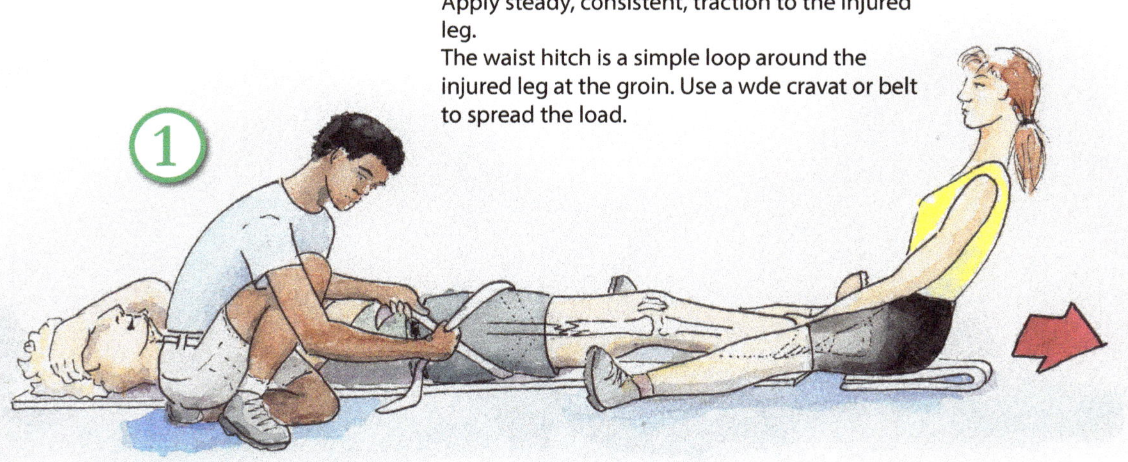

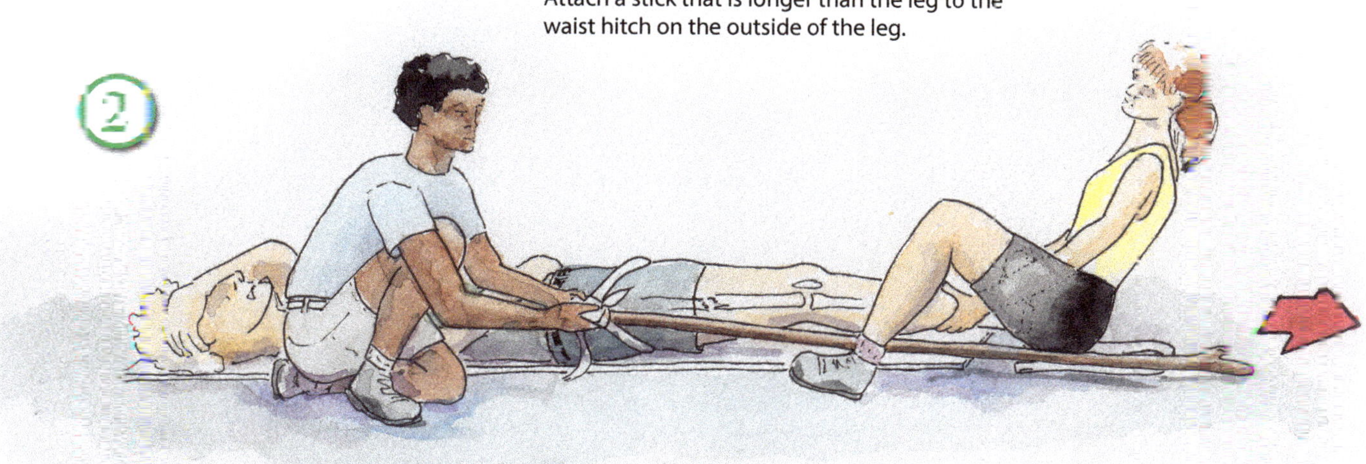

Attach a stick that is longer than the leg to the waist hitch on the outside of the leg.

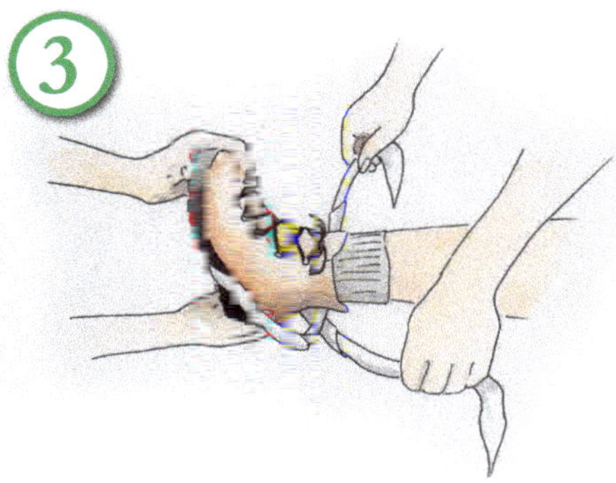

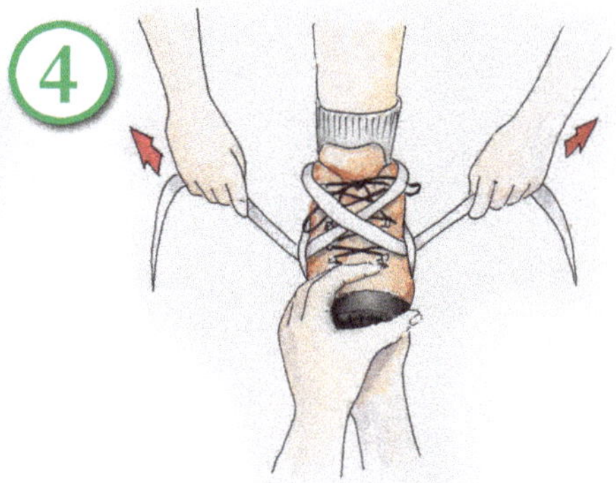

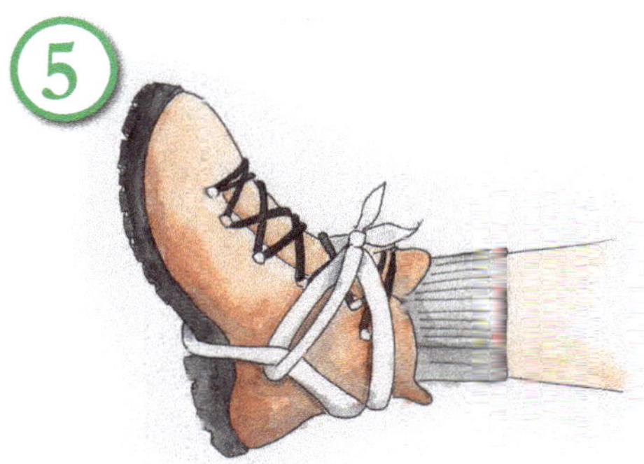

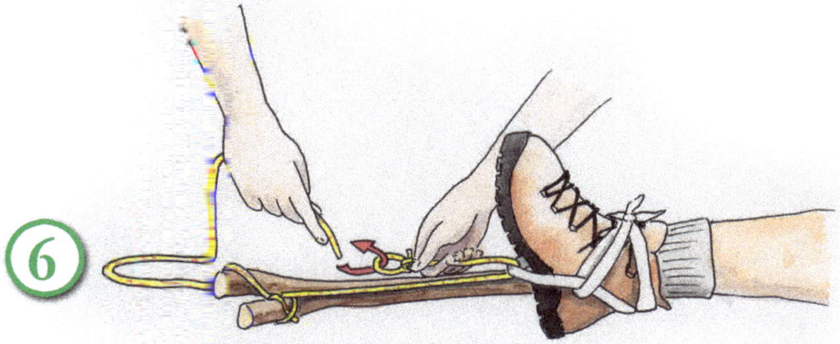

Tie a cord (or similar material) to the far end of the stick and attach it to the ankle-hitch with a trucker's hitch.

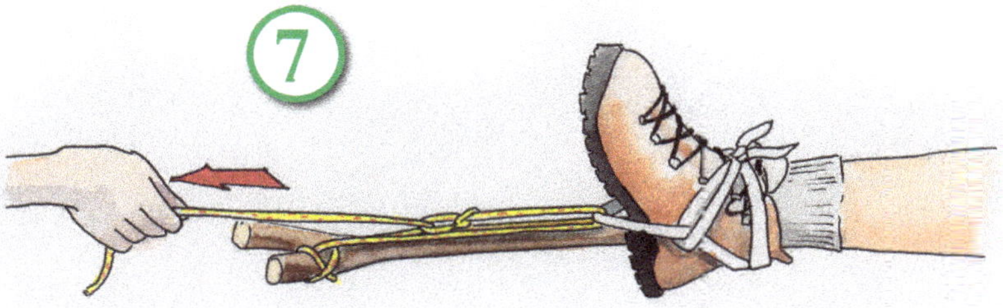

Use an ankle-hitch around the foot—this is both secure and comfortable. Boot on, or boot off? Boot-on provides stability and warmth and keeps the ankle-hitch from compromising circulation, but makes it impossible to monitor CSMs at the toes. Boot-off allows you to monitor CSMs, but provides no insulation, little stability, and can be uncomfortable. Use your judgment.

8 Make a smooth transition between manual traction and mechanical traction—any interruption can cause spasms and pain.

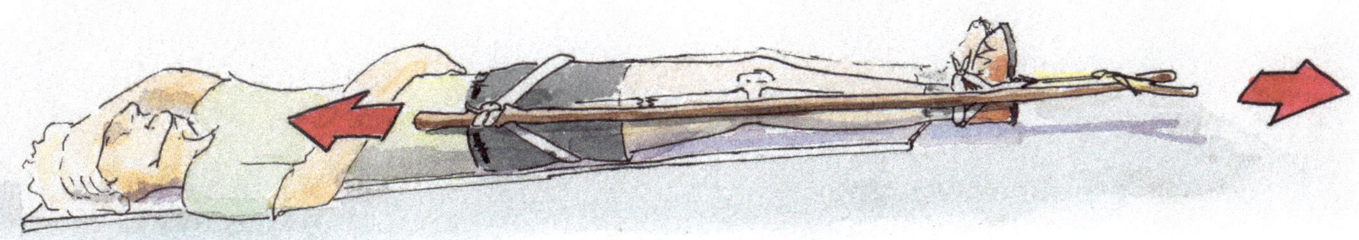

9 Secure the splint to the leg, making sure there is sufficient padding (for comfort)

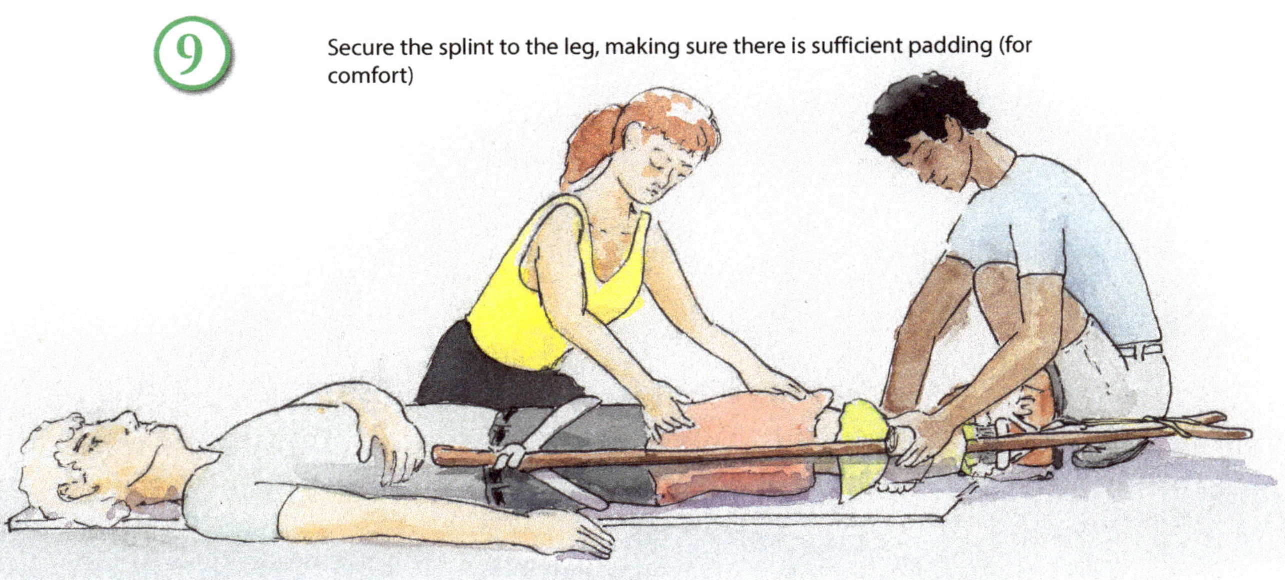

10 Wrap the leg with two 6-inch elastic bandages, beginning at the ankle and ending at the hip—this helps stabilize the splint, reduces swelling, and keeps internal blood loss to a minimum.

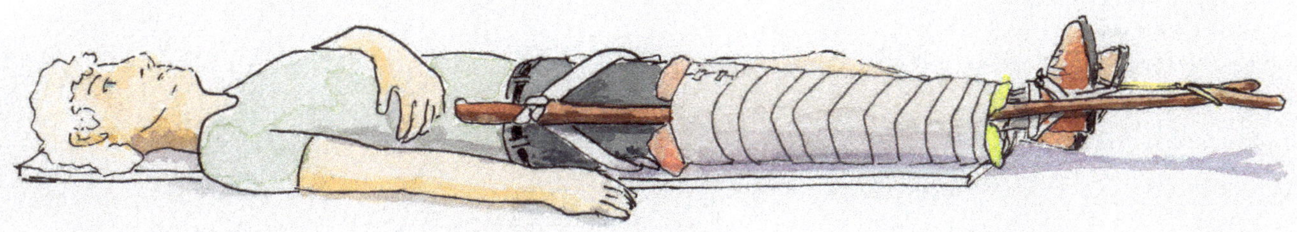

97

Dislocations occur when the bones in a joint become displaced, misaligned, or otherwise traumatized to the point where the joint pulls apart—the disruption is such that the correct anatomy is no longer maintained, and the joint's normal range of motion is reduced.

- All dislocations damage the surrounding soft tissues: muscles, tendons, ligaments, and/or cartilage.
- Dislocations can be associated with a fracture, and it can be very difficult to distinguish between a fracture and a dislocation—when in doubt, position the joint to maintain circulation distal to the injury, and splint.
- Dislocations are debilitating. They put the future function of the limb at risk because of compromised circulation.
- People who have had previous dislocations may experience less pain upon recurrence and may be more able to help you treat them.
- Dislocations sometimes reduce quickly and spontaneously. When they do not spontaneously reduce, they are often extremely painful.
- Reducing dislocations involves risk. If you attempt a reduction in the field, don't exceed the pain barrier—if what you are doing causes more pain, you are also causing more harm.

DISLOCATIONS

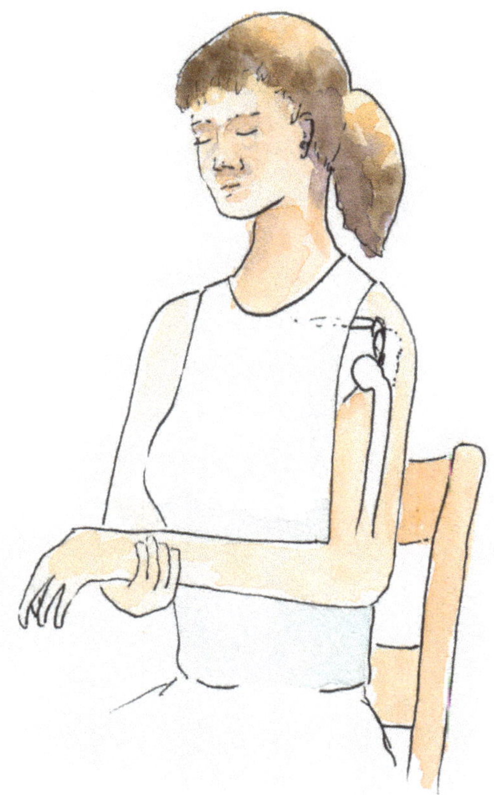

Perhaps the most common backcountry dislocation—the head of the humerus is forced forward and down out of the shoulder joint typically the result of impact (e.g., from a fall).

TREATMENT

- **Urban:** immobilize in position found and transport.
- **Wilderness**

    1. Expose and examine the joint carefully.
    2. Palpate for a possible fracture.
    3. Check CSMs.
        A. Circulation distal to the injury site.
        B. Sensation at the injury site and distal to it.
        C. Movement: by working with the patient, determine motor function and range of motion (pain will be the limiting factor).
    4. Pull traction-in-line (TIL) to reduce the dislocation.
        A. Use a steady, firm pull with slow and gentle movements (the muscles surrounding the joint will typically be in spasm, and any sudden movements will cause them to spasm anew).

B. If necessary, have someone else or a fixed object immobilize the patient to provide counter-traction.
C. The more time that goes by before a dislocation is reduced, the harder it will be to reduce—the quicker, the better.

5. Once the joint has been reduced into proper anatomical alignment, immobilize the joint with a splint.

6. RICE as appropriate.

7. Evacuate (all dislocations need to be seen by a physician).

8. Monitor CSMs distal to the injured joint every 15 minutes. If you find a compromise, carefully remove the splint, realign the joint until CSMs are restored, and re-splint.

SHOULDER DISLOCATION

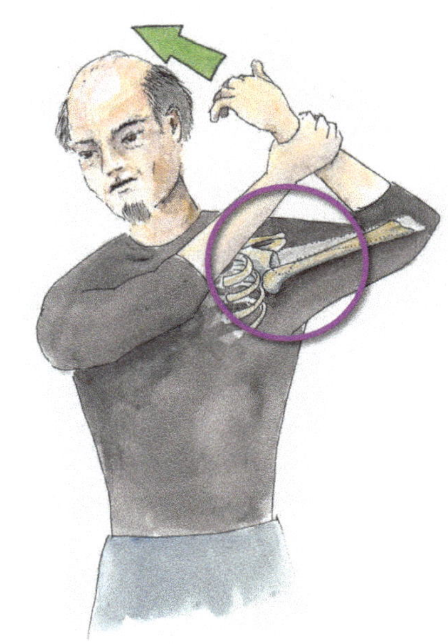

- This is the most common dislocation. Anterior (forward) dislocation is far more common than posterior (rearward) dislocation.
- The shoulder will be locked and painful, and any movement of the humerus will increase pain.
- The appropriate technique depends on the position of the humerus and the position of the patient.
- If none of the techniques listed below are successful in reducing the dislocation, immobilize in the position of comfort and evacuate immediately.

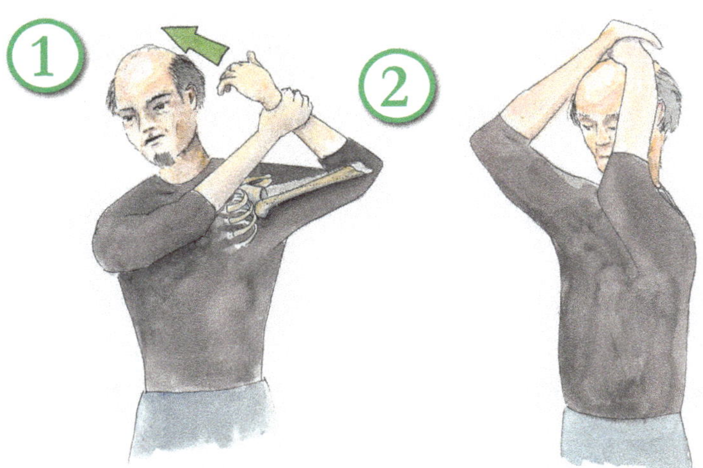

- **RELOCATION**—Use this technique if the patient is found with a dislocated shoulder, and their humerus is extended over their headHave the patient place the hand of their good arm on top of their head.
    - Then (without your help) have them place the hand of their bad arm on top of their head and interlace the fingers of both hands.
    - With their hands on their head help them to lie down on their back. As they lie flat, the elbows, via gravity, will slowly flatten out, and the shoulder will likely spontaneously reduce.
    - Once the shoulder has reduced, place the arm in a sling and swathe to support the injured shoulder.
    - Evacuate. If ambulatory, the patient may walk out.

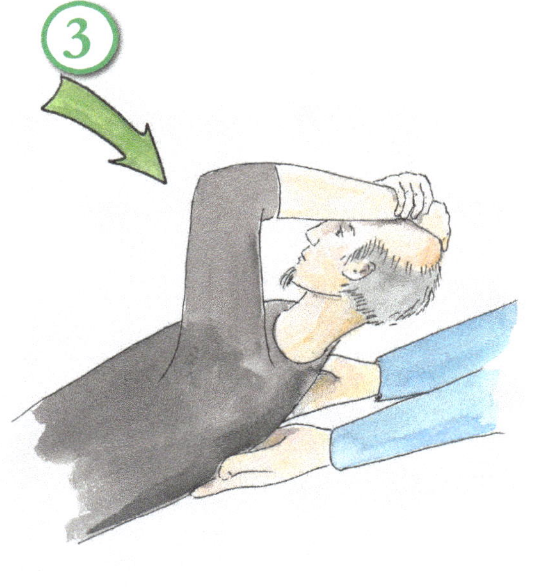

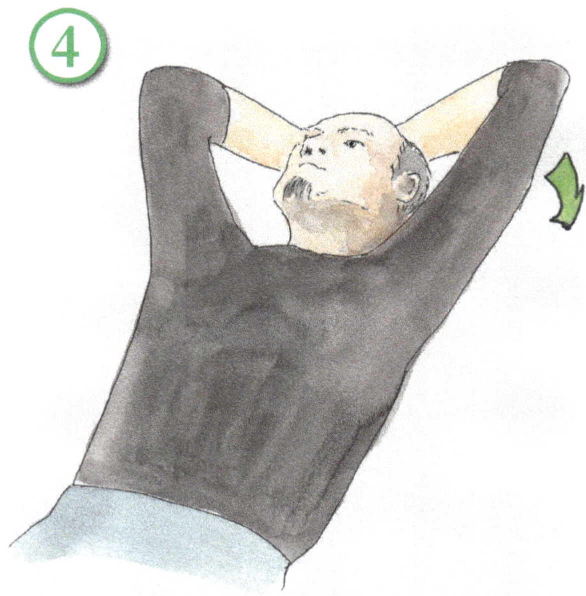

99

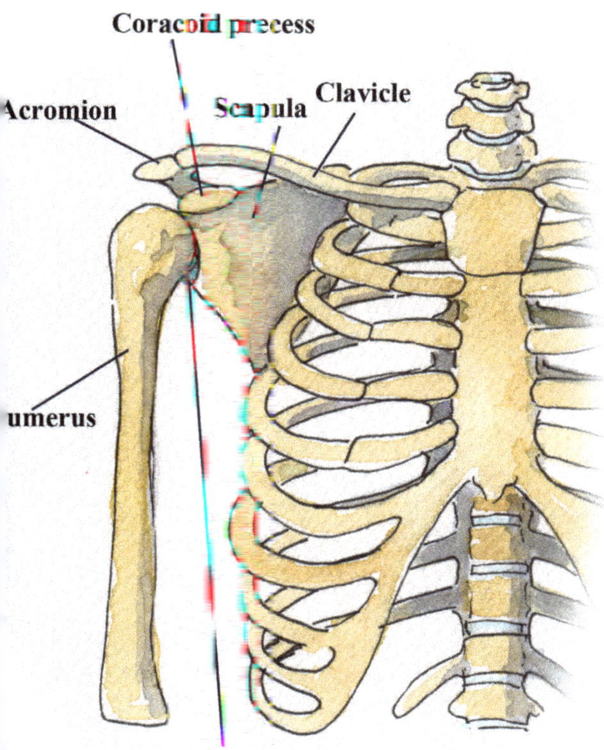

SNOWBIRD REDUCTION TECHNIQUE— Typically, the patient with a shoulder dislocation will be found sitting up with their humerus beside their chest wall and their forearm flexed across their abdomen in the "guarding position."

- Place a wide, well-padded sling in the antecubital fossa i.e. the anterior pocket of the elbow when the arm is flexed to 90%).
- Put one foot in the sling to apply downward traction.
- Slowly increase traction by pushing down on the sling with your foot, which leaves both your hands free.
- Place one hand on the opposite shoulder to keep the patient sitting up straight; have the other hand support the wrist on the injured side (or have someone stand behind them with their hands on the patient's shoulders to keep them sitting up straight).
- While under traction, as the shoulder muscles relax, externally rotate the arm.
- If the shoulder does not reduce, continue traction and retry in several minutes.
- Once reduced, support the arm and shoulder with a sling and swathe.
- Evacuate.
- If ambulatory, the patient may walk out.
- Monitor circulation every 15 minutes during evacuation.

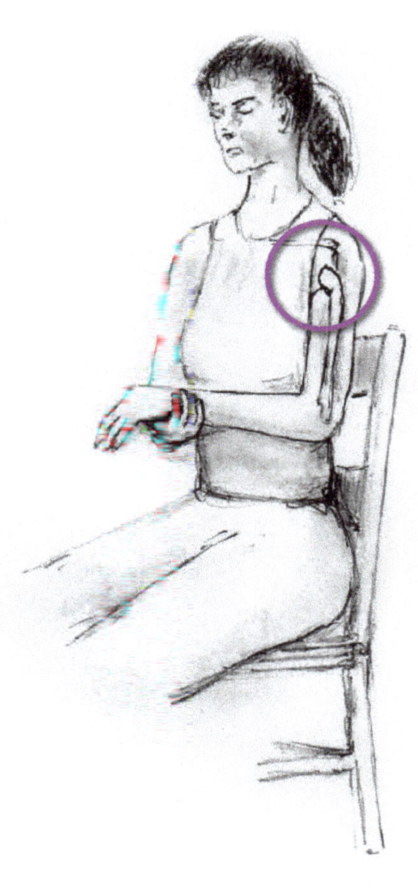

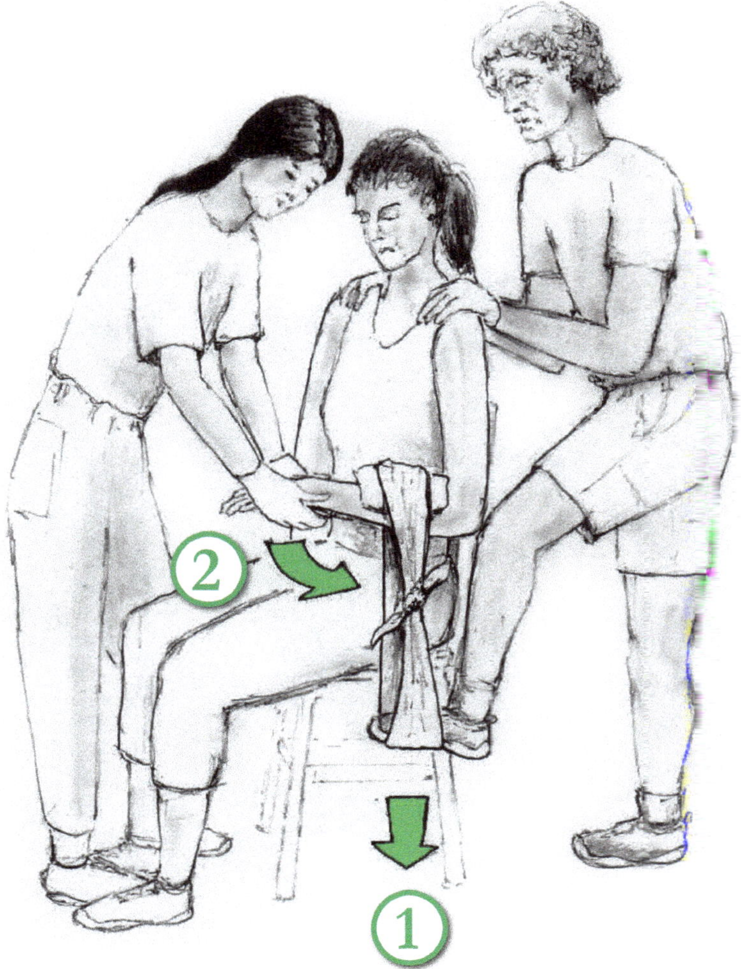

- Usually dislocates laterally (to the outside).
- The patient's leg will typically be bent.
  1. To reduce, apply gentle and firm inward pressure while slowly straightening the leg.
  2. Once reduced, splint the leg in the position of comfort.
  3. Wrap the knee with an elastic wrap to support the joint and control swelling during evacuation.

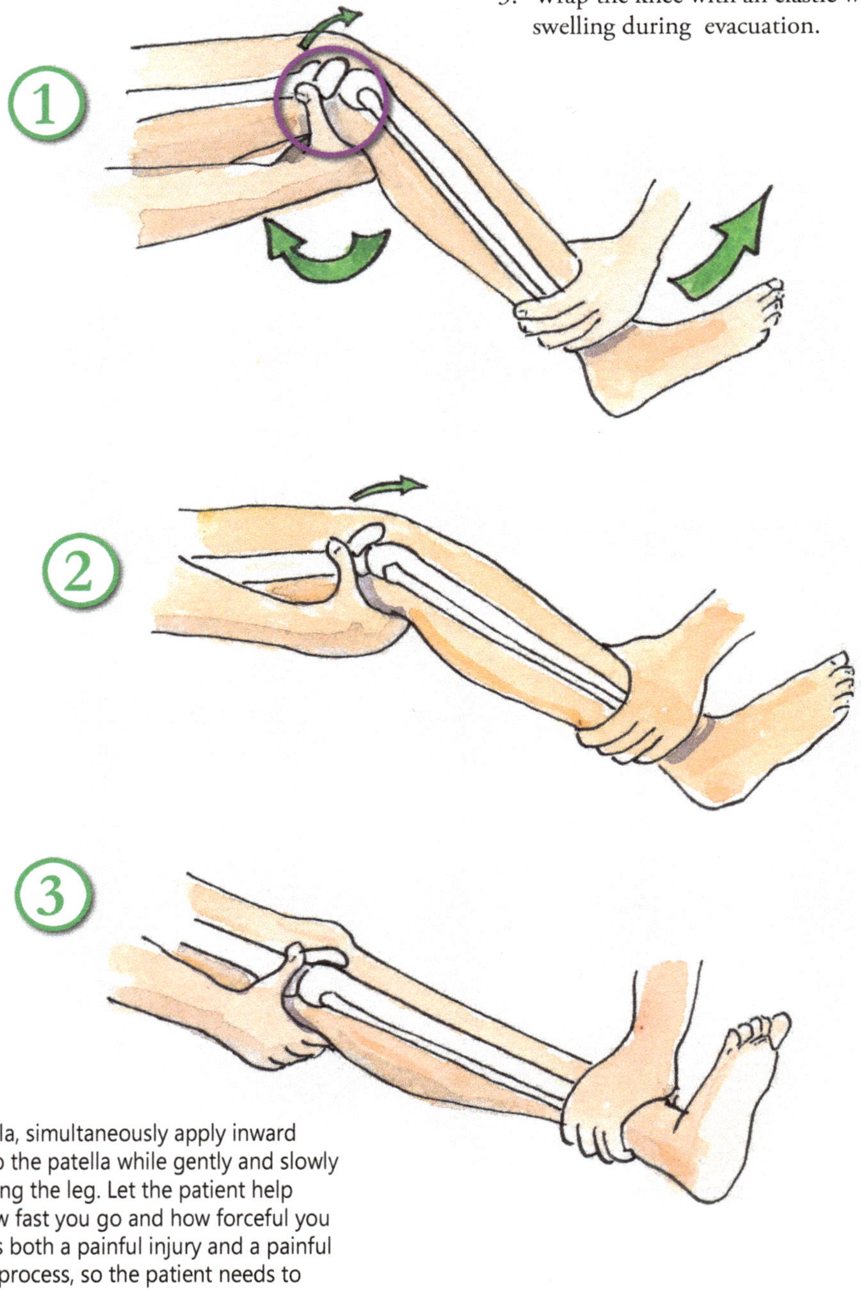

For a patella, simultaneously apply inward pressure to the patella while gently and slowly straightening the leg. Let the patient help dictate how fast you go and how forceful you are—this is both a painful injury and a painful treatment process, so the patient needs to relax!

HEAD TRAUMA

SUPERFICIAL HEMATOMA

This is the classic "egg" that quickly appears after you've been hit in the head by something (e.g., a falling coconut, a wayward fly ball in right field).

Though a relatively minor injury, it can cause dramatic swelling. Treat with a cold pack or ice to reduce swelling, and OTC pain meds.

CONCUSSIONS and TBI

A concussion is a type of traumatic brain injury (TBI) caused by a blow to the head.
A concussion may lead to a temporary loss of consciousness and they can be minor or major TBI depending on the force of the blow and the amount of damage done to the brain.

Mechanism of Injury:
A blow to the head.
Observations of the Patient:
    Amnesia – may not remember what happened.
    Appear dazed or stunned.
    Gait is unsteady, clumsy.
    Cannot follow simple instructions.
    Answers questions slowly.
    Change in level of consciousness.
    Mood or personality change.
Reported by the Patient, they are complaining of:
    Headache or pressure in the head.
    Nausea or vomiting.
    Balance problems, vertigo, dizziness.
    Blurry vision, or light of noise sensitivity.
    Confusion or memory problems.
    May fell hazy, foggy, or groggy.

SKULL FRACTURE

Every skull fracture should be considered a major medical emergency—there are just so many bad things potentially going on: the cracked bone itself, bleeding, edema (and associated increasing ICP; see next) brain injury, leakage of spinal fluid...you get the idea.

SIGNS AND SYMPTOMS

> Depression of skull area (palpable).
> Visible crack beneath laceration.
> Penetrating wound (e.g., arrow, see image caption).
> Cerebrospinal Fluid (CSF: amber-colored, sticky) leaking from nose, ears, or from around the eyes. It may mix with blood, but it does not clot and dries slower. Do not attempt to stop the flow—it is being forced out by the increasing pressure.
> Battle's sign (bruising behind the ears)—a dangerous sign indicating a basilar skull fracture.
> Raccoon eyes (bruising around eyes)—not necessarily an ominous sign.

TREATMENT

1. Monitor ABCs and for signs of increasing ICP (see next) every 15 minutes.
2. Assume spinal injury and immobilize the spine if there is significant MOI.
3. Reevaluate with any change in LOC.
4. Ventilate if respirations are inadequate.
5. Administer Oxygen, 100%, 15 liters per minute, by non-rebreather, if available.
6. Evacuate immediately and as quickly as possible.

INCREASING INTRACRANIAL PRESSURE [*ICP*]

It's common for a part of the body to swell in response to injury (or illness)—in addition to possible bleeding, this localized edema floods the affected area with various types of beneficial fluids designed to flush out damaged cells and toxins, and promote healing. Most of the time there is plenty of space for this swelling to occur (superficial hematoma), but because the volume inside the skull is fixed by the hard shell of bone, in cases of head trauma where the swelling occurs in the tissues *inside* the skull, intracranial pressure increases. Quick recognition of increasing ICP is critical.

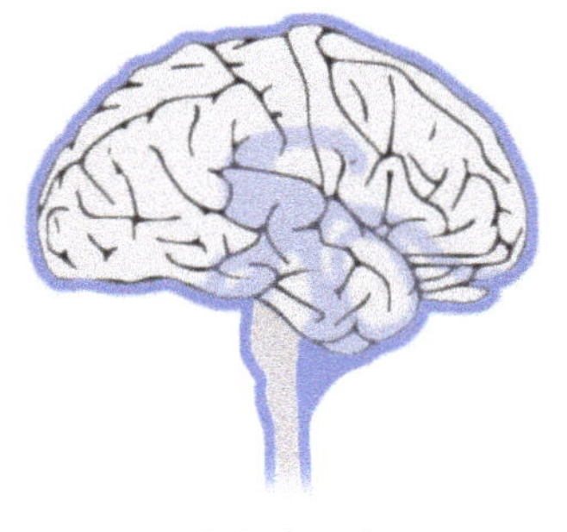

IT'S NOT ALL JUST GRAY (OR PINK) MATTER

> The brain is surrounded by cerebrospinal fluid (CSF), a clear, sticky, sweet fluid (blue in diagram) that provides buoyancy (the brain is suspended in it), cushions the brain from impact, helps supply the brain with glucose, and helps maintain intracranial pressure.

PHYSIOLGY

> Because the volume of the cranium is fixed, any bleeding or swelling inside the cranial vault will cause an increase in ICP.
> As ICP rises, the brain is compressed, in particular, the cerebral cortex and the brainstem: compression of the cerebral cortex causes behavioral changes, while compression of the brainstem causes changes to the victim's vital signs.
> If the ICP gets too high, the brainstem will herniate through the foramen magnum (the large hole in the occipital bone), resulting in death (via uncal herniation).

SIGNS AND SYMPTOMS

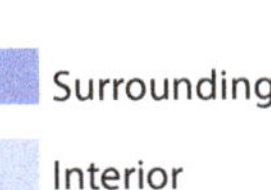

> Change in level of consciousness (deterioration).
> Headache—increases in severity with time.
> Nausea and vomiting that becomes cyclic.
> Amnesia—patient may have retrograde loss of memory.
> Seizures—risk of seizing increases with increasing ICP (late sign).
> Posturing indicates a brainstem injury (late sign).

VITAL SIGNS ASSOCIATED WITH INCREASED ICP

The vital signs do not change independent of each other—they predictably change together. When monitoring a patient with a head injury, pay particular attention to their LOC: as ICP rises, the patient's LOC will deteriorate from alert to painfully responsive. The earliest LOC changes include *uncooperativeness*, *irrational behavior* (potential refusal of care), *combatativeness* (like a "mean drunk"), and *disorientation*.

> *HR* slow, bounding
> *RR* increasing in both rate and depth, hyperventilation, or pattern breathing (see complete list, right), in order of occurrence, over time:
> > *Kussmaul's Breathing*—increasing hyperventilation, rapid and deep
> > *Cheyne-Stokes Breathing*—a cycle of breathing which gradually increases in rate and depth, followed by a gradual decrease in rate and depth, followed by a short period of apnea, then the cycle repeats
> > *Apneustic breathing*—pauses in the respiratory cycle at full respiration; this is the last stage (death follows)
> *BP* increasing, widening pulse pressure (systolic rises faster than diastolic)
> *Skin* variable based on environment and associated injuries—may be pink/warm/moist or pale/cool/clammy
> *Pupils* eventually become unequal (late sign)

TREATMENT

> Surgery is the only treatment—the only field treatment is O2.
> Evacuate immediately by the quickest means possible.
> Maintain and protect the airway from vomitus and aspiration.
> Immobilize the C-spine and place the patient in the recovery position.

SPINAL TRAUMA

THE SPINAL CORD
THE BODY'S COMMUNICATION SYSTEM

- It connects the brain to the rest of the body.
- The spinal cord is **protected** by the spinal column, which is made up of
33 individual vertebrae in five sections.
- The spinal column is very **flexible**.
- Injury to the vertebrae risks **damage** to the spinal cord.
- Damage to the spinal cord may be **debilitating** and **permanent**.

PRINCIPLES
TO KEEP IN MIND

- The **greatest risk to the neck** is when the MOI causes flexion (as if the person were ducking forward—right) and axial loading with impact on the top of the head. This can cause a burst fracture of C4/C5 and put the spinal cord at risk. When moving a patient with a suspected neck injury, keep the head and neck in the neutral position and avoid forward flexion.
- The thoracic portion of the vertebral column is the **hardest to injure** because it is so well reinforced by the ribcage. It is most often injured by direct force.
- Injuries to the transition area (T12/L1) pose the **greatest risk to the spine**—especially due to rotation, where the shoulders are rotated out of alignment with the hips. Keep the patient's hips and shoulders aligned when moving them.
- The lower back (lumbar to coccyx) is the **most common** area of the back to be injured. Approximately 85% of all back injuries occur in the lumbar spine, particularly L4/L5.
- It is always okay to move a patient into correct anatomical position (neutral position).
- **WARNINGS**
    - Unless the lack of MOI can be determined, treat **every patient as if they have a spinal injury.**
    - Remember, a person can **damage** their spinal column **without injuring** their spinal cord.

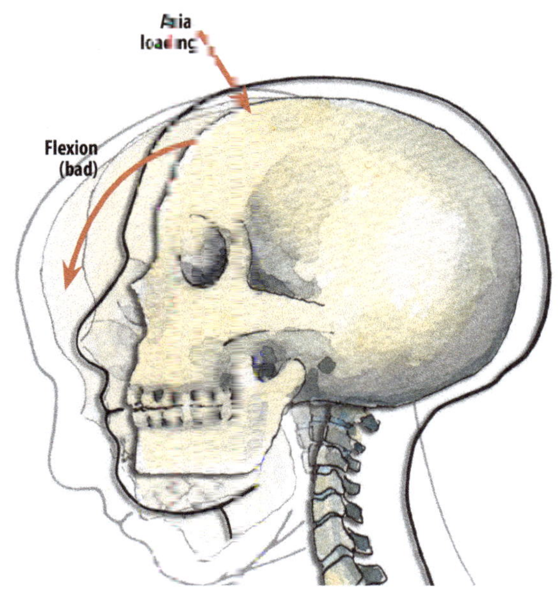

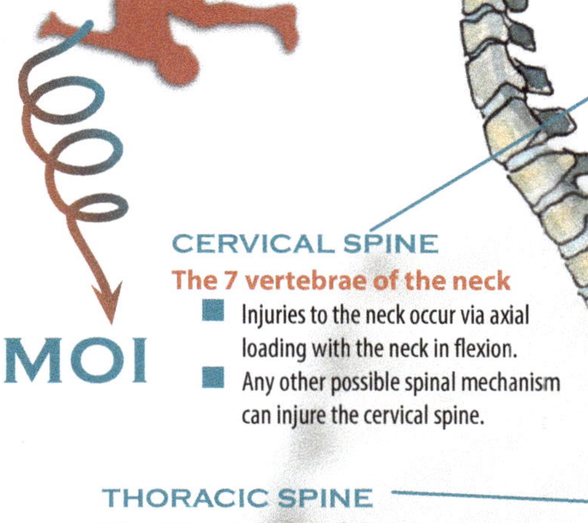

CERVICAL SPINE
The 7 vertebrae of the neck

- Injuries to the neck occur via axial loading with the neck in flexion.
- Any other possible spinal mechanism can injure the cervical spine.

THORACIC SPINE
The 12 vertebrae of the chest

- Each vertebra is associated with a rib.
- Injury almost always comes from a direct blow.

LUMBAR SPINE
The 5 vertebrae that span the rib cage to the pelvis

- The spinal cord extends down to L2. Below that is the cauda equina or "horse tail," made up of individual peripheral nerves.
- This is the most common spinal area to be injured.
- It is also the most common site of chronic injury.
- Injury occurs via a direct blow or by exceeding the range of motion.

SACRAL SPINE
A wedge-shaped bone composed of 5 fused vertebrae

- There is no risk of spinal cord damage (the cord does not extend down this far).
- Peripheral nerve trunks can be damaged.

COCCYX
The 4 rudimentary vertebra at the termination of the spinal column

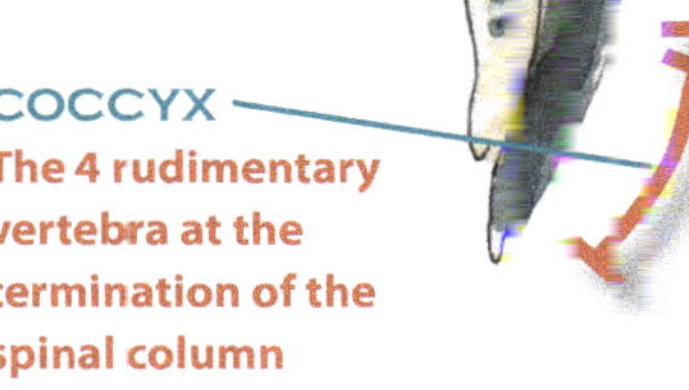

SPINAL MECHANISM OF INJURY (MOI)

- **Falls:** especially falls when high speed is involved, when the victim lands on their head or shoulders (tumbling), or any fall 3x body height or more.
- **Automobile accidents:** combinations of high speed and impact/rapid deceleration.
- **Head injury:** Any blow to the head resulting in loss of consciousness is MOI for spinal injury.
- **Diving accidents:** A blow to the head from diving into shallow water can produce a dangerous combination of axial loading and impact to the spine.
- **Direct blows:** may be the result of a fall or impact with a moving object.

MECHANISM OF INJURY (MOI)

- In most situations, **mechanism of injury** alone is enough to demand full spinal inspection and immobilization.

- In most jurisdictions, urban medical protocols have stated that all patients transported from a motor vehicle accident (MVA) or a significant fall (3x body height) **require immobilization**, even in the absence of any other signs or symptoms. (This may be changing due to evidence-based medicine.)

SIGNS AND SYMPTOMS

- **Pain** may be present in many ways and is often not spontaneous. Distracting pain may mask all pain response, making assessment unreliable until the distracting pain is reduced. Types of pain include:
  - Radiating—it shoots off in varying directions
  - Diffuse—pain is undifferentiated and ubiquitous
  - Pain with motion—it hurts when I move this
  - Point-tender upon palpation—it hurts where you poke

- **Loss of consciousness** indicates a possible head injury.
- **Guarding or muscle spasms**—my neck is stiff.
- **Paresthesia**—I feel pins and needles.
- **Numbnesss**—nope, I can't feel that.
- **Paralysis**—I'm unable to move that at all.
- **Spinal deformity**—things are out of place.
- **Swelling** along the spine.
- **Locked sensation**—it feels stuck.
- **Discoloration** along the spine.

TREATING SPINAL INJURIES

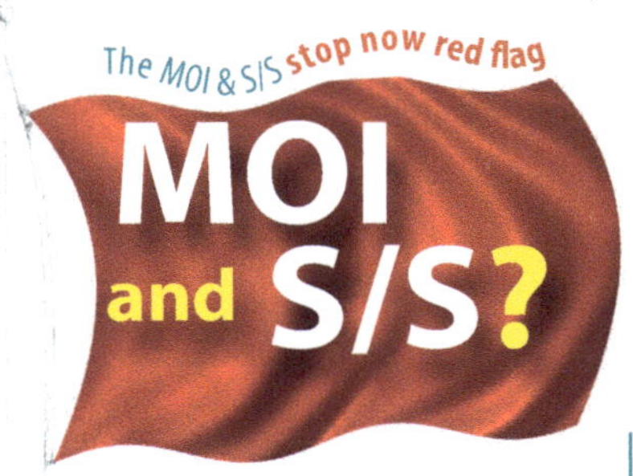

Got **ANY** of these MOI factors?

Rapid deceleration

Fall 3x body height

Direct impact

Axial loading

Head trauma

And **ANY** of these signs/symptoms?

Then you should see the spinal trauma **red flag** (above) and

1. Immobilize the **C-spine**
2. Immobilize the rest of the **spine**
3. Place the patient in a **litter**

...and then **EVACUATE**

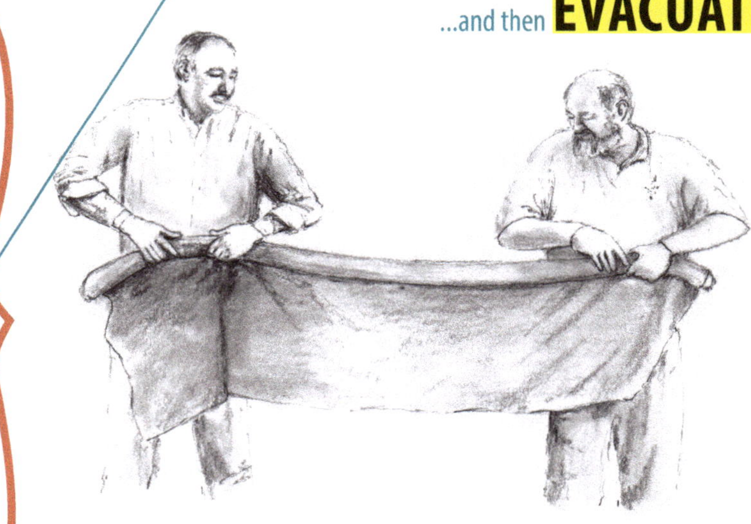

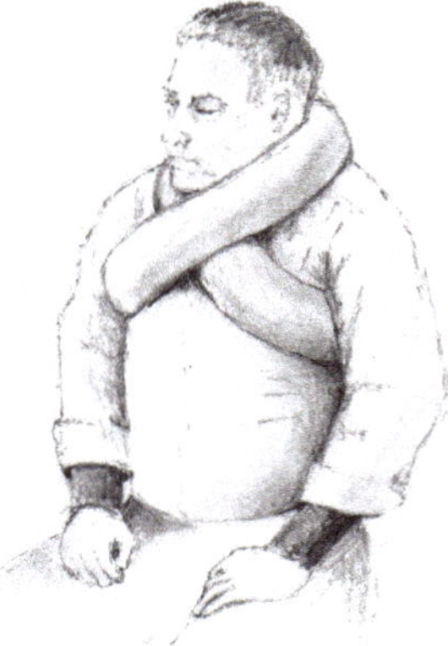

Improvised neck collar using a rolled up blanket.

LITTER PACKAGING

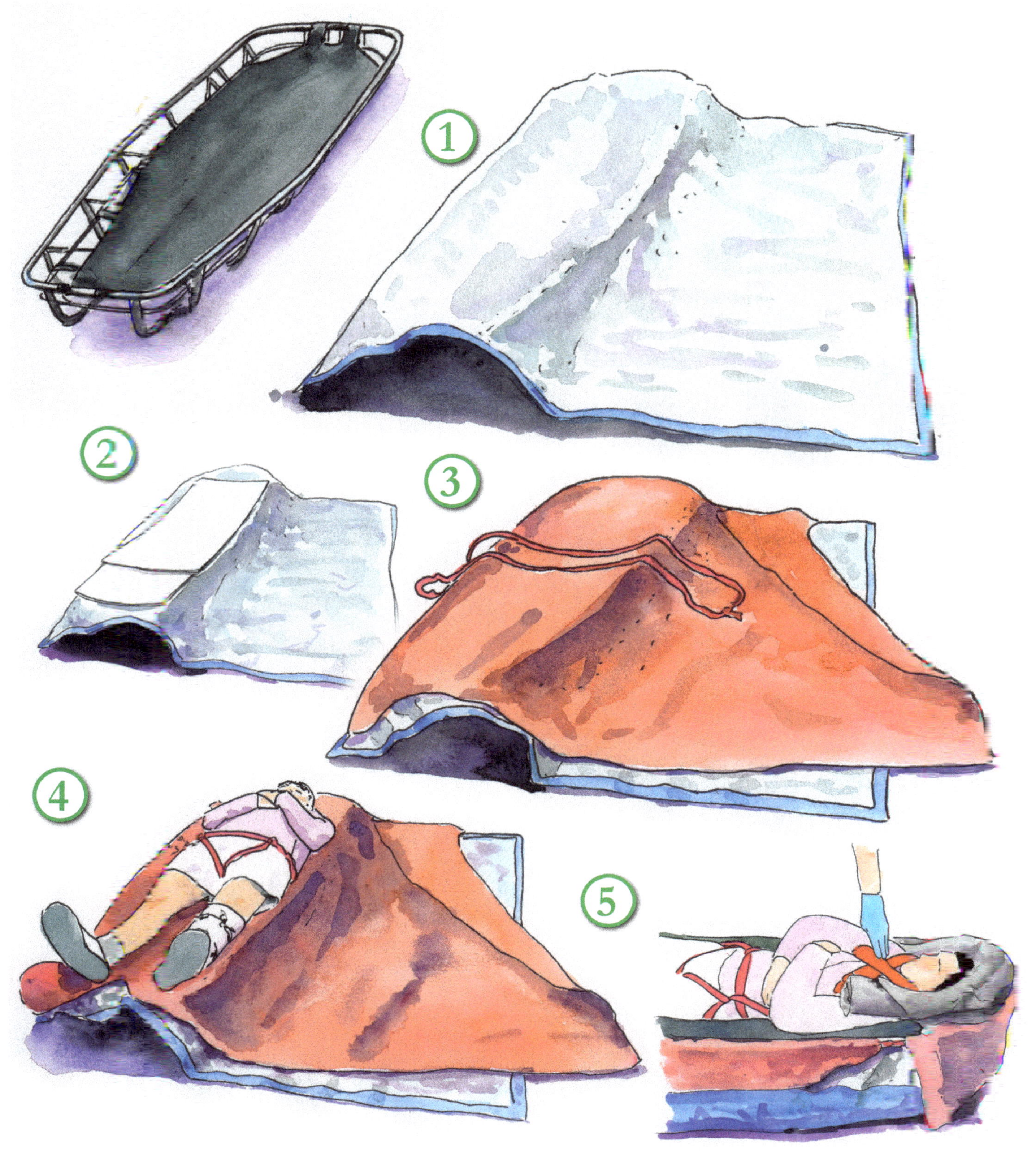

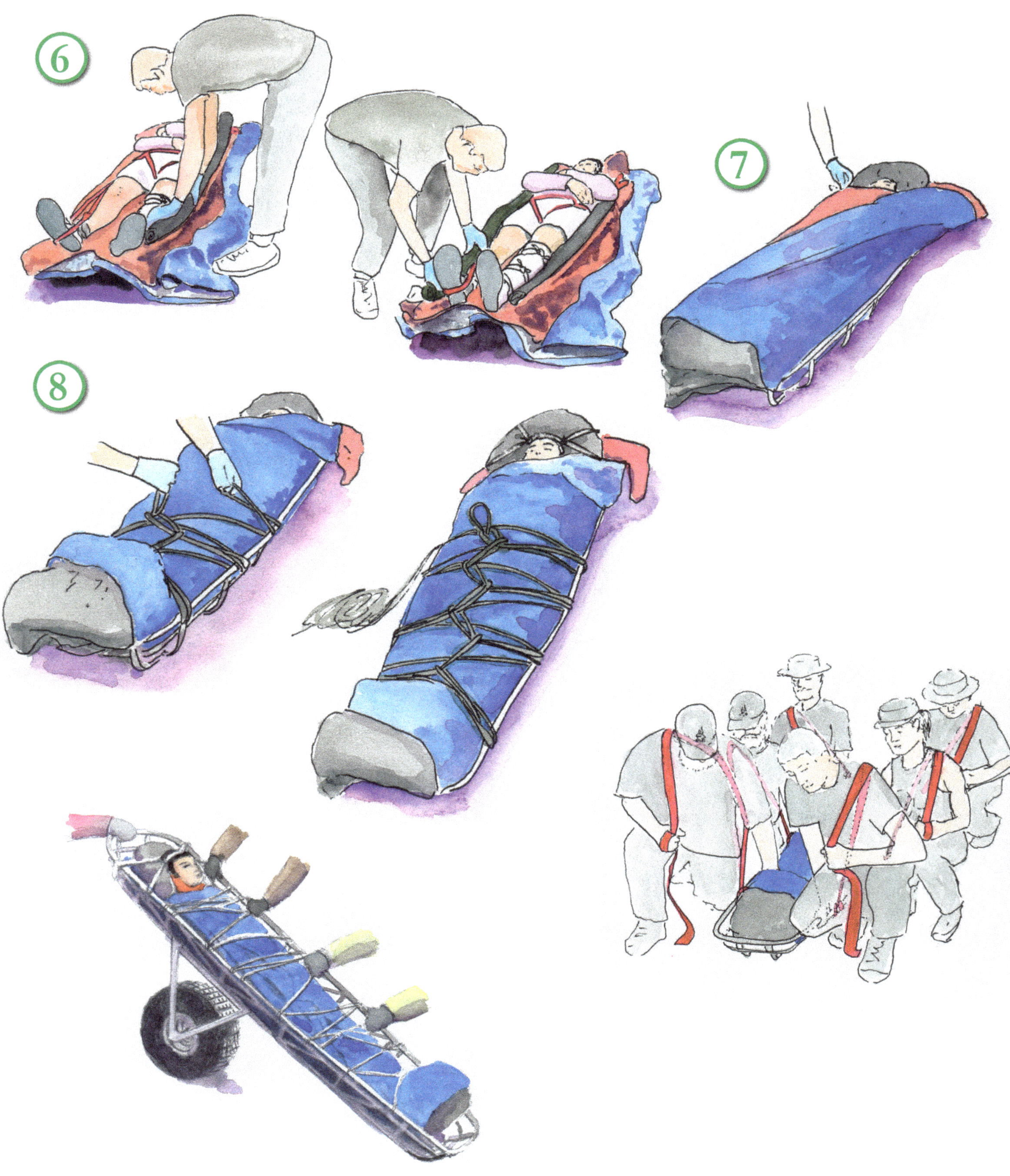

SOLO Wilderness First Responder

CLEARING THE SPINE

ALL YOU HAVE is MOI, you MAY be able to CLEAR THE SPINE allowing the person to walk out...

ADVANCED SPINAL ASSESSMENT

- Due to the risks of weather, terrain, time delays, etc., and under certain assessment circumstances, it is possible to **clear the spine** of an ambulatory patient, enabling them to walk out without immobilization.

- Clearing the C-spine is a **controversial** skill. Unless you have been trained in this technique and have practiced the skills, you should not attempt to clear an injured person's spine when there is significant MOI.

- Clearing the spine is done in the presence of **MOI only**—the following tests must be applied and the criteria must be evaluated in the following order, and the patient must meet **all criteria**—if they fail **anything**, fully immobilize them and evacuate. If they pass everything, then wave the **green flag** and go.

1. **Reliability**
   - The patient is awake and oriented x 3.
   - They are not under the influence of drugs or alcohol.
   - They are not being adversely influenced by cold or heat.

2. **No distracting pain**
   - If the patient had a distracting injury or injuries (e.g., a fractured femur), treatment must have reduced the pain to a point where it is no longer a distraction.

3. **No signs or symptoms** (yes, the redundancy is intentional)
   - The patient does not complain of pain anywhere in their back.
   - They do not have radiating pain, paresthesia (tingling), or numbness in any of their extremities.
   - They have intact circulation, sensation, and motion in all four extremities.
   - They have no tenderness the length of their spine during the physical exam.
   - They do not exhibit any guarding and there is no paravertebral muscle spasm.

4. **Range of motion test**
   - This test is performed only if the patient has been found to be reliable, is without distracting pain, and has no signs or symptoms.
   - The rescuer supports, but does not move the patient through their range of motion.
   - If during the test, the patient experiences any pain, stiffness, or locking sensations, the test is over and the patient must be immediately and fully immobilized.
   - If the range of motion is pain-free, elicits no locking sensation, and is normal, you may consider the spine to be free of injury, and the patient does not need to be collared and backboarded.
   - Performing the test: the patient should lie flat on their back and perform the following movements, in order (the patient does the work—active range of motion).
     1. They slowly rotate their head to one side, and then to the other (it doesn't matter if you start to the left or right).
     2. They slowly extend their head to look up.
     3. They slowly flex their head down by bringing their chin to their chest (Flexion).
     4. They arch their lower back off the ground.
     5. They do half a sit-up (to 45⁰).

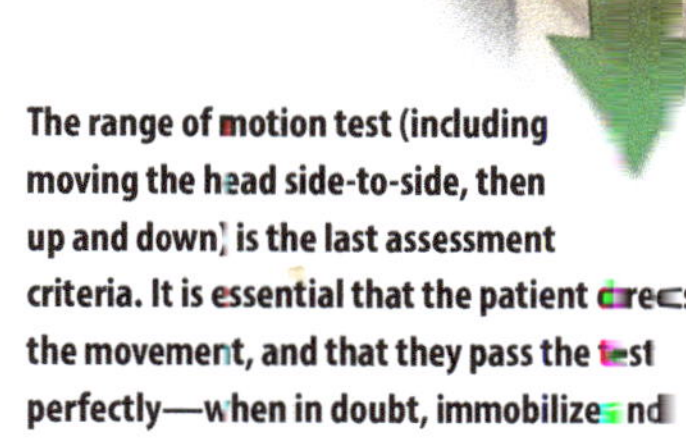

The range of motion test (including moving the head side-to-side, then up and down) is the last assessment criteria. It is essential that the patient directs the movement, and that they pass the test perfectly—when in doubt, immobilize and evacuate.

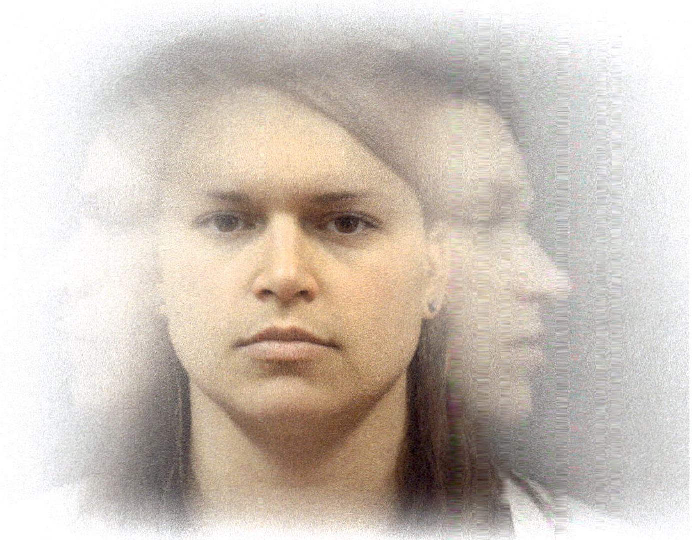

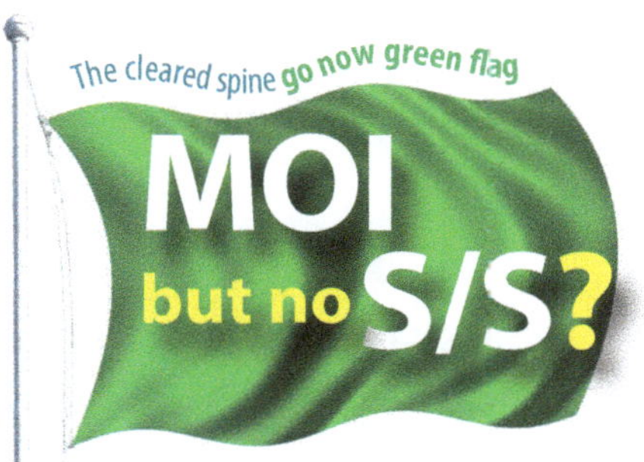

CHEST TRAUMA

Specific cardiothoracic trauma

Because so many of the signs/symptoms and treatments are shared by many of the injuries covered, we've consolidated things graphically at the end of the list—any S/S- and/or injury-specific information will be given for each condition within its description.

Chest-wall soft tissue injuries

These are simple soft tissue injuries to the superficial layers of the chest wall (skin, adipose tissue, intercostal muscles, or breasts), typically caused by a direct blow (e.g., from a fall). Although often appearing superficial, there may be more going on below the surface—examine the injuries closely and consider possible damage to the underlying anatomy (lungs and heart). You can estimate the depth of injury to be one half of the diameter of the surface injury.

Fractured clavicle

This is the most common fracture seen in emergency medicine. It is easily diagnosed because the clavicle is superficial—you can locate the point-tenderness and palpate the fracture (typically in the center to the distal 1/3). It is important to remember that just under the clavicle is a large neurovascular bundle containing a large vein, an artery, and nerves, as well as the apex of the lungs. As the clavicle breaks, a bone fragment can damage one of these underlying structures, causing bleeding, a pneumothorax, or subcutaneous emphysema. Subcutaneous emphysema occurs when air collects under the skin, indicating a tear in the trachea, airways, or the parietal and visceral pleura. A tear such as this allows air to leak out of the lungs into the pleural space and the adjoining tissues. Although this loose air is harmless, it can indicate a serious underlying injury. If this is a stand-alone injury, the patient will likely be ambulatory.

Fractured ribs

Fractured ribs are a common injury resulting from direct trauma to the chest wall. They are usually isolated injuries, which are easily managed. However, because the lungs lie directly beneath the ribs, bone fragments can pierce the chest and cause a pneumothorax, hemothorax, or both. Two treatment items are unique to this injury: first, don't wrap the ribs (this can interfere with breathing), and second, during recovery the patient should have at least four deliberate coughing sessions per day to prevent pneumonia (coughing forces air to move through all sections of the lung, removing CO_2 and reducing the likelihood of a bacterial infection).

Fractured sternum

Fractures of the sternum are relatively uncommon as they require a direct (and hard) blow to the sternum. For example, this injury can occur when an unrestrained driver hits their chest on the steering wheel during a head-on collision (where a bruise in the shape of the steering wheel may be seen). Also, avalanche victims occasionally experience sternal fractures. They are rarely serious, and do not require any specific treatment, but as always, it is important to monitor for signs of injury to the underlying structures—the heart and the lungs.

Flail chest

This is a life-threatening emergency—it is likely that there is damage to the underlying lung tissues, blood vessels, and the heart or lungs. The sternum and/or multiple adjacent ribs are broken in two or more places, creating a "free floating" segment of the chest wall (only the ribs example is highlighted at the right). There may also be extensive soft tissue damage. As the patient tries to inhale, the flail section gets drawn in by the vacuum, limiting the amount of air exchange. This asymmetrical movement of the flail section is called paradoxical motion. (Do not compress or immobilize the injured side during treatment—this will further limit air exchange.)

Pulmonary contusion

As the chest wall is injured, some energy from the blow is transmitted through the chest wall into the parenchyma (tissue) of the lungs resulting in bruising of that tissue. Over a period of hours this will cause bleeding into the lung tissue and stiffening of that area of the lung, causing a progressive worsening of dyspnea. While not an emergency by itself, over time, it will contribute to the severity of the chest trauma and respiratory distress.

Pulmonary laceration

A laceration to the parenchyma of the lung can be caused by direct blunt trauma or a penetrating wound to the chest. Both the visceral pleura and parietal pleura may be involved, and there is an obvious risk of a hemo/pneumothorax or a sucking chest wound. Monitor closely for dyspnea that worsens over time.

Pneumothorax

A simple pneumothorax is a closed injury where air collects in the pleural cavity between the lung and the chest wall. The same mechanism that causes a hemothorax can also injure the airways, leaking air into the pleural space. As the air enters the pleural space, it rises to the top of the lungs, causing them to collapse from the top down—a collapsed lung. A simple pneumothorax can develop into a tension pneumothorax—a far more serious condition—so careful monitoring is critical.

Sucking chest wound

This is also called an open pneumothorax, and yes, it's as bad as it sounds—a penetrating (open) injury has occurred allowing air to enter the pleural space resulting in a pneumothorax. This is a potentially life-threatening injury, depending upon the extent of damage to the underlying structures and lungs.

Tension pneumothorax

This is a life-threatening emergency that begins as a simple pneumothorax, but as air continues to enter the pleural space, it compresses the lungs and heart and impairs respiration and/or blood circulation. As the lung is compressed against the mediastinum, the vena cava, and the uninjured lung, it interferes with the heart's ability to refill between contractions. It also squeezes the uninjured lung, limiting air exchange. If caused by an open pneumothorax, the wound will need to be dressed with an occlusive dressing, left open on one side so that can be "burped" to reduce pressure. A patient with a tension pneumothorax will require a thoracostomy or a chest tube—immediate and quick evacuation to definitive care is needed.

Hemothorax

When the parenchyma of the lungs and the visceral pleura are injured the pulmonary vascular system will be injured, too. This causes blood to collect in the pleural space and, via gravity, settle to the base of the lungs.

ABDOMINAL TRAUMA

ABDOMINAL ANATOMY

- *Hollow organs*—these organs are most prone to penetrating trauma, and if they spill their contents into the gut, it can be very irritating and increase the risk of infection.
  - Small and large intestines
  - Bladder
  - Gallbladder
  - Stomach
- *Solid organs*—these are most prone to blunt trauma leading to blood loss.
  - Kidneys
  - Liver
  - Pancreas
  - Spleen

SIGNS AND SYMPTOMS OF ABDOMINAL TRAUMA

- Shock, from internal bleeding
- Abdominal wall rigidity (a reaction to the internal bleeding)
- Guarding, spasm of the abdominal wall muscles
- Distention from internal bleeding
- Obvious external trauma, wounds, and/or bruising
- Referred pain—pain may be referred to other areas, e.g., from the spleen to the left shoulder

TREATMENT

1. Treat for shock.
2. Wrap abdomen with two 6-inch elastic bandages to apply counter-pressure.
3. Immobilize any penetrating objects.
4. Look for associated thoracic or genitourinary injuries.
5. Minimize food and water intake.

SPECIFIC TREATMENT FOR INTERNAL BLEEDING

Internal bleeding occurs when there is damage to the vascular system inside the body but with no open wounds. The most common internal bleeding occurs when blunt trauma to the abdomen (e.g., from direct impact from a fall or auto accident) results in damage to any of the internal organs.

1. Once bleeding is recognized, gentle pressure can be applied by wrapping the abdomen with two six-inch ACE wraps to gently compress the abdominal cavity (see pelvic trauma). This will decrease the potential space for the blood to accumulate and will apply counter-pressure to the torn vessels, slowing blood loss and allowing clots to form.

INJURIES TO EXTERNAL GENITALIA

- *Impact injuries*
  1. Examine for swelling or bleeding.
  2. Control bleeding with direct pressure.
  3. Apply cold to minimize swelling.
  4. Evacuate.
- *Lacerations*
  1. Control bleeding with direct pressure.
  2. Evacuate.
- *Burns*
  1. Cool immediately and keep cool.
  2. Apply a wet, sterile dressing.
  3. Evacuate.
- *Avulsions and amputations*
  1. Control bleeding with direct pressure.
  2. Save amputated part.
  3. Evacuate.
- *Impaled objects*
  1. Leave object in place.
  2. Stabilize with sterile dressings.
  3. Evacuate.
- *Torsion of the testes:* This occurs when the spermatic cord to a testicle twists, cutting off the blood supply.

  Signs and symptoms
  - Sudden onset.
  - Swollen, red, painful scrotum—pain increases over time.

  Treatment
  1. Apply cool compress.
  2. Give pain meds.
  3. Support the testes.
  4. Evacuate (testes may die within 24 hours).

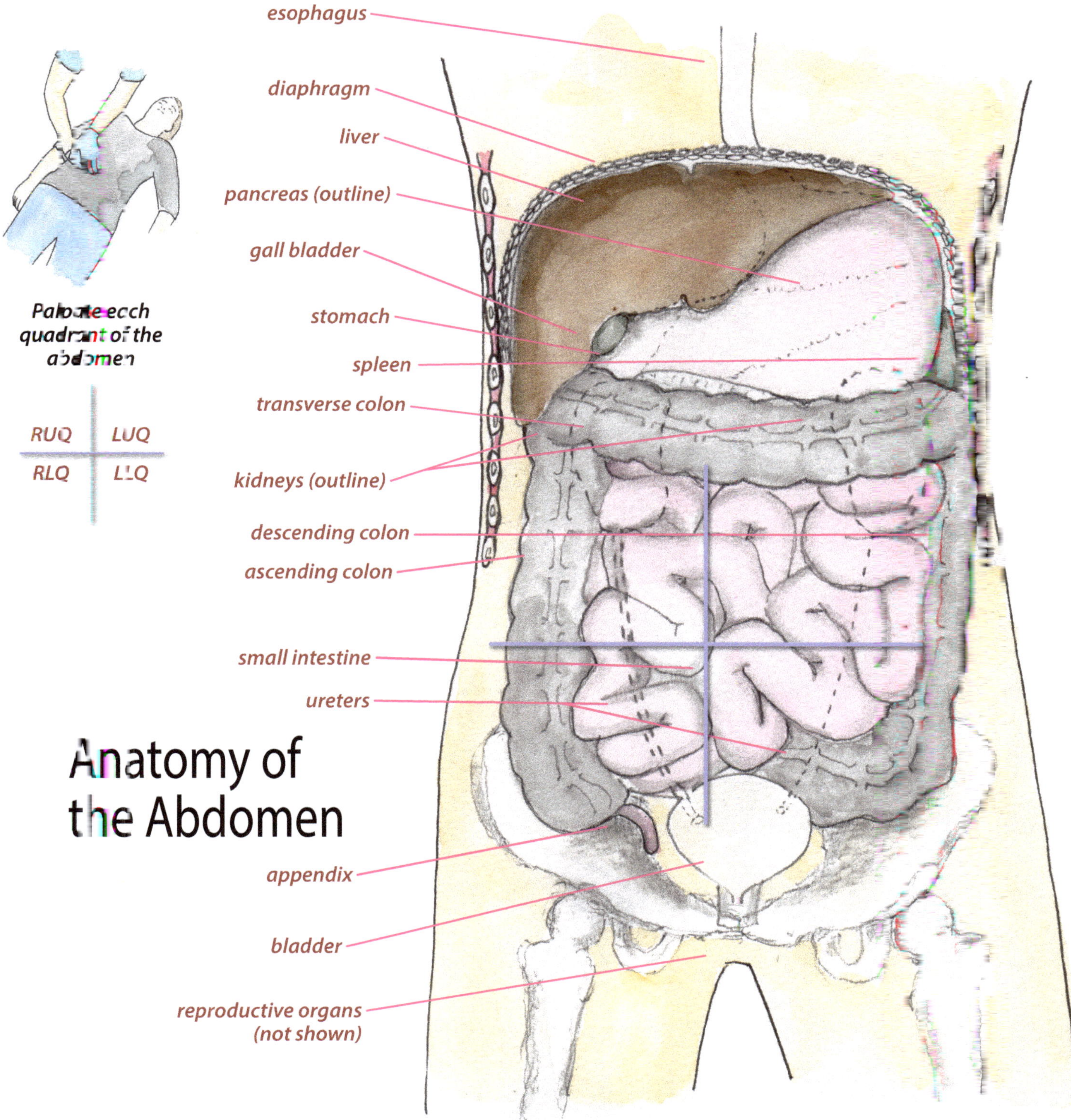

Anatomy of the Abdomen

Environmental Emergencies

ENVIRONMENTAL EMERGENCIES

WE ARE A NAKED, hairless, warm-blooded, tropical animal that must make and take a microenvironmemt with us everywhere we go so we don't die. We are not designed for the cold, yet we live in all the climates of the world—including some brutally cold places like Siberia, Patagonia, and Minneapolis. Huh...

THE HUMAN ANIMAL

Thermoregulation

Hydration

Nutrition

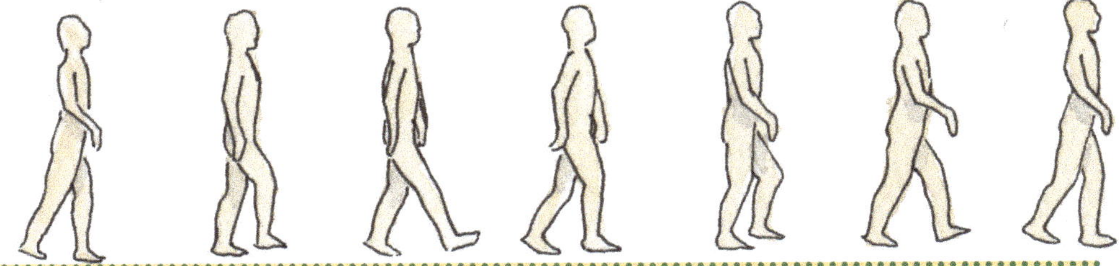

Thermoregulation **maintaining thermal equilibrium**

As the name implies, this is a balancing act between heat production, heat conservation, heat transfer, and heat loss designed to maintain the optimum core temperature of 98.6°F (37°C).

THERMOGENESIS

There are three ways to produce heat: metabolism, exercise, and behavior.

Metabolism—the set of chemical reactions that happen in living organisms to maintain life. These processes allow organisms to grow and reproduce, maintain their structures, and respond to their environments.

- Metabolism uses oxygen to burn calories which sustain life and produce heat.
- The vast majority of calories that we burn are carbohydrates or starches—sugars, glucose, and fructose.
- In order to keep the metabolic fires burning, we must keep stoking the fire with glucose and fructose by snacking often on simple sugars rather than proteins and fats—this helps maintain a higher blood sugar level.
- In a well-fed state, we maintain a 24-hour emergency supply of glucose, stored in our liver as glycogen. This 24-hour supply is at rest—on a cold winter day that store can be depleted in 5 to 6 hours.
- Metabolic activity is regulated by the thyroid, which uses the hormone thyroxine (T3 and T4) to establish the rate at which we burn calories.

- Basal metabolism is the minimum amount of energy required to maintain vital functions in an organism at complete rest.
- When the body senses a need to increase the metabolic rate (due to a cooling core temperature, or exercise) the thyroid can increase calorie consumption up to five times the normal rate.

Exercise—Muscle activity produces heat.

- Voluntary muscle activity is willful exercise: hiking, skiing, running, climbing, etc. Exercise can produce excess heat that must be vented or dissipated.
- Involuntary exercise (shivering) is a natural, involuntary response to early hypothermia in warm-blooded animals which occurs when the core temperature drops.
  - Shivering is designed to maintain homeostasis—its sole function is to produce heat. It can increase heat production up to 10 times the normal rate.
  - Shivering requires oxygen and glucose to work—you must fuel the fire. If fuel runs out, shivering will slow and eventually halt, and dangerous hypothermia will likely set in.

- Shivering begins with the muscles around the vital organs when signals from the heat center in the anterior hypothalamic-preoptic area (excited by cold signals from the skin and spinal cord) are activated when the body temperature falls even a fraction of a degree below a critical temperature level.
- Unfortunately, shivering produces no useful work, and can actually interfere with the performance of important tasks (e.g., starting a fire, walking).

Behavior—the conscious, voluntary set of actions that we take to protect ourselves.

- We feel cold, so we put on a layer.
- Feel hot? Get out of the sun and reduce physical activity.
- Behavior choices are our most important defense against becoming too cold or too hot.

HEAT TRANSFER

HEAT TRANSFER follows the laws of thermodynamics, where temperature equilibrium occurs naturally by transferring heat from a warm object to a cooler object. There are four primary mechanisms.

Conduction is heat transfer between materials in direct contact. The warm object cools and the cool object warms—nature striking a balance.

- Heat transfer ranges from 0% – 40%, depending on the type of material (foam pad versus frozen ground), and the temperature differential (the greater the differential, the greater the transfer—and the faster it occurs).

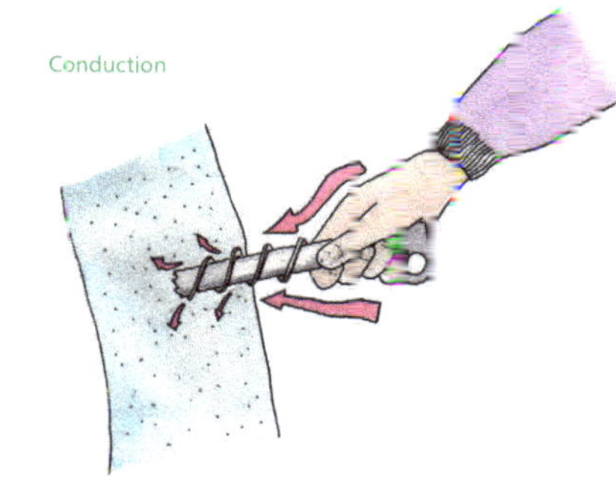

Convection is heat transfer through a fluid (both liquids and gases are fluids).

- Heat transfer ranges from 0% – 40% depending on the medium (e.g., air or water), the type of insulating material used (a windproof jacket versus open-knit sweater, or bare skin versus a neoprene suit), the temperature differential (the greater the differential, the greater the transfer—and the faster it occurs), the relative movement between the materials (wind velocity, speed of water current, etc.).
- Wind chill is an example of convective heat loss—while the ambient air temperature does not change, the rate of heat loss increases as the wind velocity increases, effectively causing heat to be lost at a similar rate as it would be at a colder temperature. Insulation can reduce the rate of heat loss, but only if there is a windproof layer over it.
- The rate of convective heat loss in water is 50 to 100 times that of heat loss in air. This helps explain why people submerged in water can become hypothermic so quickly (i.e., a naked person in 60-degree water will become hypothermic very quickly compared to the same person in 60-degree air).

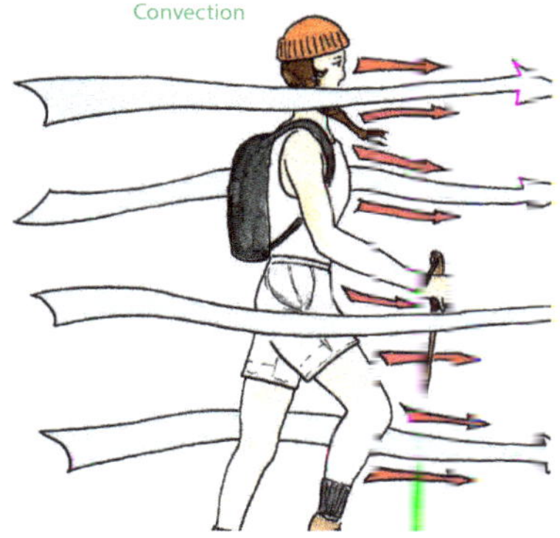

Radiation is heat transfer via the movement of molecules (infrared radiation). Any object warmer than absolute zero (0 degrees Kelvin, -273.15ºC, -459.67ºF) radiates infrared energy.

- The rate of heat transfer depends on the temperature of the object—the hotter the object, the more infrared radiation it produces. Example: a wood stove.
- Heat transfer ranges from 5% – 80% depending on the temperature differential—the greater the differential, the greater the heat transfer, and the faster it occurs.
- A warm body can lose 2% – 89% of its infrared heat into the surrounding environment.
- This form of heat loss is usually small for humans, around 2% – 5%, and is not easily controlled.
- One of the ways to recapture or preserve infrared energy is to reflect it back with a shiny, metallic surface. This is the science behind mylar or "space" blankets, (utilizing a metalized polyethylene terephthalate film). Unfortunately, it does not work very well because the molecules in the reflective material are too far apart; and, therefore, most of the infrared energy is not blocked or reflected back. Since they are often wind and waterproof, space blankets also help with conductive heat loss.

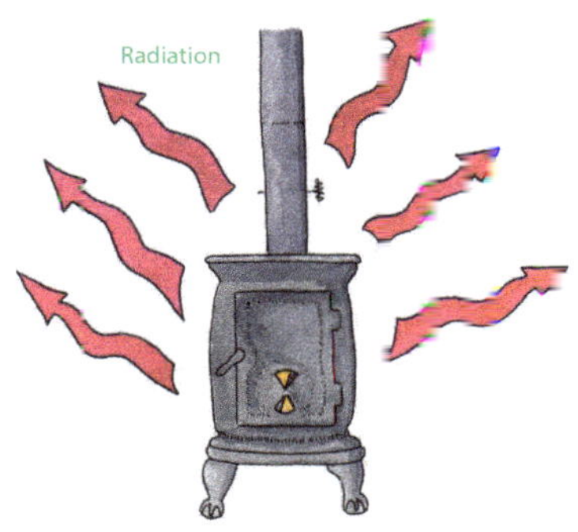

Evaporation

- Evaporation is the transfer of heat via the vaporization of a liquid. For this discussion: the evaporation of water from the surface of the skin.
  - All warm-blooded animals use the evaporation of water to cool.
  - Fur-covered mammals and birds pant, evaporating water out of their lungs, thus cooling the pulmonary circulation. Short, shallow breaths move air in and out of the upper airways without causing gas exchange in the alveoli. This avoids the risks and consequences of hyperventilation—blowing off too much CO_2. As the CO_2 level goes down, the pH of the blood goes up (see hyperventilation syndrome).

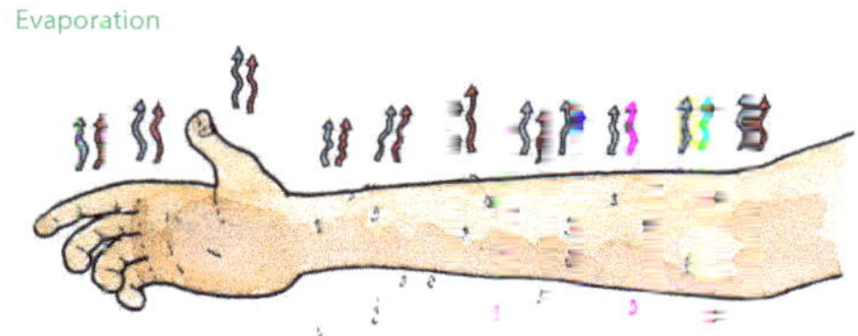

- Humans sweat, and the evaporation of water from the skin (our largest organ, accounting for approximately 10% of our body weight) cools the blood flowing in the venous circulation below it, and thus the systemic circulation, removing excess heat from the core.
- One gram-calorie equals the amount of energy necessary to raise 1 gram of water 1 degree Celsius. One kilocalorie equals the energy necessary to raise 1 kilogram (1,000 grams) of water 1 degree Celsius.
- Heat transfer ranges from 0% – 90% depending on how warm the object is, how warm the water is, the moisture content (humidity) differential, and the surrounding vapor pressure.
  - The greater the moisture differential and the lower the vapor pressure, the greater the rate of heat loss.
  - The higher percentage of humidity, the slower the rate of evaporation.
  - The lower the vapor pressure, the drier the air, the faster water will evaporate, and the greater the rate of heat loss.
- If we begin to overheat, our thermal regulatory center in the brain sends out a signal to the sweat glands in the skin, and they secrete sweat onto the surface of the skin.
- As the sweat evaporates it will remove the heat from the blood flowing through the capillaries in the skin, cooling the blood that returns to the core.
- We must stay hydrated to keep this heat pump going.

Hydration

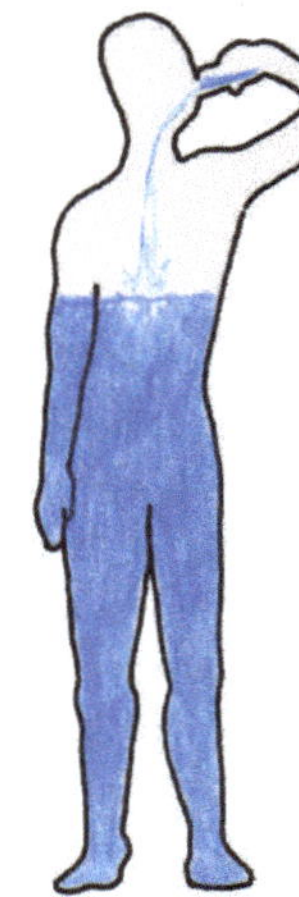

THE WET FACTS

- We live in our own sea made up of salt water and electrolytes.
- Water helps maintain homeostasis (including thermoregulation).
- Life is totally dependent upon water—you can survive three days without water (months without food).
- Water is used in the digestion and in the absorption and utilization of nutrients.

ELECTROLYTES

- Sodium (Na), chloride (Cl), potassium (K), calcium (Ca)
- Together, electrolytes help maintain cellular fluid volume and effect electrical conduction.

- Sodium, chloride, and potassium allow nutrients and water to cross cell membranes.
- Sodium is primarily found in the extracellular fluid surrounding the cells.
- Sodium chloride is table salt—so we get it in our diet by eating salty foods.
- Potassium is primarily an intracellular fluid, and is found in many fruits and vegetables, especially bananas.
- Calcium allows muscle contraction (including the heartbeat) and nerve conduction via the myocardial cells in the heart. Calcium is found in all dairy products, meats, and many vegetables. Our skeletal system is made out of a matrix of calcium—if our serum calcium level begins to drop, we absorb some out of our bones.
- Electrolytes are maintained in our body in exact quantities and proportions—too little or too much causes problems.

HYPONATREMIA

Hyponatremia, also called "water intoxication," occurs when free water (plain water, without electrolytes) is over-consumed.

The excess water dilutes the existing sodium in the extracellular fluid, causing "dilutional hyponatremia."

The kidneys react to the excess fluid by increasing urine production.

This causes us to lose sodium, adding to the dilutional hyponatremia problem, lowering the extracellular concentration of sodium and causing a downward cascade of symptoms, which increases the severity of hyponatremia. The loss of sodium interferes with and slows cellular metabolism.

This is a potentially life-threatening problem.

PREVENTION

Hyponatremia is easy to prevent.

Don't over-consume free water—drink fluids with electrolytes in them.

Eat nuts (salted best) and fruits (bananas are great). Eat a little trail mix when you stop to drink.

Nutrition

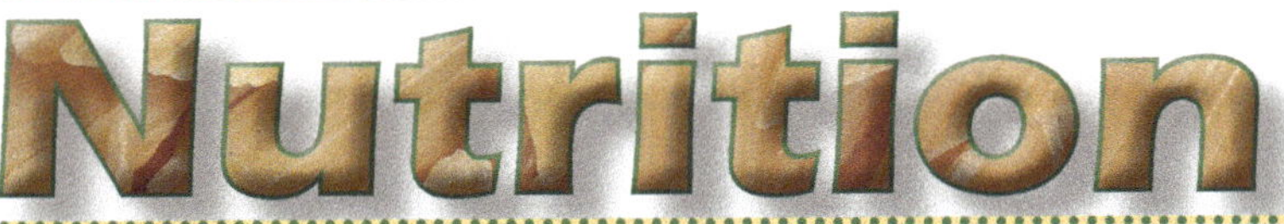

- **About 70%** of daily caloric intake is expended in the operation and maintenance of the body (metabolic processes and thermoregulation).

- The remaining **30%** is expended in movement.

- The **only fuel burned** in our cellular furnace is **glucose** or **fructose**.

- In a **well-fed state**, we maintain a **24-hour emergency supply** of glucose in our liver as glycogen.

- That 24-hour supply is at **rest**; on a cold winter day in just **5 to 6 hours** you can **deplete** that store.

CARB/FAT/PROTEIN		
Carbohydrates	Fat	Protein
60% of daily nutritional requirements	10% of daily nutritional requirements	30% of daily nutritional requirements
4 calories/gram	9 calories/gram	4 calories/gram
200 – 400 grams/day (800 – 1600 calories/day)	20 – 60 grams/day (180 – 540 calories/day)	30 – 55 grams/day (120 – 220 calories/day)
Typical Daily Calorie Needs		
Normal daily activity: 2000 – 2500 calories/day		
Winter outdoor sports: 3000 – 4000 calories/day		
When exposed to the cold, we can increase our basal metabolism—our fuel consumption—five times		
High-altitude mountaineering: 4000 – 6000 calories/day		

HEAT RELATED INJURIES

Dehydration
Heat Cramps
Heat Exhaustion
Heat Stroke

Heat-related injuries

are some of the most common emergencies seen in the outdoor setting, and in virtually every circumstance they can be prevented because they are so often related to behavior. An understanding of the risks and preventive measures can go a long way in reducing the frequency and severity of these emergencies.

Causes

- Excessive dehydration from sweating and salt-loss (without replacement) in a warm environment to the extent that the sweating mechanism can no longer function.
- A high-humidity environment where sweat cannot evaporate off the skin—causing the cooling effect to be lost.
- Failure to take precautions or recognizing early warning signs while exercising in a hot environment.

- Contributing factors include:
  - Age (the very young or very old are more susceptible)
  - Poor health
  - Fatigue
  - Prior history of heat illness
  - Use of certain medications
  - Alcohol consumption
  - Heart disease
  - Over-exertion in a hot environment
- Heat illness is a continuum—if unrecognized and untreated, mild illness can progress to a life-threatening emergency.

Dehydration — SIGNS AND SYMPTOMS

- Headache and mild nausea
- Irritability
- Dark urine
- Thirst

TREATMENT

1. Rehydrate with water and electrolytes (e.g., Gatorade).
2. Improvise: 1 liter of water, 1 teaspoon salt, 8 teaspoons sugar.
3. Pre-made oral rehydration solution (ORS).
4. ½ a banana or ½ cup of orange juice can also be added to help supply potassium.
5. Maintain hydration for the long term.

Heat Cramps — SIGNS AND SYMPTOMS

- Muscle pain and cramping, usually in the legs, caused by dehydration and electrolytes depletion.
- Usually occurs after exercise.

TREATMENT

Treatment is the same as for dehydration.

Heat Exhaustion — PHYSIOLGY

- Is caused by working in a hot environment
- Is a combination of salt and water loss secondary to sweating in hot conditions.
- Heat exhaustion typically occurs in people who are not acclimatized to heat.
- Those not used to working in a hot environment will lose salt (sodium chloride NaCl) more rapidly than someone whose physiology has adjusted to working in hot conditions. Sodium plays an important role in maintaining cell wall integrity and membrane permeability, and is essential in maintaining normal homeostasis on a cellular level. If the amount of sodium in the extracellular fluid decreases, system-wide cellular dysfunction will occur, causing flu-like or exhaustion symptoms.
- The combined loss of water and a decrease in sodium is known as hyponatremia (see Hyponatremia).
- Heat exhaustion is not a life-threatening emergency: it is relieved by rest, hydration, and electrolyte replacement.

Heat Exhaustion

- Fatigue (which can be profound)
- Thirst
- Possible dizziness
- Increased heart rate
- Increased respiratory rate
- Pale, clammy skin
- Muscle cramps
- Nausea with possible vomiting
- Level of consciousness: minor mood changes that can vary from a simple headache and slight anxiety to agitation, confusion, and syncope.
- Pulse: with dehydration and volume contraction, heat-exhaustion patients will have a compensatory increase in pulse—the greater degree of dehydration, the faster the pulse.
- Blood pressure: at rest, their BP will be stable, but they may have mild orthostatic hypotension (low blood pressure) that is quickly remedied when they are supine. Orthostatic dizziness— dizziness caused by low blood pressure (the familiar "head rush" you get when you stand up quickly after being at rest).
- Respirations: breathing rate may be mildly increased, primarily from a symptomatic hyperventilation caused by anxiety.
- Skin: the capillary beds in the skin may vasoconstrict in reaction to the hypovolemia resulting in pale, cool, and clammy skin. Alternately, the skin may be warm and flushed in reaction to the heat.

1. Even without treatment, the patient will most likely spontaneously recover on their own over several hours. With appropriate treatment, recovery will be much faster.
2. Rest in a cool place.
3. Find shade if possible.
4. Remove any excess clothing that may trap heat.
5. Apply cool cloths to body (e.g., damp bandanna on forehead).
6. Replace lost fluid and salt (see dehydration treatment). At least 1 – 2 liters of oral rehydration solution (ORS—see the dehydration section).
7. Monitor body temperature.
8. The patient should recover within 6 – 8 hours.
9. Once recovered, the patient can cautiously resume activity.
10. If the symptoms of heat exhaustion are ignored and the person continues to work and sweat hard, it can progress to heat stroke

Heat Stroke

Okay, this is a big nasty one—thankfully, it's fairly rare. In the wilderness environment, most people quit exerting themselves long before heat stroke sets in. In the urban environment, heat stroke deaths make the news when competitive athletes (marathon runners, football players) push themselves (or are pushed by others) way beyond the danger point. With understanding, preparation, and vigilance, heat stroke is *always* preventable. But once it really gets going, it's almost impossible to stop outside of an emergency department.

- **Heat stroke is a *life-threatening* emergency.**

- **If not treated immediately, it will quickly progress to *coma and death*.**

- **The time from the onset of symptoms to *death* can be as little as *15 minutes* after the sweating mechanism fails and the core temperature begins to rise.**

- **For those who survive, heat stroke can cause *permanent disability*—a number of tissues can suffer end-damage from the increased core temperature.**

Types of Heat Stroke

Classic

- Dehydration in a hot environment caused by the person "over-sweating" without replacing lost fluids, which leads to the failure of the sweating mechanism, causing the core temperature to rise rapidly.
- The patient is losing water faster than they are replacing it.
- Once the sweating mechanism fails, cooling stops and the core temperature rises rapidly.

Exertional

- Exercising in a hot and high-humidity environment where the sweat mechanism cannot function because the sweat cannot evaporate; again, the core temperature rises rapidly. The sweat, even though copious, cannot evaporate fast enough, and the

Heat Stroke *PATHOLOGY*

patient overheats.

- Brain: encephalopathy (swelling of the brain) is the norm.
- Liver: hepatic (liver-related) injury is common, and the liver is most susceptible to early damage.
- Interesting note: the liver is a biochemical factory that is so busy with chemical reactions that it is normally 1 degree C warmer (2 degrees F) than the rest of the body.
- Because it runs warmer anyway, the liver has less of a temperature buffer and permanent damage is possible (and can occur faster).
- Kidneys: Renal failure is common due to myoglobinuria (the presence of myoglobin, an iron- and oxygen-binding protein in the muscle tissue of most mammals, in the urine) from rhabdomyolysis (the rapid breakdown of skeletal muscle due to injury to muscle tissue).
- Muscles: Damage results from rhabdomyolysis (see previous bullet).
- Blood: Coagulopathy (clotting disorders) due to disseminated intravascular coagulation (DIC) is common.
- Death occurs when the core temperature exceeds 107 degrees/41.6 degrees—the point at which the tissues of the brain are destroyed.

Heat Stroke *SIGNS AND SYMPTOMS*

- The patient will be "red, hot, and mad" due to vasodilation as the body tries to deal with the increase in core temperature.
- The skin is red, hot, and may be dry (classic) or sweaty (exertional).
- The patient cannot continue to sweat because they are dehydrated, or because evaporation is impossible (i.e., high humidity).
- The patient will have a change in level of consciousness (LOC): they will be disoriented, confused, combative, and may hallucinate wildly. These changes are caused by core temperatures above 104F/40C.
- The patient may have seizures.
- The patient may not be able to urinate.
- The patient will have an increased heart rate.
- The patient will have an increased respiratory rate.

  Heat stroke needs to be recognized early and treated aggressively. The duration and degree of temperature elevation determines the level of organ damage and the ability for the patient to recover.

TREATMENT

1. Remove the patient from the heat and sun and place them in a cool, shady place.
2. Remove clothing down to underwear.
3. Cool them immediately by soaking with cool water and fanning to accelerate evaporation.
4. Vigorously massage limbs to encourage hot blood to flow to the extremities where it can cool.
5. Beware of shivering, as shivering produces heat. If they begin shivering, stop cooling them until they stop shivering then resume cooling at a less aggressive rate.
6. Hydrate once conscious.
7. Do not allow the patient to exercise.
8. Evacuate immediately to definitive care (don't let the patient walk out on their own—you may have to improvise a litter).
9. Continue cooling during transport.

PREVENTION

Prevention for · heat-related illness

- Prevention of heat-related injuries, in particular, heat stroke, is very important because of the risk of permanent injury or even death.
- Maintain adequate fluid and electrolyte (salt) intake.
- Monitor the group for fluid and electrolyte intake.
- Be aware of changing environmental conditions. Allow time to acclimate to new environments.
- Wear proper clothing, including a hat.
- Avoid overexertion in hot and humid conditions: above 90F.; at or above 70% humidity.
- Rest often, especially in extreme environments.
- Do not allow outside pressure to push you beyond safe limits.

COLD RELATED INJURIES
HYPOTHERMIA

HYPOTHERMIA **IS THE LOWERING OF THE BODY'S CORE TEMPERATURE** to a level where normal brain and muscle functions are impaired. It typically happens when several things occur simultaneously: low temperatures (<40F/4.5C), wet conditions (damp clothes), lack of fuel and hydration (food and water), and physical fatigue. This cascade of problems causes our thermo-regulatory system to fail—it just can't keep up with the heat loss (see the thermoregulation information in the Human Animal section).

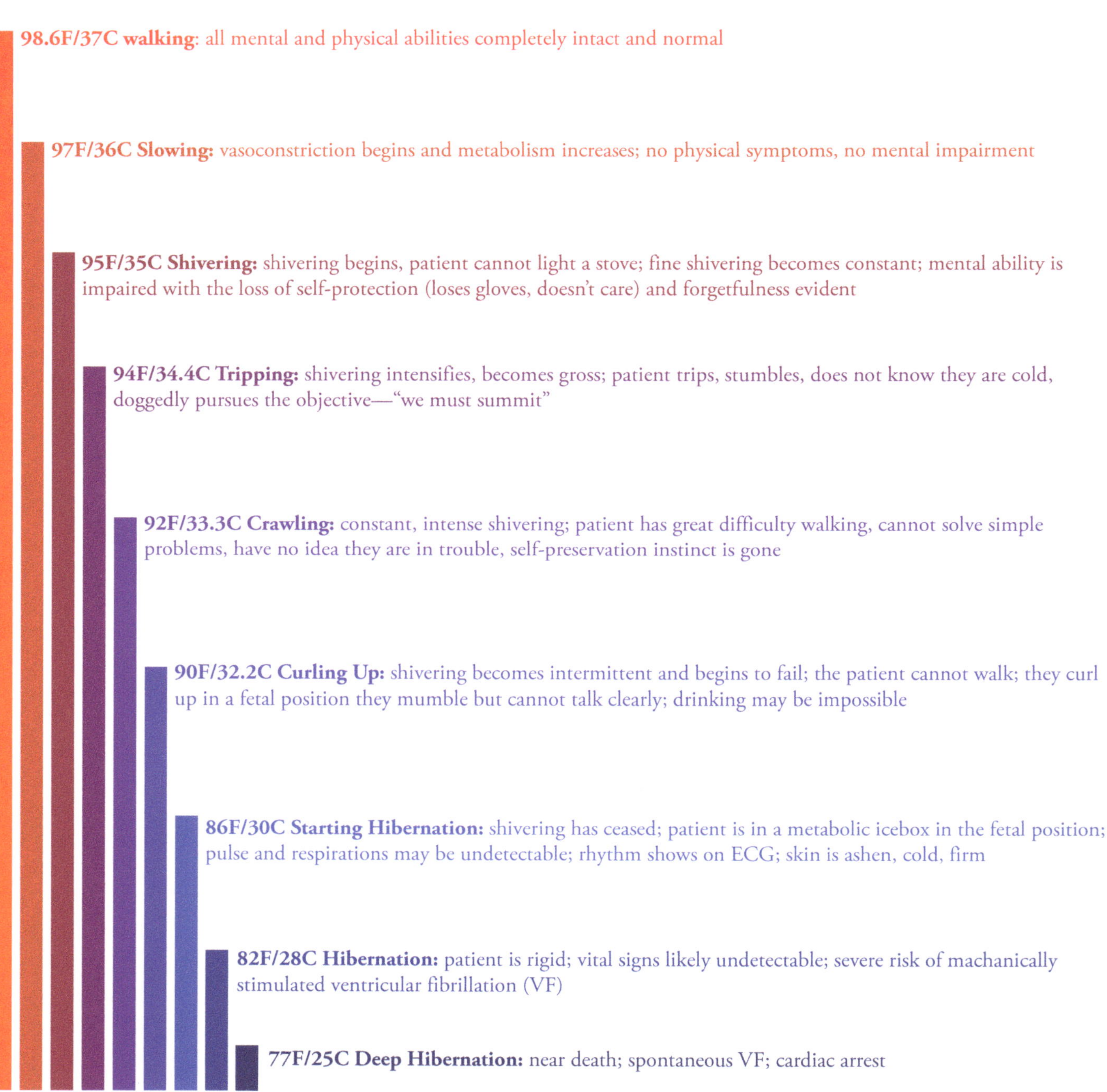

# of HYPOTHERMIA

FOR MILD TO MODERATE HYPOTHERMIA (the patient is still conscious and responsive—their core temperature has not dropped below 92F (33.3C).

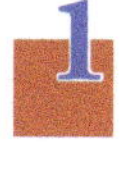 Remove the patient from immediate danger and further exposure.

 Create shelter: tent, bivouac, snow cave.

 Get them dry and keep them dry.

 Remove their wet clothing, dry them off, and re-insulate them with dry clothing.

 Place the patient in a hypothermia wrap and protect them from the ground.

 If conscious and can safely swallow, feed the patient sticky sweet fluids, such as Jell-O in warm water or warm Gatorade. Have them sip constantly. You cannot give them too much water or sugar. Hypothermia victims cannot digest solids. If unconscious, do not try to feed them orally.

FOR SEVERE HYPOTHERMIA (patient unconscious and likely in the fetal position). Do the above, plus:

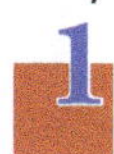 Avoid excessive movement or jarring.

 Give rescue breaths.

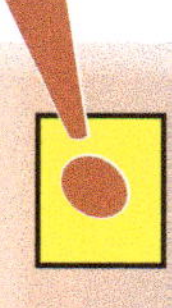 **DO NOT DO CPR!** The myocardium of the heart is very susceptible to fibrillation because of elevated potassium levels surrounding the cells. **Bumping or jostling** can cause the heart to go into **ventricular fibrillation**. It is almost **impossible** to defibrillate a hypothermia patient.

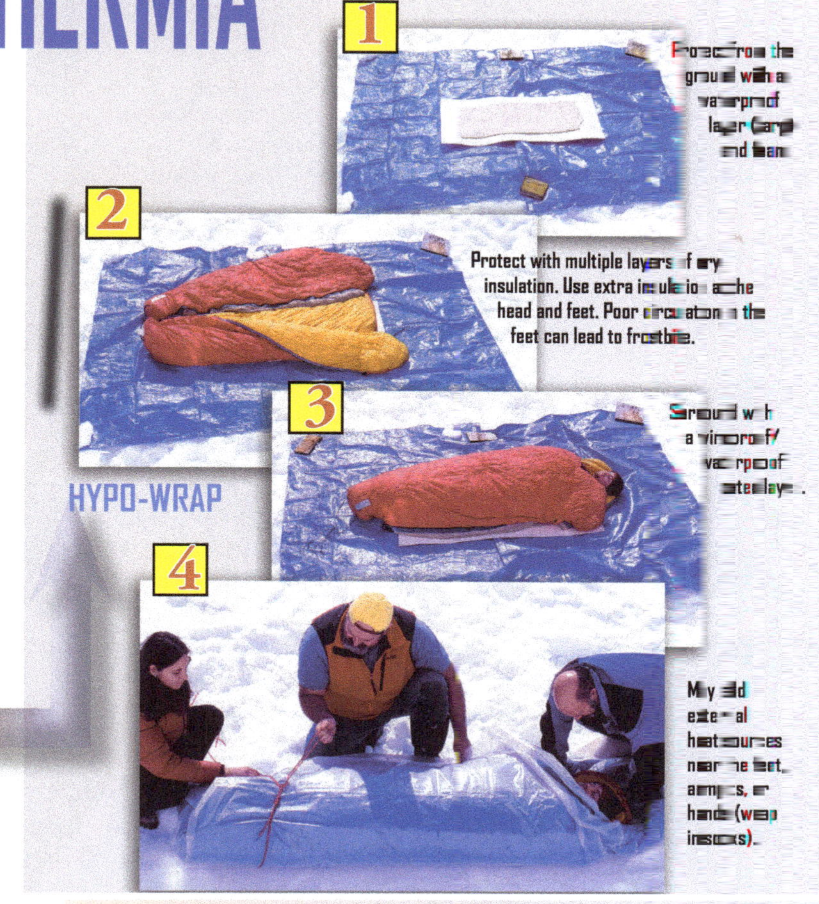

PREVENTION of HYPOTHERMIA

- Know your enemy: be prepared for wet, wind, and cold.
- Wear fabrics that stay warm when wet. Do not wear cotton—the phrase "cotton kills" really has validity: cotton loses almost all its insulating ability when wet.
- Get dry and stay dry—it can be difficult to re-warm a damp or wet person, and it can be extremely difficult to keep a damp person warm.
- Stay well-hydrated.
- Snack often on quick-burning carbohydrates (energy bars, candy, etc.).
- Carry bivouac gear and know how to use it.
- Be attentive to yourself, to your companions, and to the environment—pay particular attention to mental-status changes.
- Turn around before you get in trouble. This is a difficult point to determine, but there are almost always early warning signs.
    - Someone in the party is moving slowly or complaining of being cold and/or tired.
    - Weather/route conditions are not what you expected or are changing for the worse.
    - You fall behind the schedule of your plan for the day.
    - Someone (anyone) says something like, "I don't feel good about this."

FROSTBITE

FROSTBITE is the localized freezing of tissue caused by the combination of **below freezing ambient air temperature** and **constriction of blood vessels** which shunt blood away from cold areas of the body. Since water expands when it freezes, tissue destruction occurs when the cells freeze and burst. There are varying degrees of frostbite based on ice formation in the tissues and the extent or depth of the freeze. For wilderness medicine, the field treatment can be divided into three diagnostic and treatment categories based on ice formation in the tissues: superficial, partial, or deep. These are similar to the severity or degree of a burn.

SUPERFICIAL FROSTBITE

is localized vasoconstriction, but no ice forms in the tissues.

SIGNS AND SYMPTOMS

- The area is cold, numb, and pale, but still soft and pliable.
- Although not frozen, the tissue is still damaged.
- The tissues, while not frozen, have a decreased blood flow, and thus are not getting enough oxygen.
- If not re-warmed quickly (<6 hours) permanent tissue damage can occur (see immersion foot/trench foot).

TREATMENT

1. Inspect the area closely and inspect the insulation—determine the cause.
2. Make sure that the frostbitten area is dry.
3. Re-warm in the field using skin-to-skin contact.
   - A. Hands/feet in armpits/groin.
   - B. Never massage, rub with snow, or use an external heat source.
3. Warm the patient.
   - A. From the inside with high-carb snacks, warm Jell-O, etc.
   - B. From the outside with additional dry insulation (e.g., new mittens). If they are capable, have them do isometric exercises.
4. Hydrate the patient.
5. Correct any problems before resuming activity (e.g., change to warmer boots, dry mittens, etc.).

PARTIAL-THICKNESS FROSTBITE is

localized vasoconstriction and cooling with some ice crystal formation.

SIGNS AND SYMPTOMS

- The area is the same as 1st degree: numb, pale, but still pliable.
- There is pain with thawing.
- Fluid- or blood-filled blisters appear (blebs).

Treatment is the same as superficial, except:

1. If a bleb forms, protect it with a bandage and evacuate the patient.
2. Do not puncture the bleb.
3. Protect the frozen part from re-freezing, which can occur quickly and cause further damage.

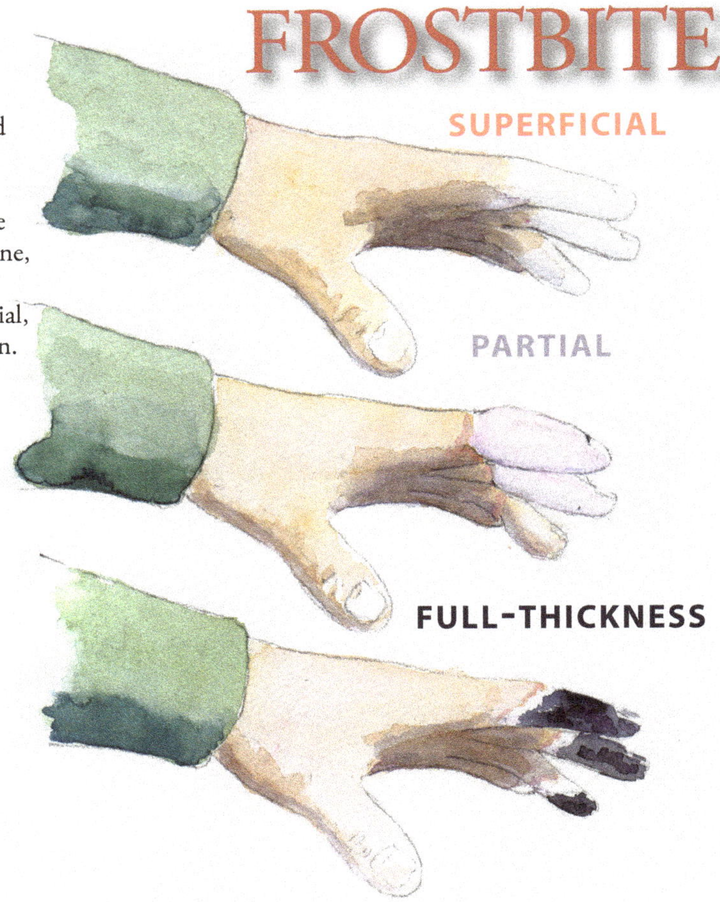

FULL-THICKNESS FROSTBITE is deep freezing

involving muscles, tendons, nerves, and other tissues.

SIGNS AND SYMPTOMS

- The area is numb, cold, white or waxy, and hard to the touch.
- Tissues are frozen solid (rock hard) and ice forms in the cells—the tissues are destroyed.

TREATMENT

1. Do not rewarm in the field—the goal is to prevent further damage.
   - A. The thawing of frozen tissue can release large quantities of proteins that can cause high fevers and renal failure.
   - B. Once thawed, the area is useless.
   - C. A deeply frostbitten foot can still be walked on—if it is thawed in the field, a litter carry will be necessary.
   - D. Thawed tissue will be extremely painful.
   - E. If thawed tissue is refrozen, additional damage will be done.
2. Inspect the area closely.
3. Remove any wet of frozen clothing or boots.
4. Dry and re-insulate the area to prevent further damage and freezing.
5. Feed high-carbohydrate foods and give warm, sweet liquids.
6. The deeply frozen person is also likely to be hypothermic—treat accordingly.
7. Evacuate to definitive care, preferably a trauma center that specializes in cold injuries (severe cases may require surgery (amputation).

123

NON-FREEZING COLD INJURIES

Raynaud's Syndrome

Raynaud's Syndrome is a peripheral vascular disorder marked by abnormal vasoconstriction of the extremities on exposure to cold or emotional stress—a hypersensitivity reaction to cold exposure.

We are tropical animals and adapt to the cold environment by creating a micro-environment around us—it may be below zero outside, but it needs to be in the 70s next to our skin. We create this micro-environment by using: shelter, clothing, and external heat sources.

- Raynaud's was first described by French physician Maurice Raynaud.
- It is fairly common, occurring in about 5% of the population.
- It is 4x times more common in women than in men.
- Raynaud's tends to worsen with age.
- Once it occurs, it will recur whenever the affected parts are exposed to cool temperature—for example, swimming in 60 degree water.
- Raynaud's may be the result of genetics and/or of a prior injury such as frostbite.
- When Raynaud's occurs, the risk of frostbite increases.

PHYSIOLOGY

Because we are tropical, we have a relatively poor protective response to cold exposure.

All the vasculature in the affected part of the extremity (e.g., the tips of fingers, toes, ears, or nose) partially closes down, not just the capillaries and small-diameter vessels.

It appears that the problem is with the sympathetic innervation of the arteriovenous anastomoses (the growth of connective collateral vessels that serve the same volume of tissue as the capillaries), which shunt blood away from the cold area. We are designed to let our fingers freeze and fall off in order to preserve our core and brain temperature—where our vital organs lie.

An aside—certain mammals, such as dogs and cats, do the opposite: they vasodilate the blood vessels going to the cold areas to keep them warm. They do this because they have fur to insulate them.

- Pale, waxy, or blueness in extremities, usually fingers or toes, which typically occurs within 10 – 30 minutes of cold exposure (see image at right).
- Numbness and/or paresthesia (pins and needles).
- Sweating ceases as the body tries to keep the core warm.
- In severe cases, blisters can form due to the production of free radicals as a result of the tissue damage.
- Each time the cycle of cold/vasoconstriction to warmth/vasodilation takes place in the Raynaud's susceptible person, the vasoconstriction seems to occur with less stimulation and re-warming symptoms seem to be worse and more painful.

ASSESSMENT

Before you can treat and manage Raynaud's Syndrome you must make a proper diagnosis—is this primary Raynaud's caused by cold exposure, or is it secondary Raynaud's where the Raynaud's is a symptom of another disease or a drug side effect?
Some possibilities:

- Scleroderma—mixed connective tissue diseases, polymyositis, dermatomyositis
- Lupus (SLE)—a systemic autoimmune disease causing the immune system to attack and damage tissue
- Rheumatoid arthritis
- Buerger's disease —recurring progressive inflammation and thrombosis (clotting) of small and medium arteries and veins of the hands and feet
- Polycythemia—a disease state in which the proportion of blood volume that is occupied by red blood cells increases
- Cryoglobulinemia—a medical condition in which the blood contains large amounts of cryoglobulins (proteins) that become insoluble below normal body temperature ($<37^0$C/98.6^{0}F)

Just because it's above 32^0 doesn't mean that we won't have problems. When our skin is exposed to cold, damp temperatures, tissue damage can result that is painful, chronic, and difficult to treat. These injuries are not life-threatening, but they can be limb-threatening.

- Carpal tunnel syndrome
- Drug-induced: beta blockers, ergotamine, methysergide, vinblastine, bleomycin, oral contraceptives
- Estrogen replacement therapy without progesterone

PREVENTION

- Avoid or limit cold exposure and protect the effected area with effective (dry) insulation.
- Avoid situations where Raynaud's could be triggered.
- If possible, avoid medications that can make Raynaud's worse: beta-blockers, ergotamine, methysergide, vinblastine, bleomycin, and oral contraceptives.
- Avoid nicotine, caffeine, alcohol, and over-the counter decongestants.

TREATMENT

- Treat the whole patient—keep them warm, fed and hydrated.
- Re-warm the tissue. When the circulation is re-established there will be a hyperemic (reddening) response in the skin with throbbing pain that typically lasts 5 – 10 minutes; itchiness sometimes occurs.
- Calcium channel blockers are considered to be the most effective pharmacological treatment. Nifedipine XL 30 – 90mg po qd, is the drug of choice. If not effective or if side effects occur, try other calcium channel blockers: diltiazem 30 – 120mg po qid, or felodipine 2.5 – 10mg po qd. Verapamil has not been shown to be effective.
- Try retraining your body to reduce the tendency to shunt blood away from your exremities using a method developed by renowned cold weather expert Dr. Murray Hamlett (below).

Hamlett's method for managing Raynaud's

This is a non-invasive, non-pharmacological method to attempt to retrain the neurovascular response to cold exposure. Remember Pavlov's dog—the dog that would have a hunger response and drool when the researchers rang a bell? Well, guess what—there is a good chance that your vasculature can be trained to vasodilate rather than vasoconstrict when exposed to the cold.

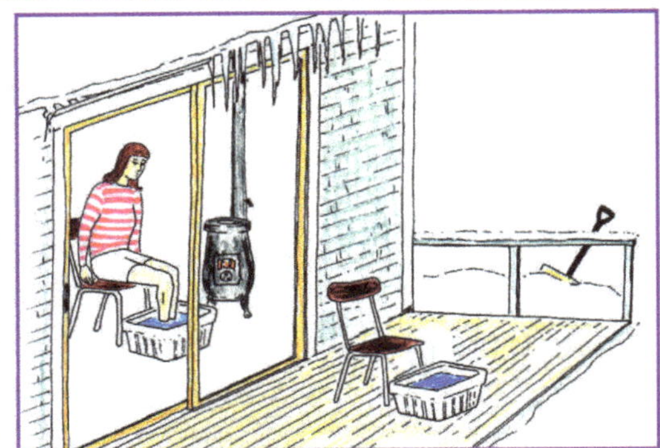

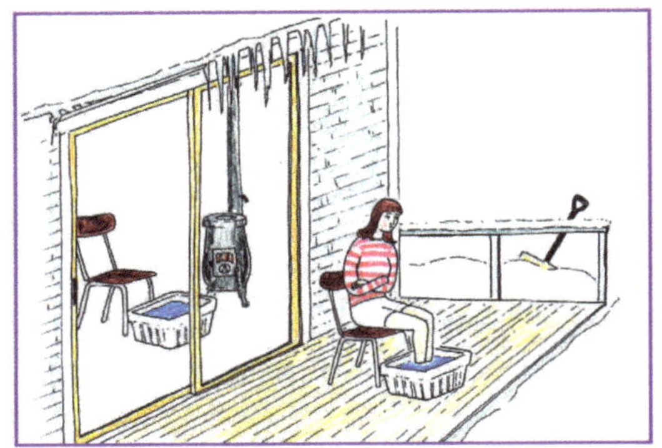

EQUIPMENT

- 2 – 4 foam coolers (depending upon whether you are doing just your hands or your feet, or all four extremities at once).
- A source of warm water.
- A cool environment: 32F – 40F (0C – 4.5C).

SETUP AND DRESS

- Dress to be comfortable for the inside environment (70 degrees).
- Do not add layers when you go outside—you want your body to cool off. You must allow your head and trunk to cool off while keeping your hands/feet warm.

STEPS

1. Fill the foam coolers with warm water, 105° – 110°F (40° – 43°C); place one set inside the house where it is warm and one set outside where it is cold.
2. Start inside: make yourself comfortable and sit down with your feet and/or hands in the warm water for 2 – 5 minutes.
3. Wrap you hands and/or feet in a towel to keep them warm and go outside
4. Sit down, allowing your head and body to sense the cold, while placing your hands and/or feet in the warm water for about 10 minutes.
5. After 10 minutes, go back inside and repeat the inside treatment.

- The process works best if you do 3 – 6 cycles per day (in for 2 – 5minutes, out for 10 minutes, then in for 2 – 5 minutes) every other day for a total of 50 cycles (i.e., 8 – 16 days).
- This method is inexpensive and very safe. If it works or helps, great; if not, you've lost nothing but a little time, and you now have some coolers for picnics.

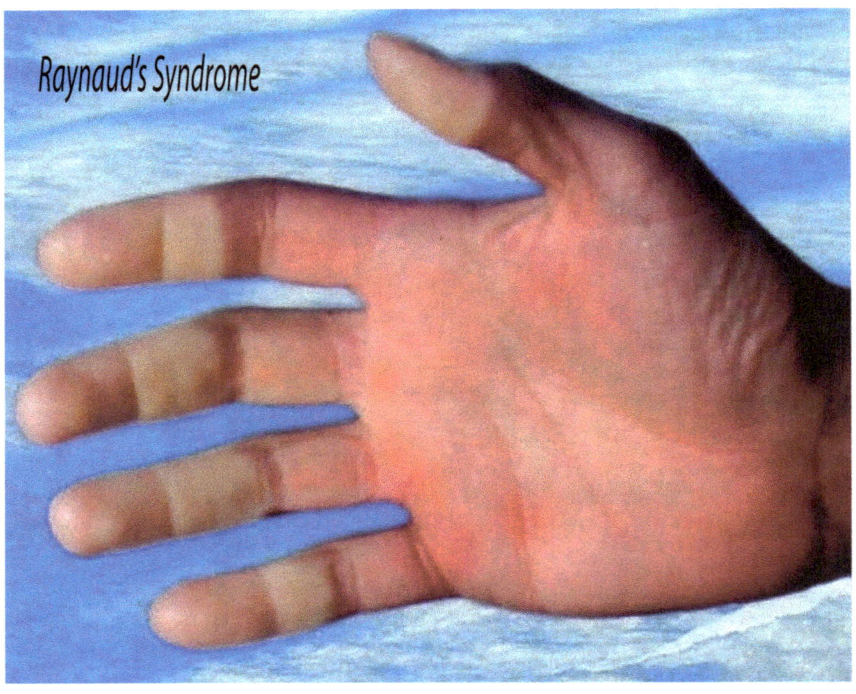

Classic Raynaud's: bloodflow shuts down and leaves tissue (often on the fingers and toes) pale-to-cyanotic, wax-like, and numb. It's more annoying than dangerous, and the rewarming process can be painful.

Chilblains

Chilblains (also known as pernio) occurs when a predisposed individual is exposed to cold, humid and/or damp conditions. The capillary beds are damaged, causing redness, itching, inflammation, and blisters (acral ulcers—ulcers affecting the extremities).

PREDISPOSITIONS

- Individuals with close family members who have/had chilblains
- People with circulation problems
- People with lupus
- People whose homes are drafty and cold (not well-insulated)
- Tobacco smokers
- Very thin individuals

PATHOPHYSIOLOGY

- The process usually starts with an initial injury, such as frostbite, and the onset of symptoms is typically 2 – 24 hours after exposure.
- Tissue damage occurs to the capillary beds and to the neurovascular apparatus that controls vasomotor response.
- As an extremity re-warms and the vasculature dilates, fenestrations (small gaps) open between the endothelial cells, allowing intravascular fluids (plasma) to leak out into the surrounding tissue.
- The immune system reacts to this fluid leakage causing blister formation, erythema, swelling, tenderness, itchiness, a burning sensation, and tender blue lumps.
- This lays the foundation for future vasoconstriction and vascular shunting of blood away from the affected cold area—chilblains will often come on faster and be worse with subsequent exposures.
- Long-term, localized, violaceous (purple) plaque forms that is thick, tender, slightly cyanotic, and with a shiny appearance.
- Chilblains typically heals within several days—but it can become chronic if environmental conditions persist.

TREATMENT

- The same as for Raynaud's.

Trench foot

Trench foot and immersion foot are synonymous. This is a nonfreezing cold injury to the extremities (typically the feet and lower legs) caused by vasoconstriction of the peripheral circulation, resulting from prolonged exposure to cold, damp, and unsanitary conditions—being cold and wet for more than six hours (e.g., standing in ice water). The term trench foot was coined during WWI when so many injuries occurred as troops in Western Europe were forced to stand for hours in trenches half-full of cold water. During WWI, WWII, and the Korean War, there were over 1 million casualties from trench foot and frostbite. Today, hunters, hikers, kayakers, construction workers, snowmakers, or anyone who works or plays in cold, wet environments are at risk.

PHYSIOLGY

- Ischemia (caused by vasoconstriction) for more than six hours leads to tissue death. This leads to gangrene, nerve damage, and loss of tissue.
- After six hours of compromised circulation, the capillaries and supporting tissues of the skin begin to die from hypoxia (lack of oxygen).
- Immersion in cold water is not necessary: wet socks, wet insoles, or wet boots can put feet at risk in temperatures between freezing and 62°F (17°C).
- Immersion foot injuries are permanent and very painful.
- The colder the water, the shorter duration is needed to cause injury.
- The injury can result in extensive tissue loss (amputation may be necessary).
- Several things can increase risk and exacerbate the injury: blunt trauma, tight footwear, nicotine and alcohol consumption.

SIGNS AND SYMPTOMS

- Initially: cold, wet, numb, macerated extremities (softened by immersion—what your skin looks like under a Band-Aid).
- There may be an obvious line of demarcation between the affected tissue and healthy tissue.
- Feet become numb and turn red (erythema) or blue (cyanosis) as a result of compromised vascular supply.
- As the condition worsens, the affected tissue may begin to swell.
- Advanced trench foot presents with blisters and open sores which can lead to fungal infections.
- If advanced trench foot is left untreated, necrosis (tissue death), gangrene (advanced and widespread necrosis), and putrefaction and liquefaction (necrotic tissue digested by enzymes, eventually becoming liquefied) will set in. Tissue will begin to slough off.
- Nerve, muscle, and epithelial cells are the most susceptible to the effects of hypoxia resulting from immersion foot.
- A permanent injury, immersion foot can cause as much tissue damage as frostbite.
- The risk of a secondary bacterial infection is very high.

TREATMENT

- If the damage is minor and appropriate treatment is done immediately complete recovery is normal—although it will be painful.
- As the extremity begins to rewarm, color will return and the feet will become red, hot to the touch, hyperhidrotic (excessive sweating, swollen, and painful. The pain can be excruciating and difficult to relieve—even narcotics may not bring relief.
1. Remove the patient from the cold and wet environment. Place them in the supine position. Get them dry and keep them dry—remove wet garments and dry the affected area.
2. Re-warm them (can be very hard, skin-to-skin contact is best. Once rewarmed keep the area warm.
3. Do not do massage and do not immerse the affected tissue in warm water—it will be too painful.
4. Elevate the feet to minimize swelling and tent any sheets or blankets over the patient's feet—even the weight of sheets on the feet will be painful. If possible, direct a fan toward the feet as they will be hot and very sweaty.
5. Evacuate the patient immediately, and keep them fed and hydrated.

PREVENTION

- Keep hands and feet dry.
- Change socks regularly, and sleep in dry socks at night.
- As with other cold-related injuries, a person who has contracted trench foot will be more susceptible to it in the future—take extra care.

BIVOUAC

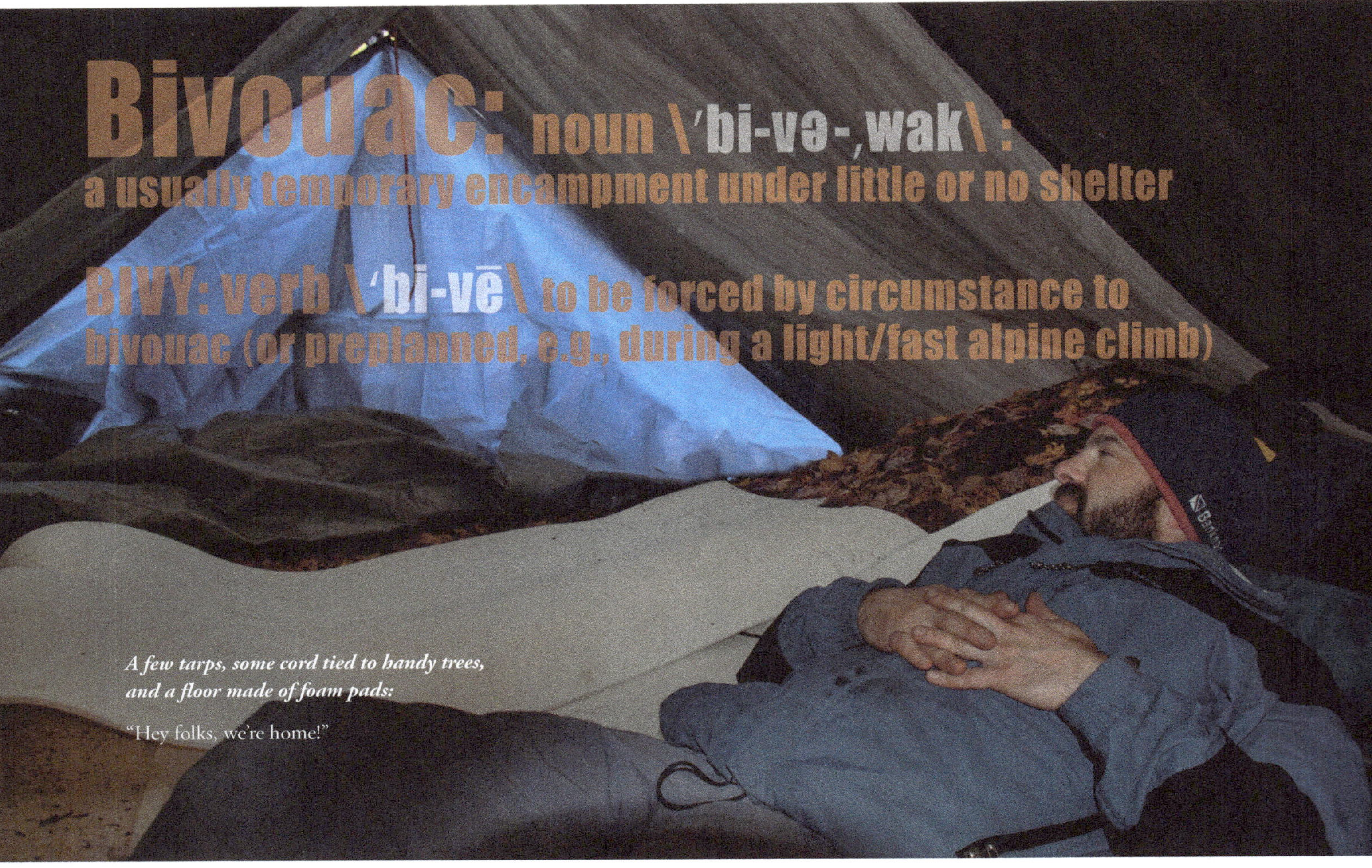

A few tarps, some cord tied to handy trees,
and a floor made of foam pads:

"Hey folks, we're home!"

When faced with the need to bivouac, you must consider things beyond the care of the injured—some of which may be out of your control.

weather

- A primary concern.
- You have no control over it.
- It can have a dramatic influence on all your decision-making.
- Know the long-range forecast before you head out.
- Understand the basics of backcountry weather forecasting.

terrain

- Although you generally control the nature of the terrain across which you choose to travel, accidents or sudden illness strike unpredictably, and you may be forced by circumstances to treat a patient and consider a bivouac on terrain that may not be well-suited to that purpose.

time and distance to definitive care

- What time of day is it?
- How soon will it be dark?
- How soon will it be light?
- How far from the road are you?
- How long will it take to get out?

127

resources and people

- What is the size, age, experience, and skill level of your group?
- What kinds and amount of food, extra clothing, and equipment are they carrying?

the patient's needs

- It may seem as if the patient's needs should be of paramount concern; however after their injuries/illness have been treated appropriately, the focus must turn back to the group's welfare and needs, and these must be balanced with those of the patient.
- How stable is the patient?
- Can they await evacuation?
- Considering these concerns, can the group "self-rescue" safely?
- If not, how will those same concerns affect the group if they have to bivouac?

The elements of effective bivouacs

All these elements increase the group's safety, wellbeing, and productivity.

basic considerations

- Protection from water
- Protection from wind
- The availability of fire/heat/warmth
- The availability of food and water

terrain considerations

Rocky

- Avoid high, exposed places.
- Seek natural shelter: caves, big boulders, cliff overhangs, depressions, talus fields (often provide small caves or protective overhangs—ensure stability).
- Enhance your site by building a windbreak.
- Remember, some of these places may become unsafe during a thunderstorm.

Woodlands

- Avoid marshy ground and drainage areas.
- Seek low trees—they often offer greater protection.
- Build lean-tos with tarps, trees, and tree limbs.
- Use pine trees as natural rain/snow shelters.
- Use dry leaves and duff or pine boughs for ground insulation.

Snow

- Avoid potential avalanche terrain and high snow deposition areas.
- Dig a deep trench and cover with a tarp.
- Dig a snow cave (into a slope is easier): keep the entrance low and the roof thin and cut an air hole.
- In proper snow conditions, cut blocks for an igloo/windbreak.
- Alternately, make a quincy: make a big pile of snow (bigger than you think), compact it (the more, the better), dig into it to form a snow cave.

EMERGENCY BIVOUAC KIT:

- Wool socks
- Two trash bags
- String
- Mylar space blanket
- Candle stub
- Small tin cup
- Lifesavers candy
- Waterproof matches

Stuff this all in a wool cap and keep in the bottom of your daypack.

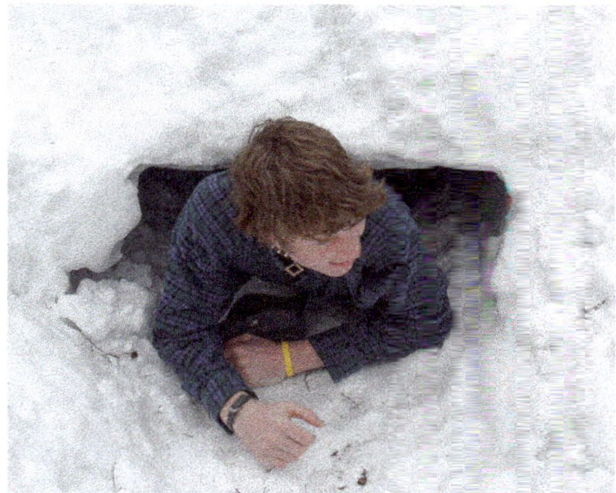

Cool, a snow cave: Cramped, damp, dark, and hard to ventilate. But they get nice and warm and are completely windproof. The flannel shirt and baseball cap are not ideal.

LIGHTNING

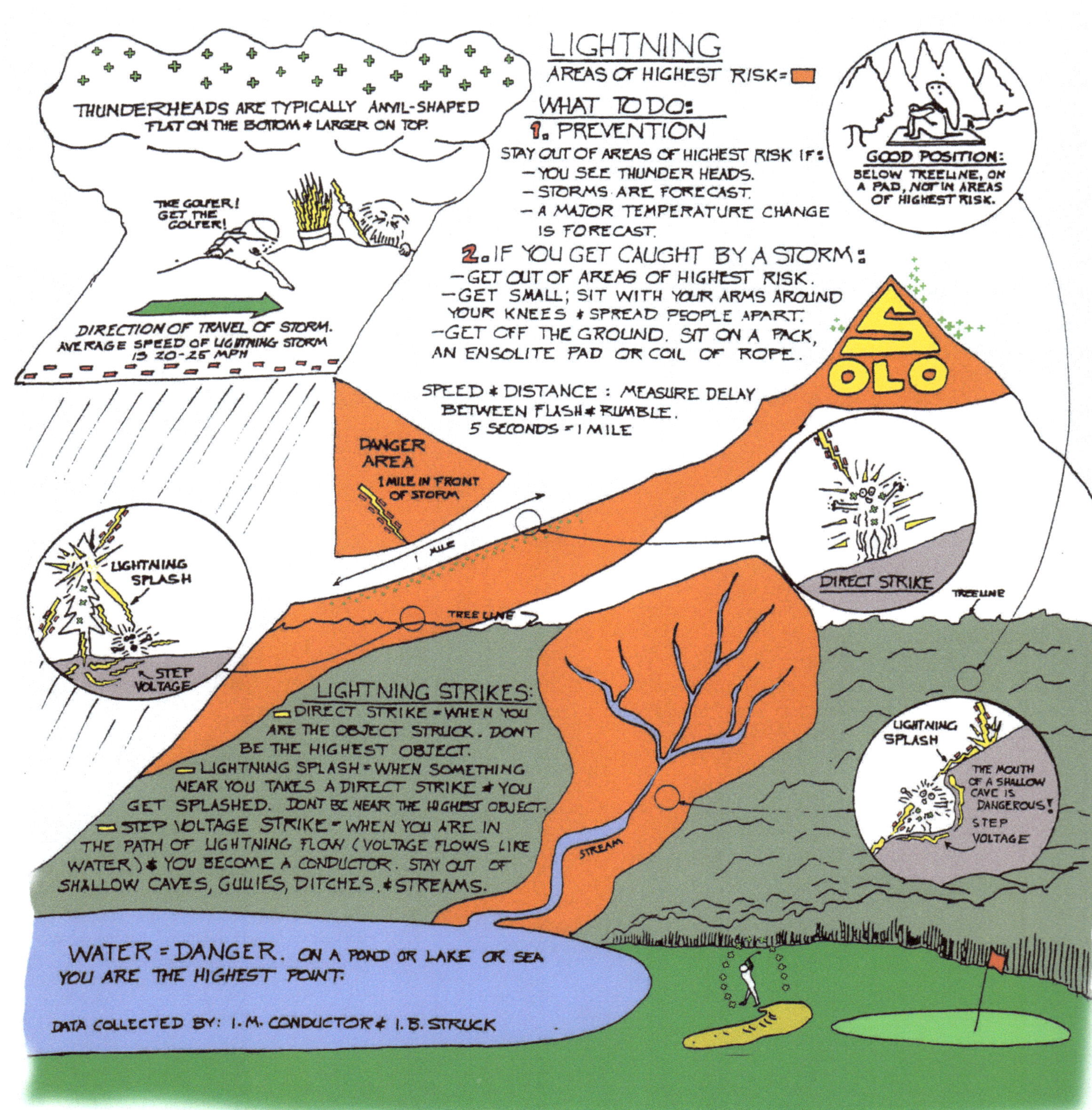

LIGHTNING
AREAS OF HIGHEST RISK =
WHAT TO DO:
1. PREVENTION
STAY OUT OF AREAS OF HIGHEST RISK IF:
- YOU SEE THUNDER HEADS.
- STORMS ARE FORECAST.
- A MAJOR TEMPERATURE CHANGE IS FORECAST.
2. IF YOU GET CAUGHT BY A STORM:
- GET OUT OF AREAS OF HIGHEST RISK.
- GET SMALL; SIT WITH YOUR ARMS AROUND YOUR KNEES & SPREAD PEOPLE APART.
- GET OFF THE GROUND. SIT ON A PACK, AN ENSOLITE PAD OR COIL OF ROPE.
SPEED & DISTANCE: MEASURE DELAY BETWEEN FLASH & RUMBLE.
5 SECONDS = 1 MILE
GOOD POSITION:
BELOW TREELINE, ON A PAD, NOT IN AREAS OF HIGHEST RISK.
THUNDERHEADS ARE TYPICALLY ANVIL-SHAPED FLAT ON THE BOTTOM & LARGER ON TOP.
THE GOLFER! GET THE GOLFER!
DIRECTION OF TRAVEL OF STORM. AVERAGE SPEED OF LIGHTNING STORM IS 20-25 MPH.
DANGER AREA 1 MILE IN FRONT OF STORM
1 MILE
LIGHTNING SPLASH
STEP VOLTAGE
DIRECT STRIKE
TREE LINE
TREELINE
SOLO
LIGHTNING SPLASH
THE MOUTH OF A SHALLOW CAVE IS DANGEROUS! STEP VOLTAGE
STREAM
LIGHTNING STRIKES:
DIRECT STRIKE = WHEN YOU ARE THE OBJECT STRUCK. DON'T BE THE HIGHEST OBJECT.
LIGHTNING SPLASH = WHEN SOMETHING NEAR YOU TAKES A DIRECT STRIKE & YOU GET SPLASHED. DON'T BE NEAR THE HIGHEST OBJECT.
STEP VOLTAGE STRIKE = WHEN YOU ARE IN THE PATH OF LIGHTNING FLOW (VOLTAGE FLOWS LIKE WATER) & YOU BECOME A CONDUCTOR. STAY OUT OF SHALLOW CAVES, GULLIES, DITCHES, & STREAMS.
WATER = DANGER. ON A POND OR LAKE OR SEA YOU ARE THE HIGHEST POINT.
DATA COLLECTED BY: I. M. CONDUCTOR & I. B. STRUCK

Lightning Drill:

If you are caught out in a storm:

-Get out of areas of highest risk

-Get small

Sit with your arms around your knees

-Get off the ground

Sit on a pad, a pack, or a coil of rope

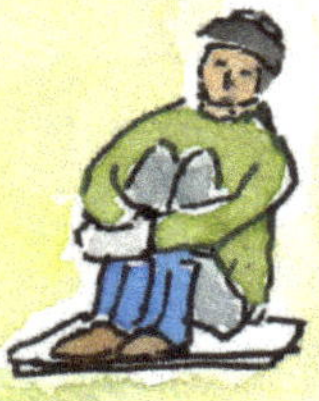

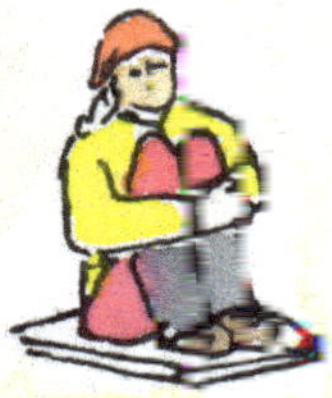

-Spread out

If one person is injured the rest should be able to help

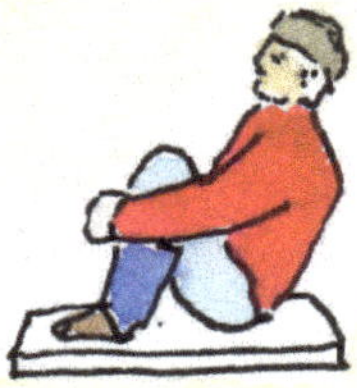

Be aware: watch the sky

Lightning storms move fast—watch for places you might get to for shelter

If someone is struck by lightning:

-Check to see if they are breathing

-Check to see if they have a heartbeat

-You may have to do CPR

If they have a heartbeat and are breathing you may have to treat for burns and soft tissue injuries

RULES TO LIVE BY

- When a thunderstorm approaches, go inside.
- If outside, stay away from the highest objects: mountain peaks, ridges, boulders, hilltops, tall trees, towers and large metal objects, utility poles, ski lift towers, bridge superstructure, fences, etc.
- Don't sit under overhangs or go into shallow caves; stay out of large open areas (fields).
- Lightning flows like water, so stay out of gullies, washes, and stream beds.
- Put on your rain gear and prepare for foul weather.
- Move at least 100 yards away from any shoreline.
- Find a low spot and sit on something insulated (foam pad) with your legs crossed.
- Spread your group out: do not hold hands or sit back-to-back; by spreading out, you minimize the risk of multiple victims if a direct strike does occur.
- **The 30 – 30 Rule:** when you see lightning, count the seconds from the flash until you hear thunder, and divide the number by five to estimate the distance in miles. Speed of light: 186,000 miles per second (visible strike instantaneous). Speed of sound: 770 mph (about 1,000 feet per second, or five seconds per mile). If the time difference between the lightning flash and the thunder is 30 seconds or less (indicating the storm is about six miles away), take all precautions immediately.
- Wait until 30 minutes after the last strike to resume your activities.
- If on water, if possible, get off the water and move at least 100 yards away from the shore. Lightning is absorbed by fresh water, however in salt water the lightning will travel along the surface longer due to the increased conductivity thus making a person on salt water at greater risk of strike.
- If you have to stay on the water, put on a personal flotation device (PFD).
- Prepare for the winds of the squall line and the potential to be capsized.
- Sit in the center of the boat and stay away from the mast and metal shrouds and stays.
- **Indications that you may be about to be struck by lightning:** hair stands on end, skin tingles, light metal objects vibrate, you may smell ozone, you may hear crackling or a "kee-kee" sound.

DROWNING

The definition: "Drowning is a process resulting in primary respiratory impairment from submersion in a liquid medium."

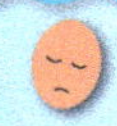 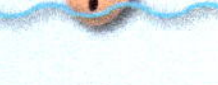 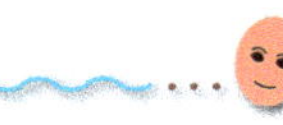

SUBMERSION

From an emergency care standpoint, submersion means to be completely under water—the airway is below the surface of the water.

IMMERSION

A person has been dunked under the water temporarily, but their head and airway are now above the surface of the water.

NEAR DROWNING

Survival for at least 24 hours after a submersion episode—there still may be serious complications.

The difference between submersion and immersion is subtle, but those few inches can make the difference between life and death.

PATHOPHYSIOLOGY

SEQUENCE OF EVENTS

- The drive to breathe can cause gasping for air, swallowing, aspiration of water, and voluntary apnea (breath-holding).
- This eventually leads to involuntary breathing and the inhalation of water, causing laryngospasm.
- If the laryngospasm eventually relaxes, water rushes in, and this is referred to as a "wet drowning."
- 15% don't relax, resulting in a "dry drowning."
- The laryngospasm leads to a loss of consciousness.
- Asphyxia follows leading to respiratory arrest, then cardiac arrest, then death.

The drowning victim will face the shore and reach a hand or hands out of the water

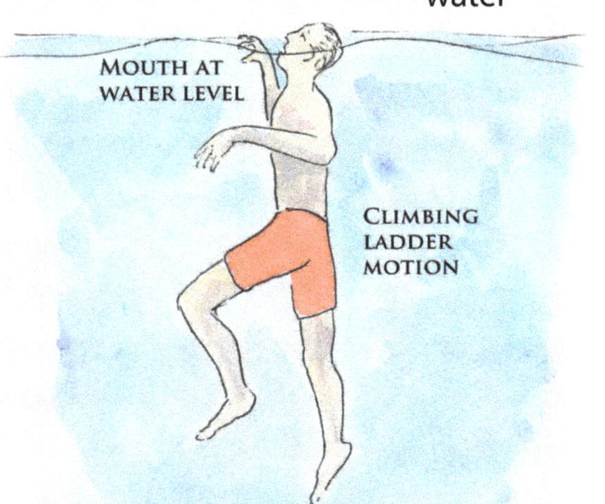

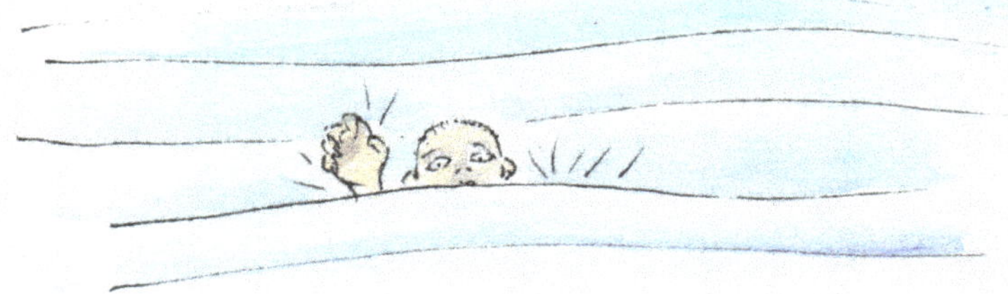

What you would see from the shore

PREVENTION

-If you are going to be near water, teach everyone that if they think they are drowning they should flip on their back and float
-Practice this if you have the chance

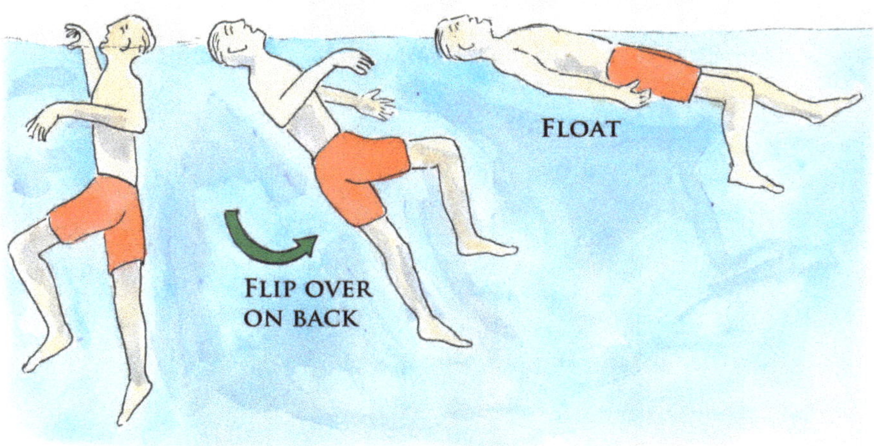

RESCUE PRINCIPLES

Reach, Throw, Row, and Go

Reach: Try and reach the victim with something long and rigid that they can grab

Throw: Try and throw a rope or something that will float to the victim

Row: Try and get to them in a boat
Don't try and get them into the boat, let them hang on

Go: If you cannot Reach, Row, or Throw, you can swim out to help the victim
This is dangerous. A drowning person is panicking and can drag you down too

TREATMENT

1. Do they have an **OPEN AIRWAY**? If not, open it.
2. Are they **BREATHING**?
   a. If not, begin artificial respirations (this can be done while still in the water).
   b. If breaths won't go in, massage throat to relax laryngospasm.
   c. Be prepared for water to come up from the lungs after breaths.
3. **CIRCULATION**—do they have a pulse?
   a. If not, begin CPR.
   b. This requires a firm surface.
   c. Expect the patient to vomit during CPR—don't let them aspirate vomitus.
4. **CERVICAL SPINE** (inspect, protect if significant MOI is suspected).
5. **HISTORY** (ask bystanders, if available).
   a. How long was the person in the water?
   b. What is the water temperature?
   c. Is the water contaminated? Take a sample.
6. Is there **RELATED TRAUMA** (e.g., neck injury from diving)?
7. Treat for **HYPOTHERMIA**.
8. **EVACUATE**. Transport all drowning victims, even if fully conscious and coherent, to the local emergency room for further evaluation and monitoring.

THINGS THAT AFFECT SURVIVAL

AGE the younger the better.

DURATION SUBMERGED the shorter the better

WATER TEMPERATURE the colder the better.

WATER PURITY the clearer the better.

TIMING OF CPR the sooner the better.

DRY VS. WET DROWNING dry drowning victims have a higher survival rate

If the victim's **LARYNX** can be relaxed quickly enough and they are resuscitated, they are more likely to survive without compli-cations. In a wet drowning, the larynx spasms and shuts after water has entered the lungs.

WET DROWNING VICTIMS even if resuscitated, face complications such as damage to the surface lining of the lungs and pneumonia. Once out of the water, these patients are not yet out-of-the-woods.

If they have **ASPIRATED WATER**, they are at risk of having some of the surfactant rinsed out of their lungs, which will cause respiratory distress and secondary drowning in minutes to hours.

SECONDARY DROWNING is death caused several to many hours subsequent to the initial incident by the damage done to the lung and circulatory system.

Additionally, wet drowning victims are at high risk of **ASPIRATION PNEUMONIA**.

ALTITUDE ILLNESS

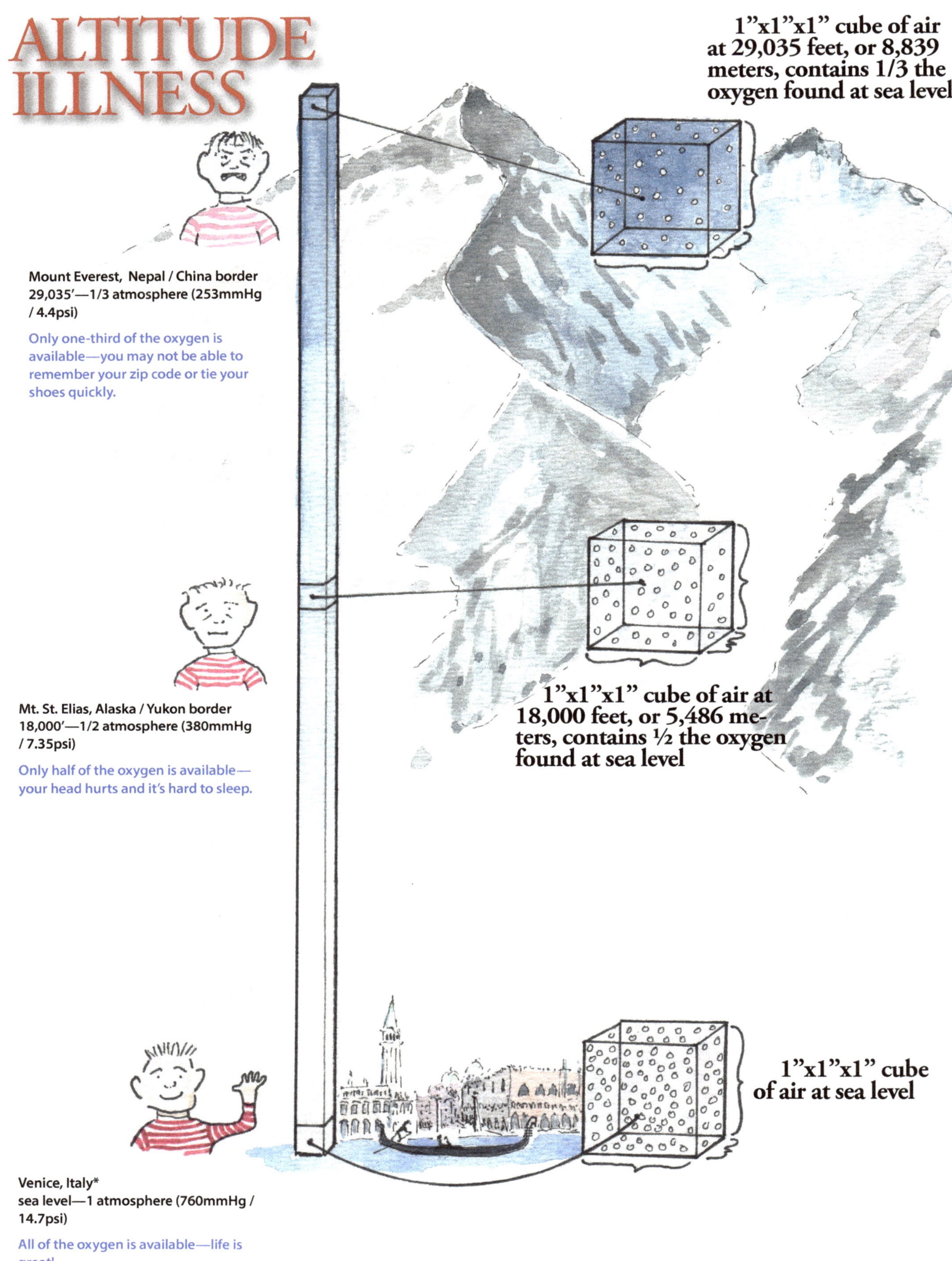

Mount Everest, Nepal / China border
29,035'—1/3 atmosphere (253mmHg / 4.4psi)

Only one-third of the oxygen is available—you may not be able to remember your zip code or tie your shoes quickly.

Mt. St. Elias, Alaska / Yukon border
18,000'—1/2 atmosphere (380mmHg / 7.35psi)

Only half of the oxygen is available—your head hurts and it's hard to sleep.

Venice, Italy*
sea level—1 atmosphere (760mmHg / 14.7psi)

All of the oxygen is available—life is great!.

ALTITUDE . . .

- It's simple: air has mass and is compressible—as gravity pulls the air down, its own weight causes it to squish and become more dense. If you take a given one square-inch column of air (left), it will become more dense as you move from the outer edge of the atmosphere to the surface of the earth.
- The pressure caused by this compression is measured in millimeters of mercury (in a barometer) and pounds per square inch (PSI).
- While the proportions of oxygen to the other gases that make up the atmosphere remain the same throughout the column (known as partial pressure: 21% oxygen, 78% nitrogen, 1% other gases), because the atmospheric pressure is lower the higher we go, and the air therefore less dense, the amount of oxygen available to us decreases.
- At 18,000 feet, your deep breath will have the same volume as at sea level, but there will only be half as many oxygen molecules available.
- As we ascend, other environmental/meteorological things change: for every 1,000 feet of ascent, the air temperatures typically crops 3°F and the concentration of ultraviolet (UV) light increases by 4%; the air also gets less humid the higher we go (because it's less dense, it cannot hold as much water).

ACUTE MOUNTAIN SICKNESS (AMS)

AMS is a pathological effect of high altitude on humans, caused by the low atmospheric pressure at higher altitude, which makes less oxygen available. It does not typically occur below 8,000' (2,500m). It is the most common and least dangerous high altitude illness (snow blindness and sunburn excepted). It can occur in anyone, regardless of experience at altitude, underlying health, or fitness. AMS presents as a set of nonspecific symptoms that resemble the flu, caused primarily by the consequences of an increase in respiratory rate and effort. As the body acclimatizes, the symptoms will clear, and once they clear, it is safe to go higher—never go up until your symptoms go down.

SIGNS AND SYMPTOMS—a headache accompanied by:

- Nausea with or without vomiting
- Fatigue or weakness
- Loss of appetite
- Dizziness or lightheadedness
- Insomnia (common at altitude—not indicative of AMS if it's the only symptom)

TREATMENT

- **Descend immediately—500m – 1,000m** is usually sufficient. Ascending with symptoms increases the risk of contracting HAPE and HACE—which can be deadly.
- Rest.
- Hydrate.
- Monitor urine color (it should be copious and clear).
- If there is no improvement over 12 – 24 hours, descend further: to the last sleeping altitude where symptoms were not present, or as far as necessary for improvement.

TREATMENT

Remember, as a Wilderness First Responder the primary treatment for altitude illness is to get the patent to lower altitude.

HIGH-ALTITUDE PULMONARY EDEMA (HAPE)

HAPE and HACE are killers. HAPE is non-cardiogenic pulmonary edema (fluid in the lungs) that occurs in otherwise healthy people, typically over 2,500m (8,200'), although is has been known to occur as low as 1,500m (4,900'). The pathophysiology of HAPE is not well understood; the pulmonary vasculature becomes leaky and serous fluid (the liquid part of blood remaining after clotting) in the bloodstream begins to seep into the alveoli—in effect, the person is drowning. Going too high, too fast, is a trigger. HAPE often results from ignoring the symptoms of AMS.

SIGNS AND SYMPTOMS—signs and symptoms of AMS, accompanied by:

- Extreme fatigue
- SOB at rest, with shallow, fast breathing
- Pulmonary crackles
- Persistent cough with or without sputum
- Dyspnea not relieved by rest
- Chest tightness, pressure, or congestion
- Cyanosis of the lips and fingernail beds
- Drowsiness
- No pain—if accompanied by pain, suspect injury (e.g., ribs), acute MI, or costochondritis (inflammation of the intercostal spaces), evaluate, and treat

TREATMENT

- Immediate descent: typically 500 – 1,000m, unless prohibited by unsafe conditions (e.g., weather). Never remain at altitude if it is possible to descend.
- If descent is impossible, use a pressure bag (portable hyperbaric chamber) if available : Gamov, Certec, or PAC (see next page).
- Administer oxygen, if available: 4 – 6 liters per minute by nasal cannula or with PEEP (Positive End-Expiratory Pressure).
- Hydrate, if the patient is conscious.

HIGH-ALTITUDE CEREBRAL EDEMA (HACE)

Fluid build-up on the brain—this is the most serious altitude-related illness. It comes on quickly and the patient (unlike the HAPE patient) may be quickly incapacitated to the point where they cannot walk. It is often caused by ascending with symptoms of AMS and can occur concurrently with HAPE. If not identified and treated immediately, the patient will deteriorate rapidly, and coma and death will follow. Like HAPE, the pathophysiology is poorly understood; in this instance, the cerebral vasculature leaks serous fluid into the parenchyma of the brain.

SIGNS AND SYMPTOMS—signs and symptoms of AMS, accompanied by:

- Change in mentation (the ability to think clearly and solve simple problems, e.g., the speed at which basic arithmetic can be done)
- Loss of coordination—ataxia (a voluntary lack of coordinated muscle movements, which can be subtle), patient will be unable to tandem gait walk (walk in a straight line with the toes of the back foot touching the heel of the front foot with each step)
- Possible hallucinations
- Drowsiness
- Coma
- Cheyne-Stokes breathing (see the compensatory changes section)
- Signs of increasing ICP
  - Increasing respiratory rate and depth
  - Increasing systolic BP (pounding pulse)
  - Decreasing heart rate
  - Change (deterioration) in LOC

TREATMENT

- The same as for HAPE: immediate and rapid descent (or pressure bag), hydration,
- The patient may not be ambulatory—a litter (or helicopter) evacuation may be necessary

135

Three primary concerns

- Tissue damage
- Infection by microorganisms (e.g., viruses, bacteria)
- Envenomation

Mammals

While bears, wolves, coyotes, mountain lions, and other large carnivores get the most press, the data shows something less dramatic—the everyday critters in our lives (including ourselves) do the most chomping—see graphic at right. Bites by wild animals are uncommon.

PREVENTION

1. Don't touch or feed wild animals.
2. Keep a clean kitchen: hang food, dispose of scraps properly.
3. Never tease or make aggressive movements toward a wild animal.
4. Back away, but don't turn your back on an animal making aggressive or predatory motions.

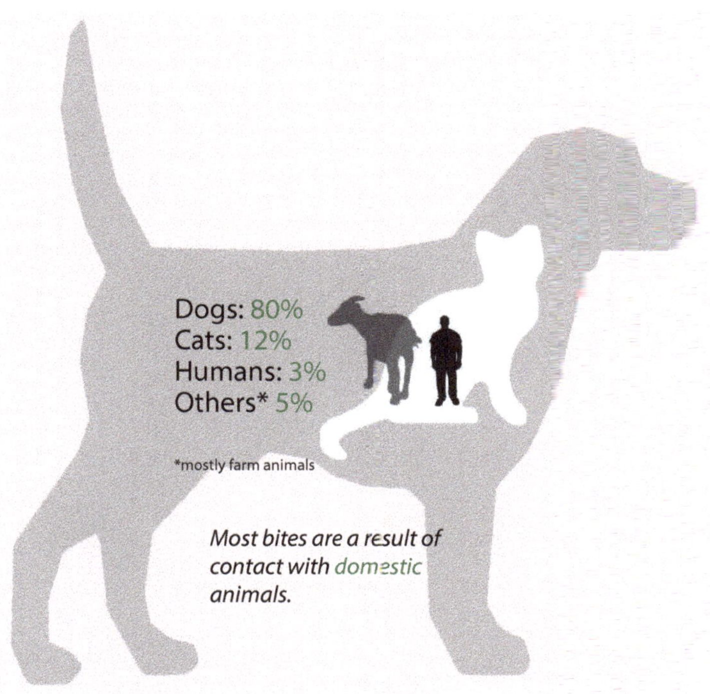

Most bites are a result of contact with domestic animals.

In __developing countries__, canid infection is the most common rabies vector (there are many feral dogs and inoculations are almost unheard of).

Data—kinds, types of venom, and distribution

- Venomous snakes in the US are of two types: pit vipers (rattlesnake, copperhead, cottonmouth), and coral snakes.
- Pit vipers inject a hemotoxin that is designed to both poison (kill) and digest prey by destroying red blood cells, disrupting blood clotting, and causing organ degeneration and generalized tissue damage. They can be locally common, are frequently found in the open and can be aggressive.
- In North America, pit viper distribution is widespread—they are found in all the contiguous states (although extremely rare in places like Maine). Rattlesnakes are found in virtually all states; copperheads are found in the eastern states to Texas; and cottonmouths are restricted to wetlands in the Southeast.
- Coral snakes inject a powerful neurotoxin that paralyzes the breathing muscles causing death by asphyxiation. They are found in the southern states from North Carolina west to Arizona. They are secretive, rarely seen, and non-aggressive—so bites (and deaths) are rare.
- There are two venomous lizards in North America: the Gila monster (neurotoxin) and the Beaded Lizard (hemotoxin). These are shy, reclusive animals that are rarely encountered. And, unlike the dart-like strike of venomous snakes, these lizards must gnaw on you for a while—bites are rare and envenomation even rarer. Both are found only in the deserts of the southwestern US and Mexico.
- People are typically bitten when they handle reptiles—approximately 70% of reptile bites occur on the hand.
- In habitats where venomous reptiles are known to live, wear protective clothing (boots, long pants), and be cautious where you put your hands and feet.

Snake and lizard bite—*TREATMENT*

1. Keep the patient calm—a high heart rate will speed the spread of the toxin.
2. Treat the wound: clean and disinfect it.
3. Monitor the pulses.
4. Monitor for anaphylaxis.
5. Do not apply cold packs; use a tourniquet, or "cut and suck."
6. Immobilize the extremity.
7. Evacuate via carry-out or walk out, as appropriate.
8. Protect yourself: try to identify the reptile, but don't risk a bite. If possible, inform the hospital of the species so they can provide the appropriate antivenom—medication for exotic species may have to be flown in.

A coral snake is identified by the rhyme "red touching yellow kills a fellow." Similar non-venomous species are identified by "red touching black, venom lack."

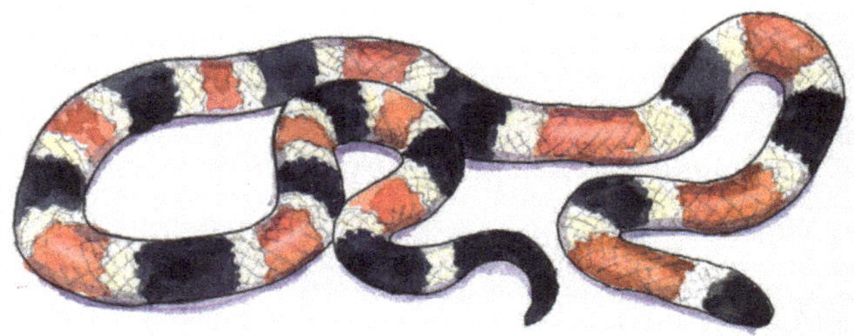

Sonoran coral snake
Micruroides euryxanthus

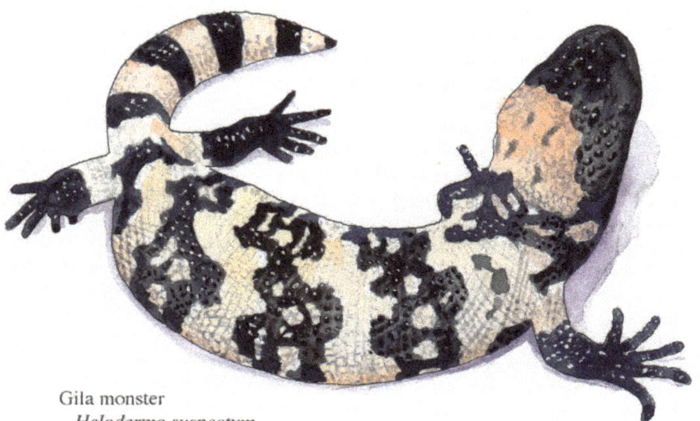

Gila monster
Heloderma suspectum

Gila monsters live in the southern parts of California, Nevada, Utah, and New Mexico, as well as nearly all of Arizona. They are listed as a threatened species and are the only venomous reptile (aside from snakes) native to the United States

There are 17 species of rattlesnake in the U.S., and 14 in the southwestern deserts. The most poisonous of these are the Mojave rattlesnake (Crotalus scutulatus), and the tiger rattlesnake (Crotalus tigris).

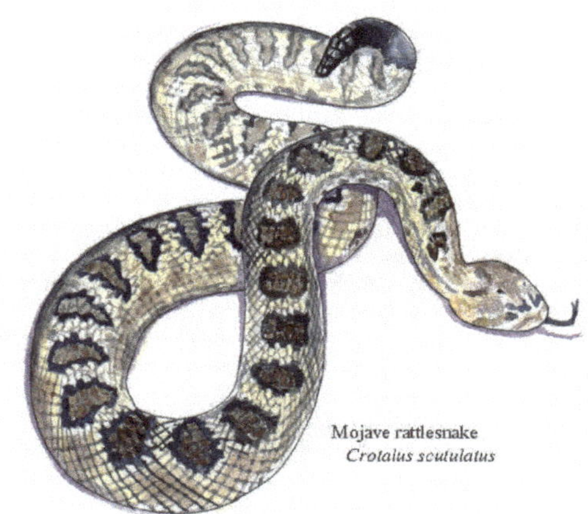

Mojave rattlesnake
Crotalus scutulatus

Hymenoptera (bees, hornets, wasps, fire ants)—*SIGNS AND SYMPTOMS*

- Pain
- Local swelling
- Redness
- Itching

Hymenoptera—*TREATMENT*

1. Remove the stinger/poison sack by scraping: do not use tweezers—if there is residual poison in the sack you will just force it into the wound.
2. Assess and monitor for anaphylaxis—if a serious anaphylactic reaction develops, take appropriate steps (see Critical Care).
3. Use topical medication for comfort.
4. Give oral antihistamine for relief of swelling and itching: diphenhydramine (Benadryl) 50mg q4 x 24 hours.

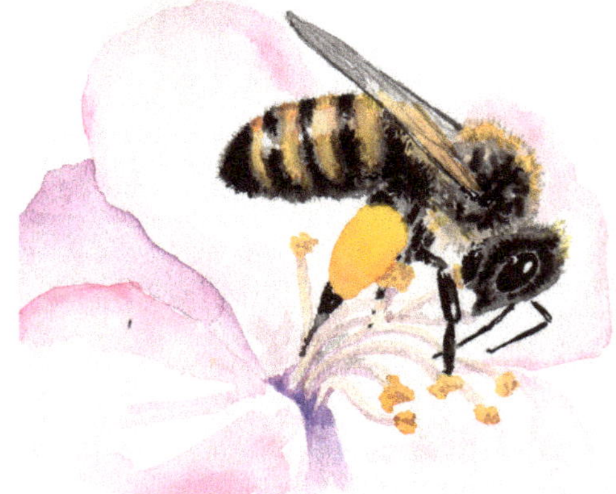

The most serious complication from a hymenoptera sting is anaphylaxis, which can cause a life-threatening allergic reaction.

Arachnids (scorpions, spiders, ticks)

SCORPIONS are small, "lobster-like" creatures with an upturned stinger in their tail. Scorpions are common in the southern tier of US states and throughout the hot parts of the world. The Arizona bark scorpion, found throughout the Sonoran Desert in Arizona, California, and northern Mexico, is the only deadly scorpion found in the US. Thousands of people are stung each year in the US, but there have only been two reported human deaths since 1968. Children and those with compromised immune systems are at greatest risk.

Scorpion—SIGNS AND SYMPTOMS

- For most species, the signs and symptoms are typically minor—pain and warmth at the sting site.
- If stung by a bark spider, the symptoms will be more dramatic. In children: pain that can be intense, numbness and tingling at the sting site, little or no swelling, muscle twitching or thrashing, unusual head, neck, and eye movements, drooling, diaphoresis, restlessness or excitability and sometimes inconsolable crying. Adults are more likely to experience increased respiratory and heart rates, high blood pressure, muscle twitches, and weakness.

Scorpion—TREATMENT

1. Immobilize the site.
2. Apply a cold pack.
3. Evacuate and monitor for anaphylaxis.

SPIDERS are eight-legged arachnids. They are extremely common—3,000 species are found in the US alone, with approximately 60 of those considered to cause medically significant bites. Only two species in the US are truly dangerous: the black widow and the brown recluse.

Black widow—Description,

Black Widow spiders are medium-sized (.5" to 1.5"), black, shiny, with long legs and a reddish hourglass mark on the underside of the abdomen. Most victims never feel the bite. Deaths are rare. Found throughout the contiguous US, more common in the south.

SIGNS AND SYMPTOMS

- Contraction of the smooth muscles of the abdomen and vasculature
- Painful abdominal cramping
- A rigid abdomen
- Elevated BP with vasoconstriction

Brown recluse—Description,

A brown, fuzzy spider typically ranging from .25" to .75" with long front legs, a large mandible, and a distinct violin shape on the back of the thorax (shared by other species, so not exclusively diagnostic). They have a painful bite that injects a digestive enzyme toxin. They are found in the southern Midwest to the Gulf of Mexico.

SIGNS AND SYMPTOMS

- A coin-sized welt which becomes a necrotic growing ulcer.

Black widow/brown recluse—TREATMENT

1. Clean the wound (and mark the margin, if a brown recluse)
2. Apply cold if the bite just occurred.
3. Monitor vital signs and watch for signs of anaphylaxis.
4. Evacuate.

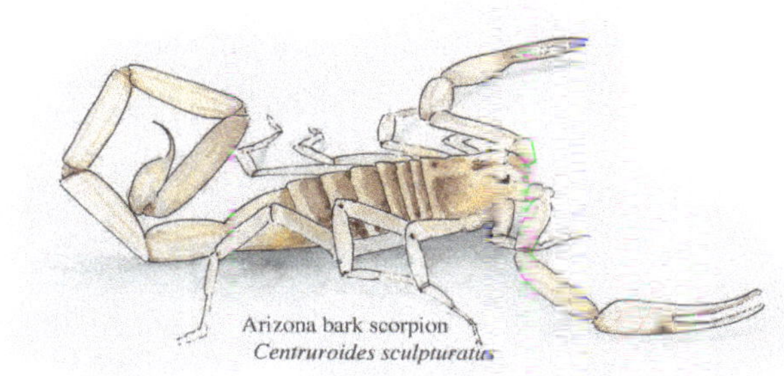

The Arizona bark scorpion stings an estimated 10,000 people in Mexico each year, with 800 deaths (annual mortality due to scorpion envenomation in Mexico is ten times higher than that due to snakebite). Worldwide, scorpions kill approximately 5,000 people annually.

Arizona bark scorpion
Centruroides sculpturatus

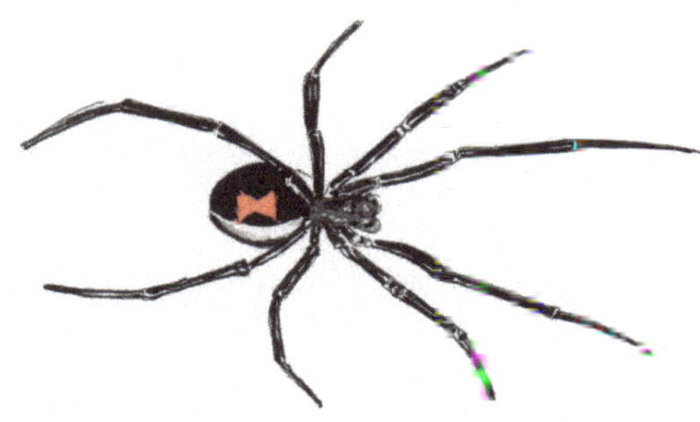

A black widow spider, its abdomen sporting the classic red hourglass, watches over it's silken ball of incubating young.

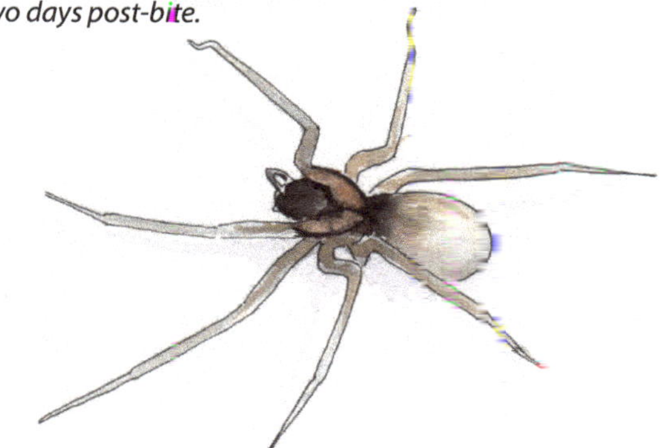

The venom of the brown recluse can cause extensive tissue damage: necrosis two days post-bite.

TICKS are small arachnids categorized as ectoparasites (external parasites). Functionally, they are tiny septic-tank vectors for several diseases, including Lyme Disease in humans, a potentially disabling disease first described in the 1970s. They vary in size from that of a speck of pepper up to a frozen pea, with large abdomens, small heads, and short legs. Colors range from tan to brown to almost black. They attach to their host by biting, then burying their heads in the skin to take a blood meal (which may take a day or more to accomplish).

Ticks—*TREATMENT*

1. Remove by pulling off as close to the skin as possible, preferably with fine-tipped tweezers. Pull upward with steady, even pressure—don't twist or jerk the tick; this can cause mouth-parts to break off and remain in the skin. If this happens, remove the mouth-parts with tweezers.

2. Clean the area well.

Lyme Disease—the most widespread tick-borne disease

Named after the small town in Connecticut, Old Lyme, where a number of cases were described in 1975, it is found in temperate climates worldwide, is the most common tick-borne disease in the Northern Hemisphere, and is one of the fastest-growing infectious diseases in the US. The bacteria is carried by several species of tiny ticks including the deer tick, and causes fever, headache, depression, and a characteristic red, bull's-eye rash. The disease can lay dormant and symptoms may take months to appear. In its early stages, Lyme Disease can be readily treated with antibiotics. Later, after the bacteria has been widely disseminated throughout the body, treatment is more difficult and complications more serious (e.g., arthritis-like symptoms).

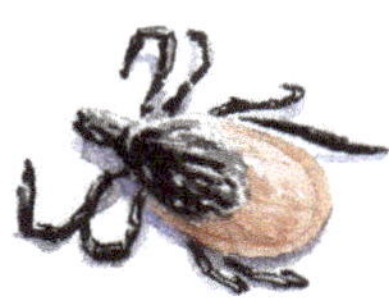

The wood tick, also known as the American dog Tick, (above) is extremely common in the eastern two-thirds of the US. It bites animals and humans with equal abandon and is a vector for Rocky Mountain Spotted Fever.

The deer tick, also known as the black-legged tick, is a notorious carrier of Lyme disease.

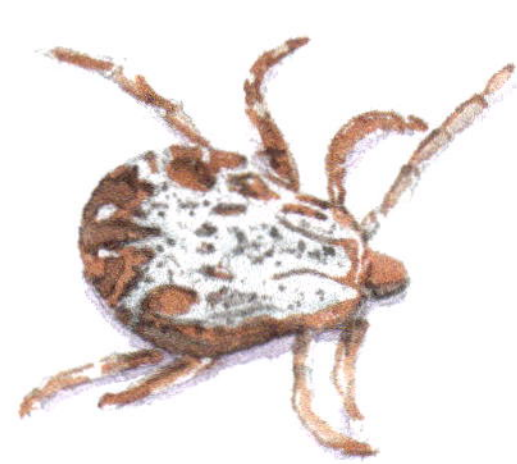

The deer tick, shown actual size next to a fishing dry fly.

The Rocky Mountain Wood tick, (upper right) also a vector for Rocky Mountain Spotted Fever.

The Bottom Line: ticks can be very small and a bite can go un-noticed; if you have been in an area where ticks are common and you start to feel ill for no apparent reason, get to definitive care and get checked out!

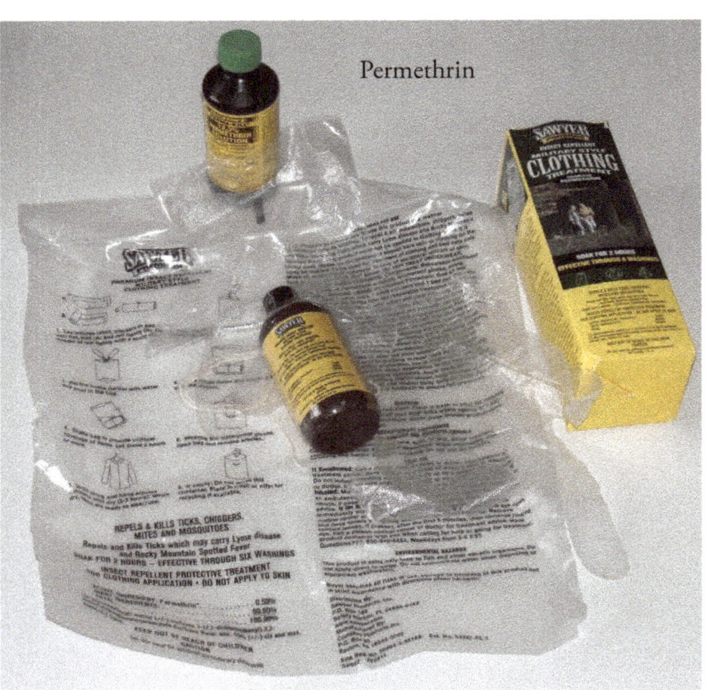

Permethrin

PREVENTION

- Use insect repellents or insecticides.
- The insecticide Permethrin is very effective. While it kills the ticks, it does not adhere well to the skin, so you have to apply it to clothing. Permethrin can also be used on tents and mosquito netting to provide additional protection while you are sleeping.
- The insect repellant DEET can be applied directly to the skin. It is a "repellent" and helps to keep the bugs away, but does not kill them. Use with caution on children.
- Wear protective clothing.
- Do frequent tick checks. Several times a day stop and check your skin for ticks remembering to check in places where the sun doesn't shine. Ticks like to be warm, dark, and moist.

ANAPHYLAXIS

Anaphylaxis is the extreme of an allergic reaction. The body's systemic release of histamine causes massive vasodilation and bronchoconstriction, bringing on the symptoms of an acute anaphylactic reaction: shortness of breath, wheezing, difficulty breathing, and shock.

SIGNS AND SYMPTOMS

- Initially, itching of the eyes and face which spreads to the rest of the body
- Swelling of the throat, lips, tongue, and face
- Difficulty breathing with a sensation of shortness of breath
- Difficulty swallowing
- Anxiety
- Wheezing
- Rash consisting of hives (urticaria) that are reddined, and itchy
- Shock

Vital signs & physical exam

RR—tachypnea (rapid breathing) with wheezing
HR—tachycardia (rapid heart rate)
BP—hypotension (low blood pressure)
LOC—anxious, may go unconscious
Skin—flushed, diaphoretic (sweaty), hives
Pupils—PERRL (pupils equal, round, and reactive to light)

TREATMENT

Keep the patient alive:

- Treat the bronchoconstriction and the vasodilation by administering Epinephrine (adrenalin) 0.3cc of 1:1,000 intramuscular (thigh) by an autoinjector or EpiPen.

Solve the problem:

- Once the patient's breathing and ability to swallow have stabilized, solve the problem of too much histamines by administering an antihistamine: Benadryl (diphenhydramine 25 – 50mg) by mouth every 4 hours for 24 hours.
- Evacuate the patient for further evaluation and treatment regardless of how quickly they recover.

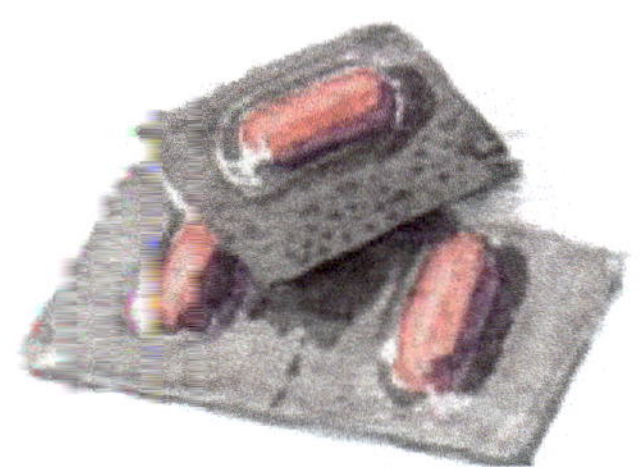

Because of significant side effects, epinephrine should be used with caution when treating acute allergic reactions. Epinephrine does not prevent or cure anaphylaxis: it reverses the potentially life-threatening symptoms. It should only be used when patients are having difficulty breathing (rapid, shallow breaths) and they are in shock (tachycardic, hypotensive, and diaphoretic). These folks may be very anxious, wheezy, have difficulty swallowing, and be turning cyanotic.

Once the diagnosis of anaphylaxis has been made, administer 0.3cc of 1/1000 epinephrine by autoinjector. Breathing will improve 30 – 60 seconds after the epinephrine has been injected. Once the patient is able to swallow, administer an antihistamine.

While the epinephrine treats the initial, life-threatening symptoms of anaphylaxis, it is the antihistamine that cures the problem by counteracting the effect of the over-abundance of histamines. Typically, 50 – 100mg of diphenhydramine is given orally and that dosage is repeated every 4 hours during the evacuation.

Even under ideal circumstances, problems can arise. Epinephrine (epi) is a naturally occurring hormone produced by the adrenal glands. Once secreted into the blood stream, it lasts about 20 minutes, and then it is broken down and eliminated. The same thing goes for the epi from the autoinjector; its effects will last 20 – 30 minutes. During that time you hope that the antihistamine has moved out of the GI tract and been absorbed into the bloodstream. If it has not, your patient will go back into anaphylaxis and require a second injection from the autoinjector. This occurs about 20% of the time.

Therefore, if you are going to carry epinephrine in the backcountry to treat anaphylaxis, you have to carry two doses of epi in autoinjectors and at least forty 25mg tablets of an antihistamine such as diphenhydramine (Benadryl). The EpiPen is one injection per autoinjector.

Who can use the drug epinephrine?

If an individual is carrying their prescription epi autoinjector, anyone can assist in administering it to them for an acute anaphylactic reaction

What if it is not their epinephrine?

Common sense dictates that you always err on the side of life. If someone is having an anaphylactic reaction, and they do not have an epi autoinjector, but someone else does, by all means use it. Just make sure that it is truly an anaphylactic reaction and that you are not risking a potentially fatal side effect for the wrong problem. When using medications, always make sure it is the right drug, for the right problem, given in the right dose, to the right person.

What is the proper use of epinephrine?

Epinephrine is often used incorrectly—for instance, to prevent an allergic reaction from becoming life-threatening anaphylaxis. This doesn't work. epi only treats the symptoms—it does not cure the underlying problem. That is the job of the antihistamines.

POISONOUS PLANTS

PATHOLOGY — what causes the rash?

- The sap, or juice, of the poison ivy, oak, and sumac plants causes the rash.
- Their sap contains an organic oil—urushiol, which causes the allergic reaction and resulting skin rash.
- The rash is an immune response, an allergic reaction, to the urushiol oil caused by the release of histamines from the body's mast cells.

SIGNS AND SYMPTOMS

- Initially, the rash is red, itchy, flat, and typically presents in stripes where the plant dragged across the skin, depositing the oil as it went.
- Over time, small blisters (vesicles) may also form.
- It is a common myth that the fluid contained in the blisters can cause the rash to spread—it cannot; the urishiol oil that caused the initial allergic reaction is gone.

TREATMENT

Antihistamines
Diphenhydramine: Benedryl, short-acting
Meclizine: many trade names, short-acting
Promethazine: many trade names, short-acting
Chlorpheniramine: many trade names, short-acting
Cetirzine: Zyrtec, long-acting
Loratadine: Claritin, long-acting
Over-the-counter (OTC) steroid cream (hydrocortisone): Cortaid, Hydrocort.

- Apply sparingly to the rash three times a day.
- Not recommended for use on the face because they can cause thinning and scarring of the skin.
- With any medication, OTC or prescription, make sure you are familiar with the possible side effects

With any allergic reaction, if you begin to experience shortness of breath or wheezing, or if the rash begins to spread systemically, body-wide, seek immediate medical attention—you may need prescription-strength antihistamines or steroids

The big three

POISON IVY (*Toxicodendron rybergii*)

- **Plants** grow erect, typically 2 – 5 feet tall, but can also climb as vines (*T. radicans*) with aerial rootlets (which cling to tree bark).
- **Leaves**: trifoliate with 3 leaflets, long-stalked—the leaves exhibit a wide range of shapes and textures; they can be stiff, leathery, or thin, hairy or hairless, shiny or dull, toothed or not, and reddish when young, 4 – 14".
- **Habitat**: young woodlands, roadside, field/forest edges, thickets, path edges, sand dunes, walls.
- **Range**: northern Quebec to Florida, Nova Scotia to Texas, Arizona.

POISON OAK

- There are two varieties in North America: Atlantic (*T. pubescens*) and Pacific (*T. diversilobum*). Both varieties appear very similar—differences will be noted.
- **Plants** grow as low shrubs (when growing in direct sun) or climbing vines (when growing in shade).
- **Leaves**: trifoliate with typically 3 leaflets (sometimes 5); the Atlantic variety's leaves are shiny. Leaf shape resembles that of an oak tree, with toothed or lobbed edges.
- **Habitat**: they are widespread and adapted to many habitats—typically below 5,000 feet.
- **Range** (Pacific): west coast of the US and Canada—one of California's most common woody plants; the Atlantic variety is found in all the US coastal states from New Jersey south to Florida and west to Texas, plus Arkansas, Illinois, Kansas, Missouri, Oklahoma, Tennessee, and West Virginia.

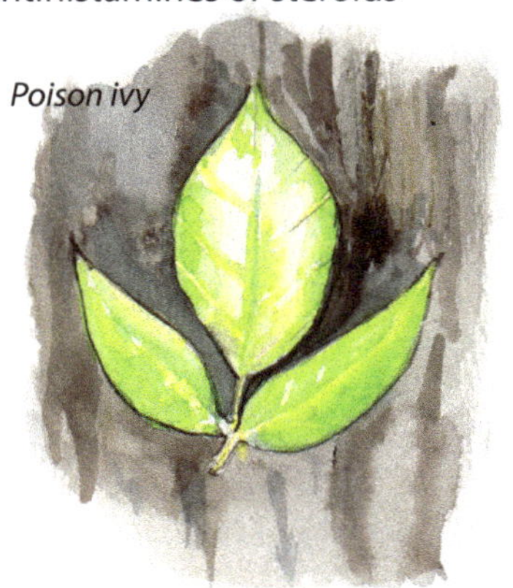

Poison ivy

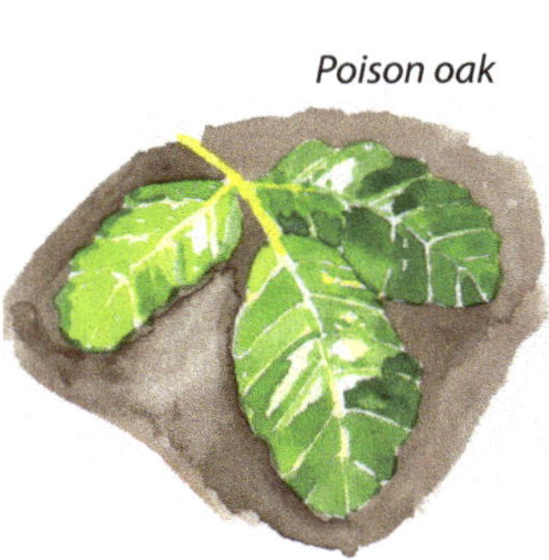

Poison oak

Poison sumac

POISON SUMAC (*Toxicodendron vernix*)

- **Plants** grow as a coarse, woody, rangy shrub typically 5 – 6 feet tall, but occasionally up to 25 feet. It does not grow as a vine.
- **Leaves**: has compound leaves with 7 –13 smooth-edged leaflets.
- **Habitat**: prefers boggy areas.
- **Range**: Quebec to Florida and west to Texas; most common in the Southeastern states.

Medical Emergencies

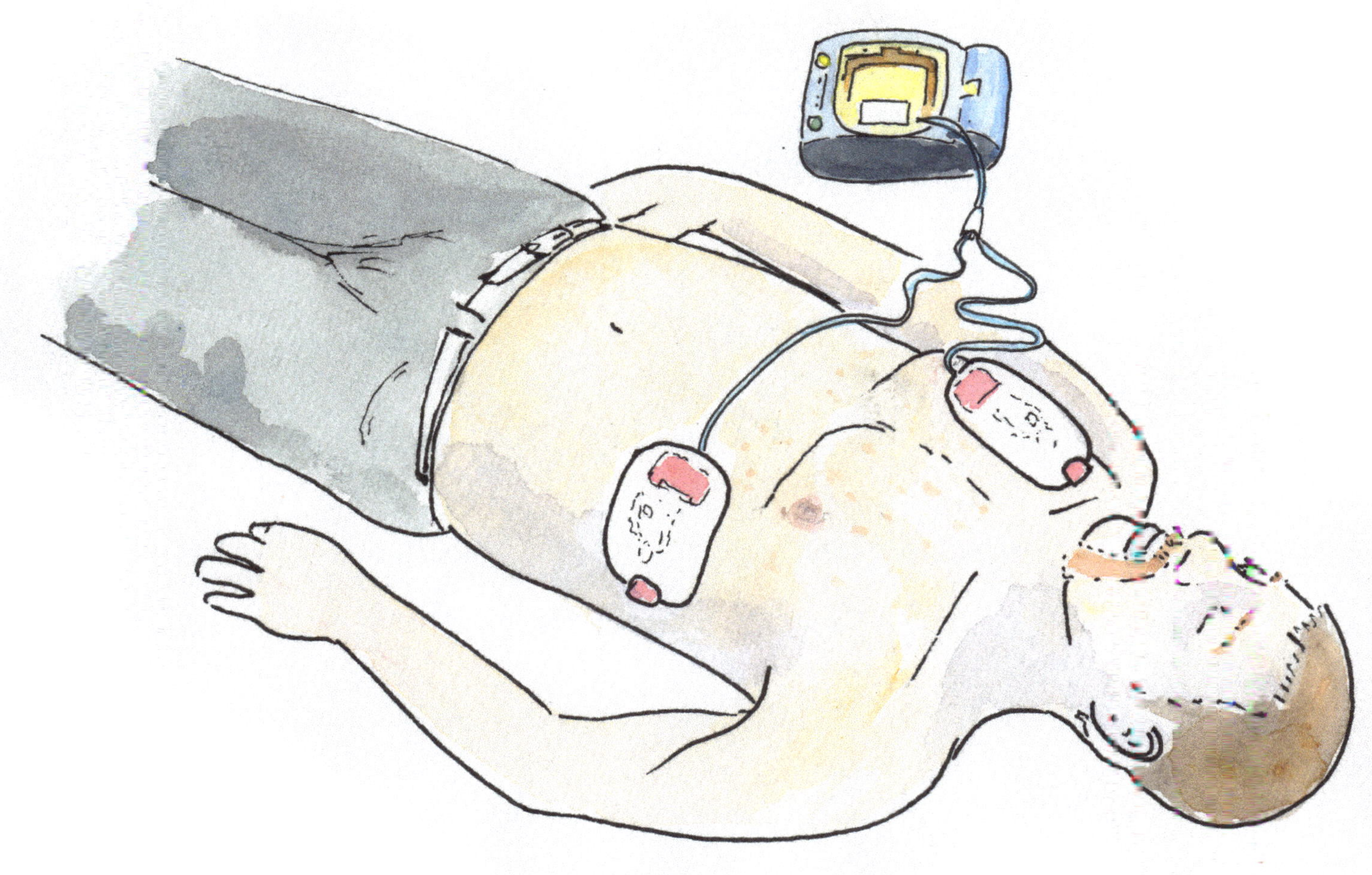

MEDICAL EMERGENCIES

What is a medical emergency? A medical emergency is when someone suffers an sudden onset of sickness, symptoms, or change in level of consciousness that is not the direct result of trauma

The **patient interview** is key . . .

EXPLORE THE CHIEF COMPLAINT (C/C)

Common Chief Complaints (C/C) associated with a medical emergency:

- A change in level of consciousness (LOC)—neurologic
- Shortness of breath (SOB)—respiratory
- Chest pain—cardiovascular
- Acute abdomen—digestive/genitourinary

MAKE A DIFFERENTIAL DIAGNOSIS

The possibilities associated with the C/C:

- A change in LOC—hypoxia, poison, diabetes, seizure, stroke, behavioral, fever
- Shortness of breath—asthma, COPD/emphysema, pulmonary emboli, lung disorders (pulmonary edema, spontaneous pneumothorax, hyperventilation syndrome)
- Chest pain—coronary artery disease (angina, acute MI, hypertension) congestive heart failure, indigestion/acid reflux
- Acute abdomen—constipation, bowel obstruction, gallstones/ kidney stones, peritonitis, genitourinary emergencies

HISTORY OF PRESENT ILLNESS AND AMPLE HISTORY

The question sequence to explore the C/C
The patient's current and past medical history

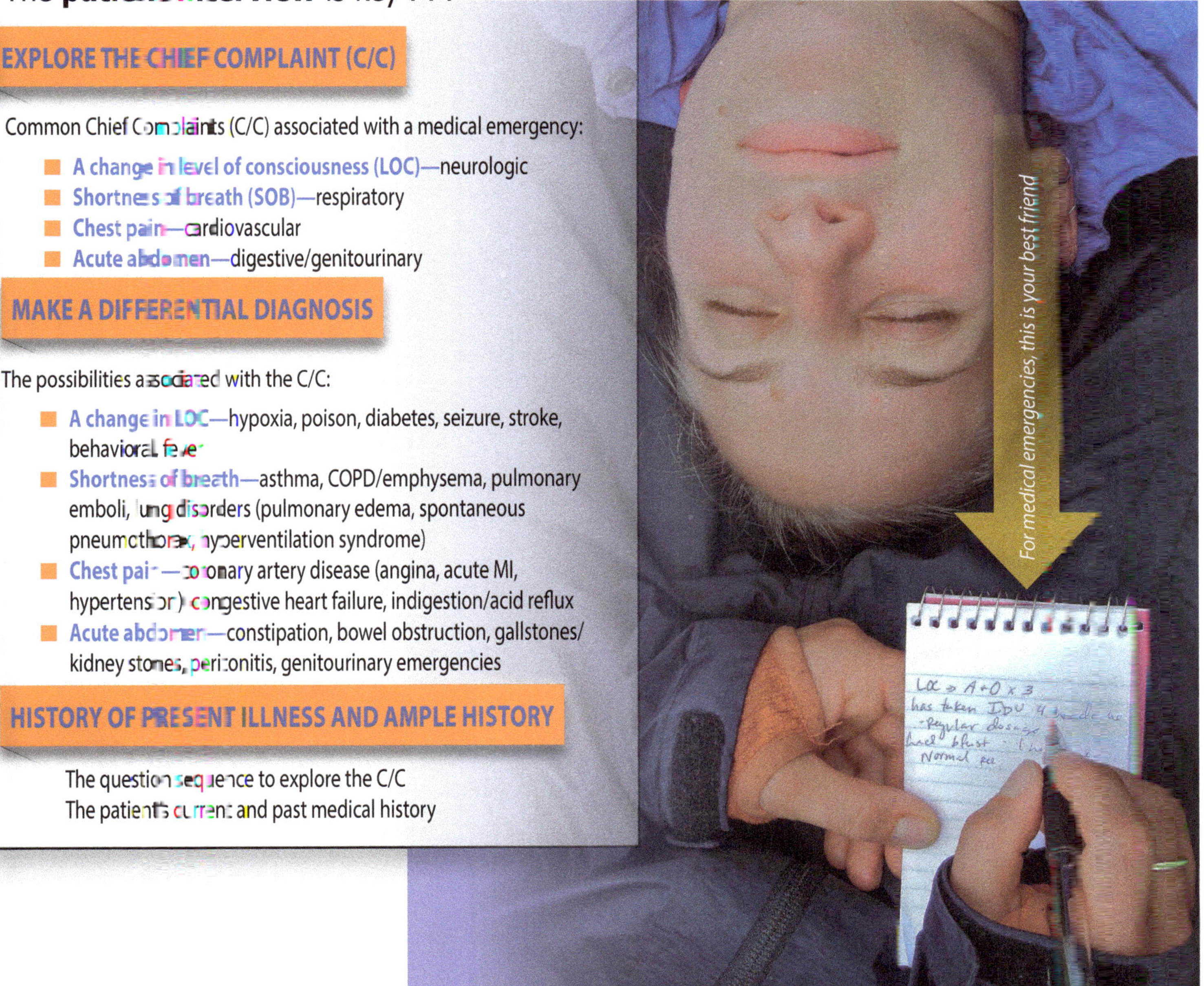

PERSON WITH A DETERIORATING LOC

presents one of the most disconcerting and challenging problems in emergency medicine. In an urban setting, the standard is to maintain the airway, place the patient in a safe position, give oxygen, transport immediately, and do your best to try to find out what's going on. Fortunately, the patient will typically not deteriorate much more during the trip to the emergency department. This is one of the few areas where there may not be a lot that can be done in the prehospital setting, but early recognition and rapid transport can and will save brain cells.

By contrast, in the extended-care environment, with prolonged evacuation times, there is ample opportunity for the patient to get worse. To make things even harder, there may be little or no clue as to the underlying cause of their change in level of consciousness (obvious trauma or a cardiac event aside), and the patient may not be able to provide you with a chief complaint or medical history.

To be able to appreciate the various threats to our mental status, and to discern what happened and where the problem is, requires an understanding of the normal physiology and function of the human brain; familiarity with brain structure, circulation, metabolism, and the role of cerebral spinal fluid is crucial to recognizing, diagnosing, and managing some of the most difficult problems in medicine: the neurological emergencies. We will often refer you to other places in this book for additional and supporting information.

AND THE PROBLEM TYPICALLY STARTS WITH THE LETTER H

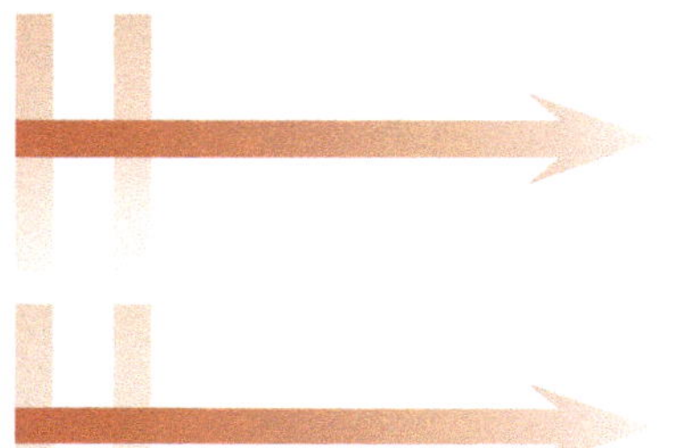

HYPOXIA

Too little oxygen getting to the brain—lack of O_2, poor O_2 exchange, heart failure, hypovolemia, cellular metabolic failure

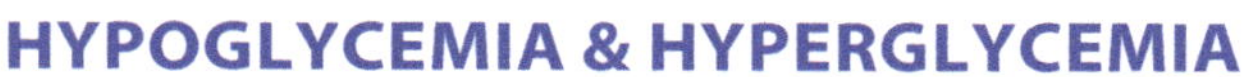

HYPOGLYCEMIA & HYPERGLYCEMIA

Too little or too much blood glucose—diabetes

HYPOACTIVITY & HYPERACTIVITY

Too little or too much neuronal activity in the brain—seizures

HALLUCINATIONS

Illness (fever), abuse (alcohol, drugs), environmental emergencies, or trauma (esp. head) leading to behavior issues

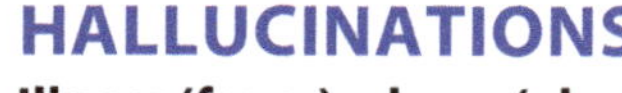

HEAD TRAUMA

increasing intracranial pressure (ICP)—covered in the Trauma section

HYPOTHERMIA & HYPERTHERMIA

Too cold to think or too hot to function—covered in the Environmental Emergencies section

SOLO Wilderness First Responder

HYPOXIA

Hypoxia is a condition where not enough oxygen is getting to the brain and other vital tissues. The neuronal cells of the brain require a constant supply of oxygen—the brain does not store glucose or oxygen. If the supply is interrupted, a person will have changes in their LOC almost immediately: consciousness can be lost in 10 seconds and irreversible brain damage and death in as little as 4 – 6 minutes.

Causes of hypoxia

1

Lack of oxygen in the air—little or no O_2 available

Carbon monoxide poisoning
Methane and other gases that displace oxygen

2

Poor oxygen exchange—little or no oxygen exchange in the lungs (alveoli)

Airway failure—oxygen can't get to the lungs
Obstructed airway
Asthma/COPD
Pulmonary edema

Circulatory failure—there is 0_2, but no blood flow
Pulmonary emboli

Stroke

Respiratory failure—loss of the ability to fully inhale and exhale
Flail chest
Sucking chest wound
Pneumothorax
Hemothorax
Drug overdose (respiratory suppressants)
Spinal cord injury

3

Heart failure—decrease in blood flow to the brain

Acute myocardial infarction—decreased blood flow to the brain

4

Hypovolemia—decrease in blood flow to the brain

Hypovolemic shock from bleeding, dehydration, vomiting, diarrhea, burns

5

Cellular metabolic failure—inability to utilize 0_2 in the cells

Cyanide poisoning

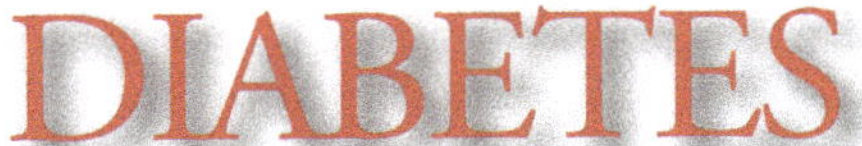
DIABETES

Diabetes is a group of diseases in which a person has a high blood glucose level, either because their pancreas does not produce enough insulin, or because the cells in their body don't respond properly to the insulin that is produced. Diabetes decreases the glucose supply to the cells and causes cellular starvation. While diabetes can typically be controlled by careful dietary monitoring and medication, emergency situations can still arise, and they can be serious, even life-threatening.

Key definitions

Insulin A hormone (beta islet cells of Langerhans) produced by the pancreas that transports glucose from the blood into the cells. Insulin lowers the blood sugar level.

Glucagon A hormone (alpha islet cells of Langerhans) produced by the pancreas which stimulates the release of stored glucose (glycogen) in the liver (glycogenolysis). Glucagon raises the blood sugar level.

Blood glucose level The amount of glucose in the blood. Blood glucose is measured by a glucometer. The level of blood glucose increases after a meal, then decreases as glucose is used by the cells.

Hyperglycemia Decreased insulin production results in high glucose levels in the blood and low levels in the cells.

Hypoglycemia Excess insulin production creates low glucose levels in the blood and low levels in the cells.

Normal physiology

1. As food is consumed carbohydrates are broken down into glucose molecules.
2. Glucose is absorbed into the bloodstream, elevating blood glucose levels (glycemia).
3. The rise in glycemia stimulates the pancreas to secrete insulin from its beta cells.
4. Insulin binds to specific cell receptors and facilitates entry of glucose into the cells: mitochondria uses O_2 to burn glucose and the resulting energy is used to produce adenosine triphosphate (ATP)—which transports chemical energy within the cells for metabolism.
5. As the pancreas secretes insulin and the cells burn glucose, the blood glucose levels in the blood decrease—which results in decreased insulin secretion.
6. This cycle repeats as a constantly self-adjusting metabolic balance: creating, storing, and releasing energy.

The diabetic's physiology

Type I

- The immune system destroys the pancreas's insulin-producing cells—little or no insulin is produced.
- Insulin injections are a lifelong necessity to control blood sugar—without supplemental insulin Type I diabetes will eventually be fatal.
- It tends to occur at a young age (as a child or young adult).
- About 5% of all diebetics have Type I.
- Symptoms: increased urination (the body is attempting to get rid of excess blood sugar) and accompanying increased thirst, increased hunger (the cells are starving because of limited glucose), fatigue and weakness, blurred vision (elevated blood sugar causes the lenses of the eyes to swell).

Type II

- The pancreas loses it's ability to effectively produce and release insulin.
- The body becomes resistant to insulin and blood sugar levels rise.
- Onset is later in life and can be linked to lifestyle behavior choices (e.g., obesity, alcoholism).
- Typically managed with oral hypoglycemics, which lower blood sugar—Type II may not require insulin injections.
- About 95% of all diabetics have Type II.
- Symptoms (many are similar to Type I): increased urination, thirst, and hunger, fatigue, blurred vision, weight gain, frequent infections (e.g., UTI), slow healing of cuts or sores (there is little fuel for repairs).

Diabetic emergencies

- Diabetic emergencies occur primarily in diabetics that are insulin-dependent (Type I). Due to their dependency upon injectable insulin, they can find themselves with either too much or too little blood glucose.
- The organ that is most affected by too little blood sugar is the brain.
- The level of consciousness and the ability of the brain to function normally is dependent upon oxygen, glucose, temperature, pressure, and neuronal activity. Altering the proper levels of any one of these factors will result in a change in Level of Consciousness.
- Without a glucometer to determine the blood glucose level, the ability to differentiate between hyperglycemia and hypoglycemia can be difficult. Fortunately, emergency care for both conditions is the same until the blood glucose level is determined.

Hyperglycemia

Hyperglycemia is elevated blood glucose due to lack of available insulin—also known as diabetic coma or diabetic ketoacidosis (DKA). There are two primary causes:

- The patient has not taken their insulin
- The patient has an infection such as a UTI or kidney infection that prevents the absorption and proper utilization of injectable insulin.

Hypoglycemia

Hypoglycemia is a low blood glucose level also known as insulin shock. The condition is caused by either too little blood glucose or too much insulin—patients have either taken their insulin and not eaten enough to meet the energy demands, or they have taken too much insulin, and the blood glucose is quickly used up. This condition can also be brought on by over-exercising, excessive alcohol consumption, or aggressive dieting.

TREATMENT
for **hyperglycemia** and **hypoglycemia**

Initial treatment for a patient you suspect of having a diabetic emergency is the same: give them glucose immediately. If their blood glucose level is high, giving them additional glucose will not do any harm—and if they are hypoglycemic, it will help.

1. If the patient is conscious and can swallow, they should drink a sweet liquid such as orange juice with several teaspoons of sugar dissolved into it.

    - Liquids are preferred to solids because they are passed through the stomach and into the small intestine faster, allowing the glucose to be absorbed more quickly.

    - Any form of glucose and fructose can be used: sugar, honey, hard candy (dissolve in warm water)—anything sweet that can be put into a liquid form.

    - Obviously, NutraSweet and other sugar substitutes are of no value, as they do not contain any glucose or source of energy.

2. If the patient is unconscious, they obviously cannot swallow. In this case, the best method for sugar administration is to utilize the absorptive surface of the oral mucosa—gently rub any sugary paste onto the patient's gums—some of the glucose will be absorbed through the buccal mucosa of the lining of the mouth.

3. If the patient's LOC returns to alert (A&O x 3), **and** if it can be determined through taking patient history what caused the emergency, **and** the patient is able take over the management of their situation (e.g., has insulin and can inject), then you're done—however, if they do not rouse, or if their is **any** doubt about their recovery, transport the patient immediately for further medical evaluation and treatment.

4. **Never** give insulin—although this is the cornerstone of treatment for hyperglycemia, administering insulin must be done in a hospital environment where the patient's blood chemistry can be monitored closely.

SEIZURE (i.e., convulsion): a temporary disruption of the electrochemical impulses in the brain resulting in a change in level of consciousness or behavior.

POSSIBLE CAUSES OF SEIZURES

- Neglecting to take anti-seizure medications
- Congenital—patient born with a pre-existing condition
- Traumatic Brain Injury (TBI)
- Meningitis, stroke
- Tumor (space-occupying lesion)
- Alcohol or drug withdrawal, alcohol or drug overdose
- Fever—febrile seizures, usually in children
- Metabolic disturbances
- Sleep deprivation
- Hypoglycemia or hypoxia

SEIZURE TERMS

Aura

- A peculiar sensation (taste, smell, sight, feeling) that immediately precedes a seizure (moments to minutes)
- Can occur as long as an hour prior to the seizure, or just seconds before onset
- Seizure sufferers who experience auras typically experience the same type of aura each time they have a seizure
- Auras can help the patient protect themselves from injury by allowing them time to sit, lie down, pull over to the side of the road, etc.

Postictal

- Period of altered consciousness which occurs immediately following the termination of a seizure
- Typically lasts between 5 and 30 minutes—sometimes longer in severe cases
- Characterized by one or more of the following: • exhaustion • altered ability to think clearly or concentrate (confusion) • short term memory problems • decreased verbal and interactive skills • other cognitive defects

Classic seizure presentation: supine, with body movement, typically most pronounced in the limbs.

TYPES OF SEIZURES

- **Generalized motor seizure (grand mal)**
  - Frequently preceded by an aura prior to onset of seizure activity
  - Tonic-clonic movement (uncoordinated muscle contraction and relaxation)
  - Postictal state may run the gamut of symptoms (left)
- **Absence seizure (petit mal)**
  - Most common in children
  - Very brief loss of consciousness—"staring off into space"
  - May be associated with eye blinking, lip-smacking, or jerky motions
  - Postictal state
- **Focal motor seizure**
  - Tonic-clonic twitching usually involving just one body part
  - May progress to a generalized motor seizure
  - Postictal state
- **Psychomotor seizure** (temporal lobe seizure)
  - Sudden alteration in personality
  - May be preceded by dizziness
  - May include hallucinations of sight, taste, sound, or smell
  - Postictal state
- **Status epilepticus**
  - More than 30 minutes of continuous seizure activity, or two or more seizures not separated by a period of consciousness
  - This is a medical emergency—transport to a hospital ASAP

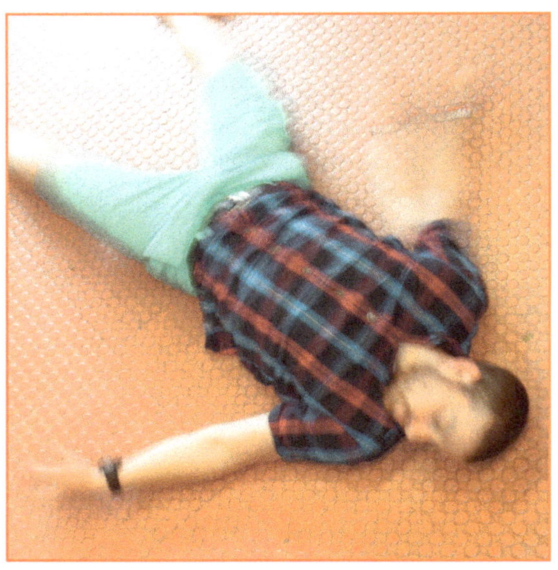

TREATMENT OF SEIZURES

- Protect the patient from harm, but do not restrain them.
- Contain the patient in an area, if necessary.
- **Do not** place a bite-stick in the patient's mouth.
- Place the patient in the recovery position to maintain an open airway (below).
- Check for other injuries.
- Take a good history: talk with patient, relatives, bystanders.
- Be prepared to describe the seizure activity, including the direction of movement of the patient's eyes, to medical personnel.
- Administer oxygen, at a rate of 4 – 6 liters per minute by nasal cannula, if available.

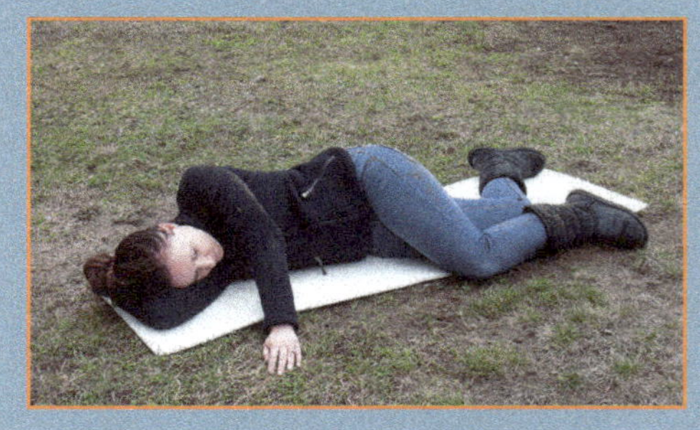

STROKE
CVA and TIA

WHAT IS A CVA?

CEREBROVASCULAR ACCIDENT

A CVA occurs when there is an interruption of blood supply to part of the brain due to a sudden vascular catastrophe caused by a blood clot (emboli) or hemorrhage (aneurysm).

SIGNS AND SYMPTOMS

CVA signs and symptoms vary depending upon which part of the brain is affected. The symptom complex may include one or more of the following:

- Loss of memory
- Inability to speak
- Facial paralysis
- Incontinence
- Frustration
- Headache
- One-sided weakness
- One-sided paralysis
- Unequal pupils

TREATMENT

1. Maintain ABCs.
2. Place the patient in a position of comfort and be prepared to manage a seizure.
3. Reassure the patient.
4. If unconscious, place the patient in the recovery position.
5. Evacuate.
6. Administer oxygen at a rate of 10 – 15 liters per minute by non-rebreather mask, if available.

WHAT IS A TIA?

TRANSIENT ISCHEMIC ATTACK

This is a "temporary stroke" caused by insufficient blood flow to the brain that spontaneously resolves within 24 hours.

- The signs and symptoms are identical to those of a CVA, but they disappear in less than a day.
- The treatment is the same as for a CVA.

stroke / assessment

F **Face:** *is their face symmetrical when they smile?*

A **Arms:** *do they have bilateral symmetry, strength, and control?*

S **Speech:** *are there impairments: inability, slurrying, decreased vocabulary?*

T **Time:** *if positive for any of the above (FAS), "time is tissue"—evacuate ASAP.*

the one chief complaint that gets everyone's attention in emergency medicine, for one simple reason—it may indicate that the person is having a HEART ATTACK and may truly be in significant trouble. Time is of the essence. Treat all chest pain as cardiac until you rule it out.

CHEST PAIN

Typical cardiac chest pain indicating acute coronary syndrome—*SIGNS AND SYMPTOMS*

- Left-sided, substernal chest pain, pressure, or tightness.
- The discomfort may radiate into the left arm, right arm, both arms, the lower jaw, etc.
- Discomfort is frequently associated with a sensation of shortness of breath.
- Discomfort is frequently associated with a cold sweat (diaphoresis).
- The chest pain or shortness of breath worsens with exertion.
- Vital signs indicate shock: rapid and shallow respirations, rapid and weak heartbeat, falling blood pressure, and the skin is pale, cool, and clammy.
- The patient may also have nausea, GI upset, and heartburn.
- In the case of angina pectoris, there may be some relief of symptoms with rest.

Principles of management

- The primary goal is to minimize the workload on the heart.
- Unless you are absolutely certain that the pain is not cardiac, evacuate ASAP.
- The patient should be kept at rest; exertion will make it worse.
- Transport them in position of comfort.
- Keep them calm and reassure them.
- If you have aspirin with you, give them one adult, 325mg or four 81mg aspirins.
- If they have a history of angina pectoris and they have sublingual nitroglycerin (NG) with them, you may assist them in taking their medicine as long as their systolic BP is >100 (radial pulse present).
- GET HELP—this patient needs to be evacuated ASAP (walking out may be appropriate).

ASPIRIN, whether round or capsule-shaped, is a medical wonder—working in so many ways that modern medicine wouldn't be the same without it. When a person is having a heart attack, fatty acid deposits in the blood vessels (atherosclerosis) can burst, and the body responds by sending platelets to the scene to form a clot—blocking the vessel and causing pain and tissue death. Aspirin reduces the clumping action of the platelets, helping to keep the vessel open and buying the patient precious time. It is a strong drug, not to be taken lightly.

Not all chest pain is caused by the heart. Other structures of the thoracic cavity can also be a source of chest pain.

What if the pain isn't caused by cardiac trouble?

MUSCULOSKELETAL CHEST WALL PAIN

- Sprains, strains, contusions, costochondritis, or rib fractures
- This is a diagnosis of exclusion.
- **C/C:** The pain can be a dull ache to a sharp, stabbing pain.
- **HPI:** They may have a history of trauma.
- **PE:** Palpation of chest wall reproduces the pain exactly. Deep breathing will also increase the chest wall pain. Fractured rib will have point tenderness at the fracture site.
- **Dx:** Non-cardiac musculoskeletal chest wall pain.
- **Rx:** Reassure, moist heat, aspirin-based cream, oral NSAID.

PULMONARY CHEST PAIN—PLEURISY

- Inflammation of the parietal and visceral pleura.
- Pain occurs with breathing as the two inflamed pleura rub.
- May be able to hear a friction rub over the area of pain with a stethoscope.
- **Dx:** Pleurisy.
- **Rx:** Reassurance, moist heat, aspirin-based cream, oral NSAID.

GASTROINTESTINAL DISEASE

- GERD and esophageal spasm.
- The chest pain can be very similar to an MI.
- Initially treat as an acute MI.
- As with an MI the chest pain may be relieved by NTG.
- Possible history of heartburn and acid reflux.

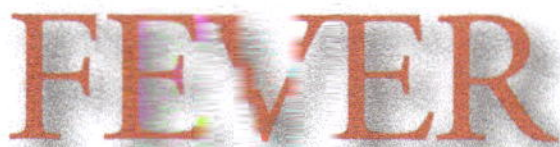

FEVER

is one of the most common medical signs—a clear signal that the body is fighting something. And it can cause a deterioration in LOC. Although a natural body defense, if a fever becomes severe enough (at or above 40°C/104°F)—regardless of the underlying cause—it must be controlled. Extremely high temperatures can cause permanent brain damage and death.

FEVER-CAUSING conditions

1. **Infections** (bacterial or viral)
2. **Tissue damage** (e.g., crush injuries)
3. **Alcohol** or **drug** withdrawal
4. **Environmental**: dehydration, heat exhaustion
5. **Other** (less common) causes: cancer, toxins, drugs such as amphetamines or MDMA (ecstasy)

TREATMENT

PHYSICAL COOLING

Tepid sponge baths (with warm, not cool water), is an old-fashioned technique that works very well. Gently sponge the water onto exposed skin and let it air dry—evaporation cools the peripheral venous blood flow (simulating sweating) and helps lower core temperature.

MEDICATIONS

OTC non-steroidal anti-inflammatory drugs (NSAIDs) help to alleviate pain and control inflammation by direct action on prostaglandins, which are the chemical mediators of inflammation—NSAIDs are also very effective at lowering fever.

- Aspirin (acetylsalicylic acid)
- Acvil and Motrin (ibuprofen)
- Aleve (Naprosyn)
- There are also many prescription NSAIDs.

Used in appropriate dosages, NSAIDs are very safe medications; however, as with any medication, it is important to know the potential adverse reactions and the warnings. Always ask about allergies before giving any medication—if the patient has had a bad reaction the past, do not administer the med.

POSSIBLE ADVERSE REACTIONS TO NSAIDs

- Anaphylaxis
- Gastrointestinal upset and gastritis. Gastrointestinal (GI) upset can be minimized by taking the NSAID with food. Reactions can vary from mild nausea or diarrhea to bleeding ulcers and a life-threatening GI bleed. Avoid giving NSAIDs to anyone who has a history of ulcers, irritable bowel syndrome (IBS), Crohn's Disease, ulcerative colitis, or any sort of inflammatory bowel disease.
- Asthmatics can be sensitive to NSAIDs (particularly aspirin). Their properties can exacerbate or precipitate an asthma attack.
- Renal or kidney problems can be made worse by NSAIDs. Avoid the use of NSAIDs in individuals with a history of renal insufficiency, kidney failure, or any form of kidney disease.

SHORTNESS OF BREATH

airways
Moving air in and out of the lungs

The trachea, bronchi, and bronchioles are smooth muscles held open by cartilaginous, C-shaped rings.

The airways are lined with cilia and goblet cells. The goblet cells secrete mucus which keeps the airway moist and sticky, trapping dirt particles, pollen, and other debris. This debris is swept up and out of the airway by the cilia in a rhythmic sweeping motion, referred to as the mucociliary escalator.

During inhalation, the air on the way to the alveoli is warmed by the surrounding tissue to core temperature, becomes 100 percent humidified, and is scrubbed clean by the mucus lining the airways.

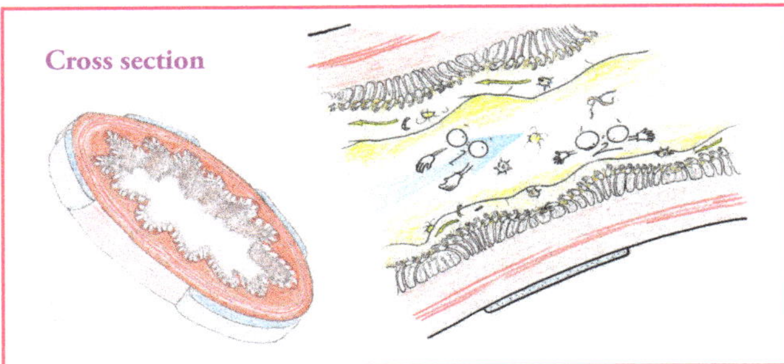

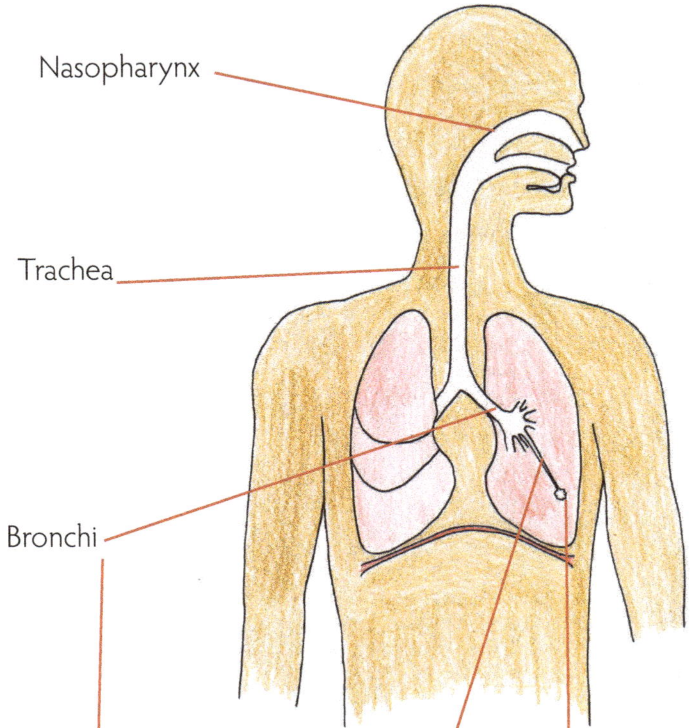

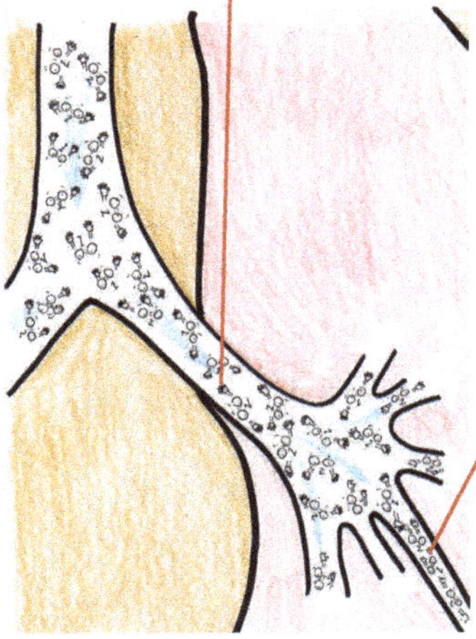

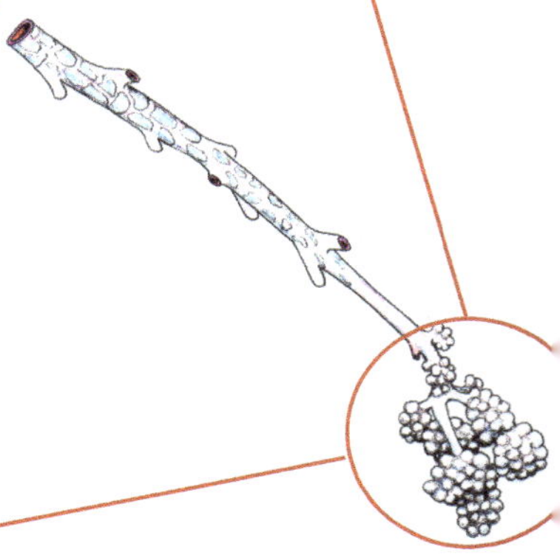

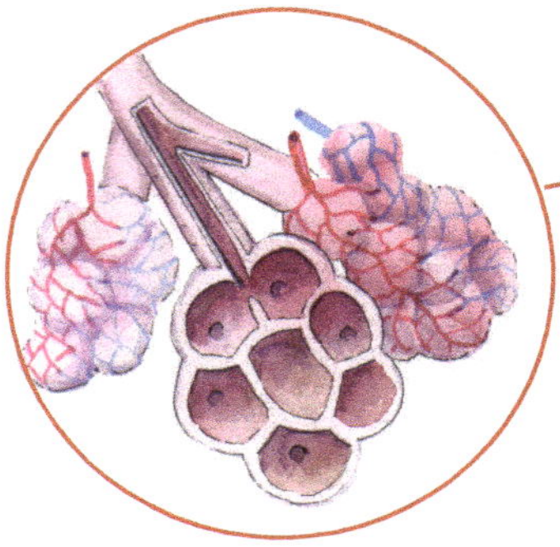

MUCOCILIARY ESCALATOR
This remarkable structure faithfully keeps our airways clean during the approximately 600 million breaths that each of us takes in our lifetime.

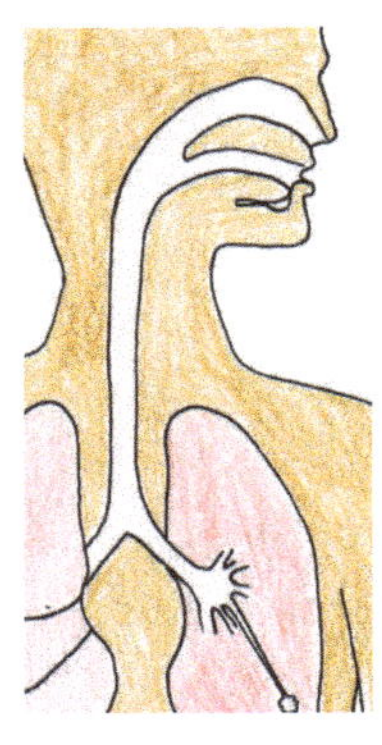

DEAD AIR SPACE
The space occupied by air in the oropharynx, nasopharynx, trachea, bronchi, and bronchioles (approximately150ml) is dead air space where no gas exchange takes place. Therefore, you must move at least 150ml of air for fresh air to reach the alveoli—where the oxygen (O_2) and carbon dioxide (CO_2) exchange occurs.

Only when air reaches here—the alveoli—is O_2 transferred to the blood and CO_2, removed.

Asthma

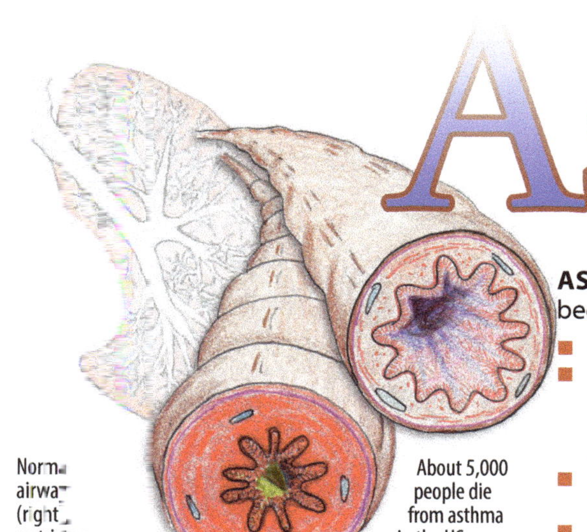

ASTHMA AND OTHER RAD DISEASES occur when the airways become narrowed, causing a restriction of airflow.

- Asthma is recurrent and reversible with medication.
- Allergens in the airway cause swelling (bronchospasm) and increased mucous production, especially noted in the terminal bronchioles, which narrow before entering the alveoli, causing air to be trapped in the alveoli.
- When the air is trapped, the patient can inhale but cannot exhale, resulting in worsening shortness of breath (SOB).
- Asthma affects approximately 9% of the US population.
- Asthma accounts for about 25% of all emergency room visits per year in the US, or about 2 million visits per year (5000[+/-] deaths)

SIGNS AND SYMPTOMS

- Coughing
- Shortness of breath
- The patient has difficulty speaking: word dyspnea—the patient is unable to count to ten on one breath
- Expiratory wheezing—audible initially with auscultation
- Tripoding—the patient sits up and leans forward with their arms braced out in front to facilitate the use of their accessory muscles to aid in respiration
- Hyperinflation of the chest
- Cyanosis
- Shock
- Status asthmaticus—an asthma attack that won't stop; may be life-threatening

ASSESSMENT OF SEVERITY

Stage 1: Minor
- Sensation of shortness of breath
- No word dyspnea; the patient can count to 10 in one breath
- Little or no wheezing

Stage 2: Moderate
- Shortness of breath and wheezing
- Word dyspnea; the patient can count between 6 – 9 words in one breath
- Air trapping, and expiratory wheezing

Stage 3: Severe
- Rapid shallow respirations
- Anxiety, and tripoding
- Word dyspnea—the patient can only count to 5
- Air trapping, rapid, shallow breathing
- Cyanosis
- Faint wheezing or no wheezing at all (not moving enough air to wheeze)
- Hyperinflation of the chest
- Shock
- Status asthmaticus

TREATMENT

1. Calm the patient, and remain calm yourself.
2. Place the patient in position of comfort (usually sitting or semi-sitting).
3. Take a good history—find out which medications, if any, the patient has taken.
4. Encourage pursed-lip breathing to create back-pressure and open the bronchioles.
5. If the patient has a rescue metered dose inhaler (MDI) albuterol or Xopenex, you can assist them in using it.
6. You can give the patient some relief and improve their breathing by gently helping them to exhale. This is an old-fashioned technique that was used before the days of the modern bronchodilator medications.
   - Have the asthmatic patient lie down and place your hands on the sides of their rib cage.
   - As they exhale, gently compress the chest wall. This helps to force out some of the air trapped distal to the bronchoconstriction.
   - As they inhale, hold the chest wall compressed.
   - Maintain compression as they exhale and inhale through a total of three cycles.
   - After the third cycle, gently release the chest wall and allow them to take a deep breath.
   - This can be repeated as often as needed to aid in forcing out the trapped air and improving the depth of respirations.
7. Consider evacuation.
8. In the backcountry—use epinephrine for status asthmaticus, and always evacuate.

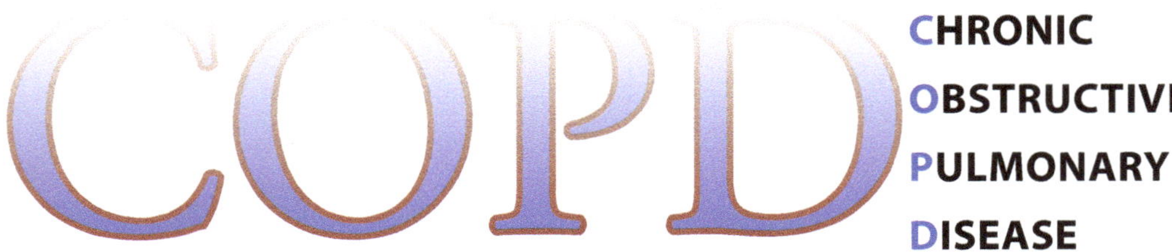

COPD

CHRONIC
OBSTRUCTIVE
PULMONARY
DISEASE

OBSTRUCTIVE AIRWAY DISEASES ARE IRREVERSIBLE because they destroy the alveoli, which decreases the available surface area for oxygen exchange. COPD refers to a group of lung diseases that restrict airflow and cause shortness of breath.

- The combination of emphysema and chronic bronchitis is the most common cause of COPD (asthma may also contribute).
- It is chronic, progressive, and irreversible—but symptoms can be controlled and minimized with medication, including supplemental O_2.
- It is commonly found in patients with a history of cigarette smoking.

EMPHYSEMA
DESCRIPTION

- This disease is characterized by deterioration of the alveolar walls, leading to decreased surface area for gas exchange.
- It is caused by smoking, smoke inhalation, or inhalation of lung irritants.
- The alveolar damage is irreversible.
- Smoking cessation or avoiding lung irritants can arrest the destructive process.
- If the destruction of the alveolar walls continues, eventually patients with emphysema will not have enough surface area for gas exchange and will have to live on supplemental oxygen—they will have to live with a nasal cannula in their nose to increase the concentration of O_2 above the 20% concentration in the air. Each additional liter (per minute) of O_2 adds 4% O_2.
- Anything that further compromises surface area, such as bronchitis, pneumonia, or pulmonary edema, will exacerbate a patient's symptoms and increase demand for supplemental O_2.

EMPHYSEMA *SIGNS AND SYMPTOMS*
- Weight loss
- Dyspnea on exertion
- Barrel chest

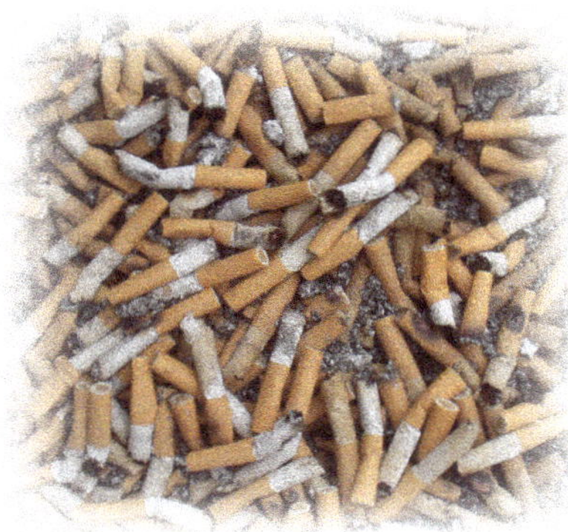
Intentionally pulling tobacco smoke into your lungs is a major cause/contributor to many major ailments (e.g., various cancers).

CHRONIC BRONCHITIS
DESCRIPTION

- This is a disease of the mucosa of the lower airway characterized by excessive mucus production.
- It is chronic when it occurs more than three months a year and has been going on for two years or more.

CHRONIC BRONCHITIS
SIGNS AND SYMPTOMS

Dyspnea on exertion
- Pulmonary edema
- Wheezing
- Associated heart disease (in some cases)

COPD CRISIS
DESCRIPTION

- This is a flare-up or exacerbation of a pre-existing COPD condition.

COPD CRISIS *SIGNS AND SYMPTOMS*

Increasing dyspnea, which may include paroxysmal nocturnal dyspnea—shortness of breath that comes on at night when a patient lies down to sleep and which forces them to get up to breathe

- Altered Level of Consciousness (LOC)—confusion, lethargy, combativeness, agitation
- Cyanosis
- Tripoding to allow use of accessory muscles in breathing
- Change in color of sputum from white to green or brown, which may indicate underlying bronchitis or pneumonia
- Cardiac dysrhythmias

COPD CRISIS *TREATMENT*

Place the patient in the position of comfort—usually sitting up.

ABDOMINAL PAIN
Acute abdomen

This term refers to the sudden onset of severe abdominal pain without clear cause that is less than 24 hours in duration. The most common cause of gut-wrenching pain and discomfort is constipation or spoiled food—but there are several <u>other causes</u>* that feel just as bad but are much worse, so much worse, in fact, that you better take them really seriously. This can be a true medical emergency requiring quick and accurate diagnosis, and the patient may need surgery.

ETIOLOGIES

Constipation: by far the most common cause of abdominal pain and discomfort

Food poisoning: also very common, associated with vomiting and diarrhea

Gynecological: menstrual cramps or ectopic pregnancy

* **Obstructions:** gallstones, kidney stones, or intestinal blockage

* **Infection:** peritonitis from an acute appendicitis or cholecystitis (infected gallbladder)

* **Bleeding or perforations:** a bleeding ulcer or diverticulitis, a puncture wound or a ruptured organ from blunt trauma

* **Ruptures:** acute aortic aneurysm, ruptured appendix or gallbladder

SIGNS AND SYMPTOMS

Location: Where is the pain? Generalized or localized?

O **Onset:** Did the pain come on quickly or slowly?

P **Palliates/Provokes:** What makes the pain lessen; what makes it worse?

Q **Quality/Quantity:** What does the pain feel like: sharp, dull, stabbing, crampy? How bad is the pain, 0 – 10? (0 is no pain; 10 is the worst pain the patient has ever experienced)?

R **Radiation:** Does the pain radiate anywhere?

S **Severity:** When the pain comes on, how long does it last? How frequently does the pain occur?

T **Time:** How long has the pain been happening?

Last in/Last out: When did the patient last eat? When was their last bowel movement?

Appearance: What is their general appearance? Are they diaphoretic (sweating) or feverish?

POC: What is their position of comfort?

Shock: Do they show the signs: pale, cool, and clammy skin, rapid and weak pulse, nausea, diminished LOC? Is there nausea, **vomiting, or constipation**?

Do they have **fever or chills**?

Are there signs of **internal bleeding:** blood in vomitus, stool, or urine, rigidity or guarding?

Is there **bruising** (may indicate organ trauma)?

EXAMINATION

1. Listen for bowel sounds.
2. Gently palpate all four quadrants, noting rigidity, tenderness, or distension—palpate the quadrant of complaint last (see graphic in abdo trauma sector).
3. Look for bruises on abdomen—especially discoloration (ecchymosis) around the umbilicus (belly button) or flanks.

TREATMENT

1. Place patient in a position of comfort.
2. Treat for shock from suspected internal bleeding
3. Give nothing by mouth (NPO).
4. Clear fluids are okay if the evacuation will be long.
5. Handle gently.
6. Evacuate.
7. The general rule is: appetite + bowel sounds = no surgical abdomen.

SPECIFIC SIGNS AND HELPFUL HINTS

If the patient has an appetite and bowel sounds, this is not a surgical abdomen.

Constipation: colicky, cramping pain that comes and goes, typically builds in intensity and then relaxes and diminishes

Peritonitis: patients typically have rebound tenderness that localizes to the lower right quadrant, where the appendix is located—we diagnose the patient with peritonitis, and the surgeon makes the final diagnosis of the source of the infection (e.g., appendicitis)

Cholecystitis: acute cholesystitis is an infected gallbladder caused by gallstones. These patients will have what is referred to as Murphy's Sign. To check the gallbladder, you ask the patient to exhale. As they do, you gently compress the right upper quadrant and hold or continue to push in and ask them to inhale. If the gallbladder is infected or inflamed, intense pain will occur as they attempt to inhale, and they will not be able to inhale until you release the pressure. This is a positive Murphy's Sign indicating cholecystitis—gallbladder disease.

Nausea and vomiting

Two of the most common symptoms associated with illness and stress are nausea and vomiting. Nausea is that vague uneasy sensation that you are going to vomit. Vomiting is the action by which the stomach contents are expelled out of the mouth.

The causes of nausea and vomiting are many and include infections, viruses, food poisoning, appendicitis, and peritonitis, as well as motion sickness, intestinal blockage, concussion, migraines, and anxiety. The symptoms can also indicate very serious life-threatening illnesses such as a heart attack, meningitis, encephalitis, kidney disease, liver disease, brain tumors, or cancer.

The sensation of nausea and the action of vomiting are controlled by the vomiting center in the brain, the area postrema. The area postrema receives signals from four locales around the body—three are in the gastrointestinal tract: the mouth, stomach, and intestines. These react to taste as well as toxins in food, which can cause food poisoning. The fourth locale is the brain, which constantly monitors the bloodstream for the chemicals of infections as well as certain medications that can cause nausea and vomiting.

The vestibular (balance) apparatus in the ears, when out of kilter, can also cause dizziness, nausea, and vomiting. And the brain can even induce nausea and vomiting from unpleasant sights, smells, and even thoughts.

Nausea and vomiting are symptoms of an underlying problem. Fortunately, the problem is usually benign and self-limiting.

The primary concerns are the risks of dehydration from not drinking enough, and electrolyte depletion from vomiting. If associated with diarrhea, the loss of electrolytes becomes an even greater risk.

PRINCIPLES OF MANAGING NAUSEA AND VOMITING

1. Try to prevent dehydration by taking small sips of a clear fluid often (ginger ale, fruit juices, or electrolyte drinks like Gatorade). This is preferred to drinking a larger volume less frequently because an upset stomach will only tolerate small amounts of fluid. Cold fluids are tolerated better than hot fluids.
2. Herbal remedies: Solutions of a ginger, peppermint, or chamomile tea will help to control nausea.
3. Over-the-counter (OTC) medications:
   - Pepto-Bismol® (bismuth subsalicylate) will help to calm the stomach and control diarrhea. Pepto-Bismol® cannot be used in someone who is allergic to aspirin. It should not be used in children and teenagers younger than 18-years-old if there is a chance that the illness is associated with viral influenza or chickenpox due to the risk of Reye's Syndrome, a left-threatening encephalopathy.
   - OTC antihistamines such as dimenhydrinate, diphenhydramine, and meclizine may help with nausea and vomiting caused by motion sickness.
4. Prescription drugs for nausea and vomiting:
   - A variety of medications for nausea and vomiting are used depending on the underlying diagnosis and cause. Two of the most common drugs for treating nausea and vomiting are phenergan and compazine. Both are available as suppositories so they will not contribute to the problem of nausea.
     → Phenergan (promethazine) suppository 25mg, one per rectum every 12 hours as needed for nausea and vomiting.
     → Compazine (prochlorperazine) suppository 5mg, one per rectum every 12 hours as needed for nausea and vomiting.
5. Once the patient is feeling better and their appetite has returned, advance the diet slowly with small quantities of bland food, such as the BRAT diet—Bananas, Rice, Applesauce, and Toast. Avoid greasy, hard-to-digest foods for 24 hours.
6. When to seek help:
   - Although nausea and vomiting are typically benign and self-correcting, you should seek help if they are associated with:
     → A fever greater than 102.5°F/39°C
     → A change (deterioration) in level of consciousness
     → Seizure activity
     → Bright red blood or digested blood (the latter looks like coffee grounds) in the vomitus
     → Vomiting that is frequent and copious and causes the patient to become progressively dehydrated
     → Symptoms lasting more than 24 hours that are not easily controlled

157

IMMEDIATE EVACUATION

Seek outside medical assistance immediately if they have abdominal pain **plus** any one of the following . . .

- S/S of shock
  - Rapid, weak pulse
  - Rapid, shallow, respirations
  - Pale, cool, clammy skin
  - Delayed capillary refill

- Rebound tenderness on physical exam

- The abdominal wall is rigid and tender to deep palpation

- They have obvious distention and tenderness of the abdomen

- They have blood in their vomitus

- They have blood in their stool (bright red blood or black tarry stools)

- High-volume watery diarrhea

- A fever greater than 103°F (40°C) with shaking rigors

- They are pregnant, with abdominal pain

CONSIDER EVACUATION

Consider evacuation if they have abdominal pain **plus** . . .

- The pain has lasted, without improvement, for more than 24 hours

- The pain suddenly increases in intensity over several hours

- The pain has gone from generalized to localized

- Vomiting has lasted for more than 24 hours

- Diarrhea has lasted, without improvement, for more than 24 hours

DURING EVACUATION

Care while seeking medical assistance

- Handle the patient gently and transport the patient in the position of comfort

- Do not give them anything to eat or drink unless they are dehydrated

- If dehydrated, give them frequent small sips of clear fluids as tolerated

- Treat them for shock if necessary

- May control a high fever, temperature above 104°F (40°C), by using tepid water sponge baths

FIELD TREATMENT

If evacuation and outside medical assistance is not needed . . .

- Allow them to rest in a position of comfort

- Complete stomach rest—nothing by mouth for 2 hours

- After 2 hours, give small amounts of clear liquids every 10 – 15 minutes

- If tolerating fluids well, may slowly increase for the next 24 hours

- Do not feed them until they develop an appetite—once they have an appetite advance their diet slowly, with bland, easy-to-digest food—the BRAT diet (bananas, rice, applesauce, toast, etc. for the next 24 hours

- Evacuate if symptoms worsen

Right Upper Quadrant – RUQ:
Liver
Gallbladder
Right Kidney and Ureter
Small Intestine
Large Intestine
Pancreas (midline – in both the LUQ and RUQ)
Stomach (midline – in both the LUQ and RUQ)
Aorta (midline)
Inferior Vena Cava (midline)

Left Upper Quadrant – LUQ:
Spleen
Left Kidney and Ureter
Small Intestine
Large Intestine
Pancreas (midline)
Stomach (midline)
Aorta (midline)
Inferior Vena Cava (midline)

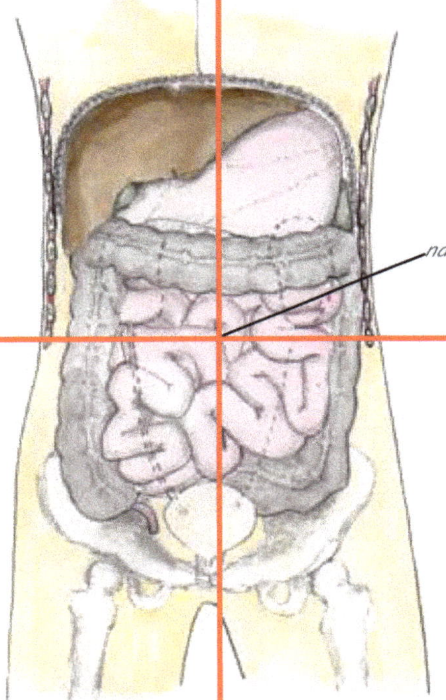

Right Lower Quadrant – RLQ:
Small Intestine
Large Intestine
Appendix
Right Ovary
Bladder (midline)
Uterus (midline)

Left Lower Quadrant – LLQ:
Small Intestine
Large Intestine and Sigmoid Colon
Left Ovary
Bladder (midline)
Uterus (midline)

158

BEHAVIORAL EMERGENCIES

BEHAVIORAL EMERGENCIES: THE BIG FOUR

MAJOR DEPRESSIVE DISORDER (MDD)

A pervasive and persistent low mood that is accompanied by low self-esteem and a loss of interest or pleasure in normally enjoyable activities.

Clinical presentation

A person's current mood and thought content, in particular, the presence of themes of hopelessness or pessimism, self-harm or suicide, and an absence of positive thoughts or plans.

Treatment

1. Evaluate the patient's risk to themselves or others.
2. If there is a belief or an actual attempt at suicide, transport the patient immediately for evaluation.
3. If the patient is an adult that is A+Ox3, and they do not want to go to the hospital, remember that the police are a useful resource in the urban environment.

SCHIZOPHRENIA

Characterized by a breakdown in thinking and poor emotional responses.

Clinical presentation

Common symptoms include delusions, such as the feeling that someone is out to get you; seeing things that are not there; disorganized thinking; a lack of emotion and a lack of motivation.

Treatment

1. Reassure the patient.
2. Attempt to determine the cause of the emergency.
3. If it is a true behavioral emergency, transport immediately.

ACUTE STRESS REACTION

Occurs immediately after an emotionally traumatic incident.

Clinical presentation

Dyspnea, anxiety, irritability, nausea, guilt, isolation, and loss of concentration, appetite, interest in life, and carpal/pedal spasms

Treatment

1. Keep the patient calm.
2. Place the patient in the Fowler's position.
3. Transport if necessary or if you are unable to control the patient.

DELIRIUM TREMENS

An acute episode of delirium (severe confusion and disorientation) that is usually caused by withdrawal from alcohol.

Clinical presentation

Nightmares, agitation, global confusion, disorientation, visual and auditory hallucinations, fever, hypertension, diaphoresis, and tachycardia

Treatment

1. Keep the patient calm.
2. Transport for further care and evaluation.

Use caution with all behavioral problems— the patient may become violent!

POISON

Poisoning ranks second to motor vehicle accidents as a cause of unintentional injury death in the US—and among people 25 to 64 it is the leading cause of death (with over 90% of cases involving drugs).

General treatment

1. Verify that the scene is safe—especially important in cases of airborne poisons, e.g., CO_2, CO, cyanide, methane, chlorine, sarin, soman.
2. Identify the poison—what was the substance?
3. Identify the exposure method:
   - Ingested
   - Inhaled
   - Airborne
   - Injected
4. Identify the time of the poisoning:
   - When were they exposed?
   - How long have they been exposed?
5. Identify the dose:
   - How much were they exposed to?
   - How much did they take?
6. Determine the patient's last food and drink:
   - What did they last eat or drink?
   - How much did they last eat or drink?
   - When did they last eat or drink?
7. Find out if alcohol or drugs was involved.
8. Get a physical description:
   - Gender
   - Age
   - Size (obese?)
9. Determine the cause:
   - Was the poisoning accidental or deliberate?
   - Was it a suicide attempt?
10. Call the emergency department and give them all the information.
11. Call the poison control center and give them all the information.
12. Follow their instructions until help arrives.

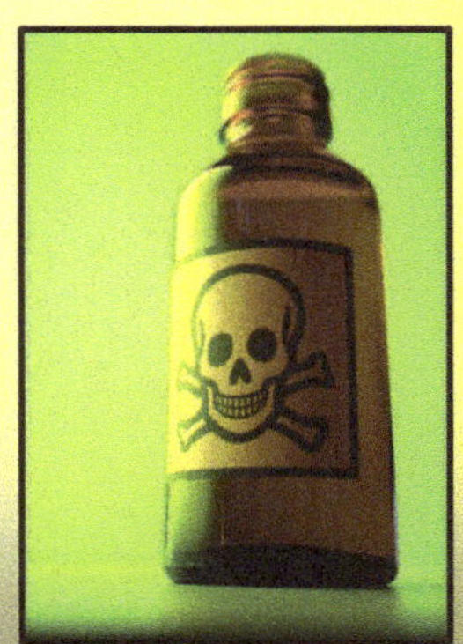

INGESTED (most common)

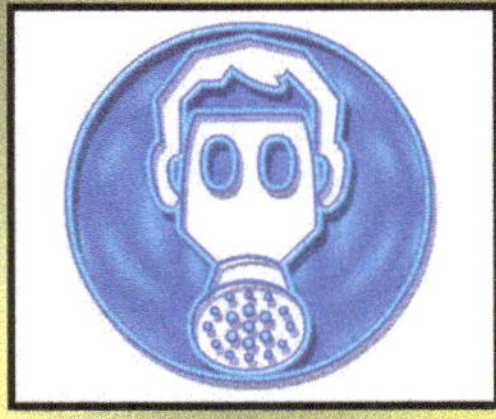

INHALED (airborne)

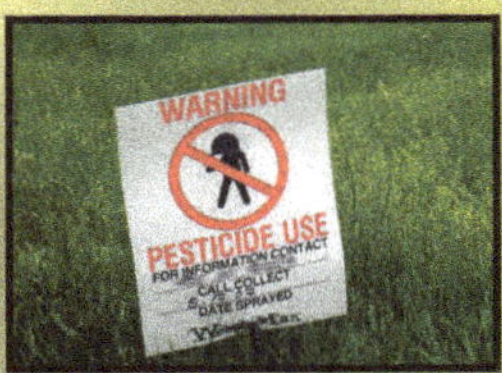

ABSORBED (skin)

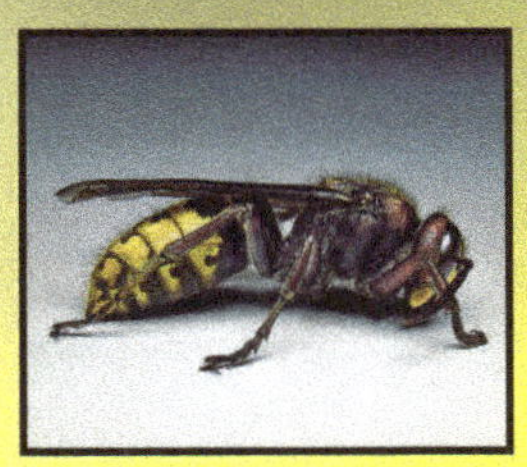

INJECTED (envenomation/needle)

Specific Treatment

INGESTED Drugs are most common.

1. Activated charcoal is the preferred treatment. It comes pre-mixed. Typical dose is 25 – 50ml.
2. Dilute the poison with water or milk.

INHALED e.g., CO_2, CO (most common, methane, chlorine, cyanide.

1. Ensure scene safety.
2. Remove the patient from the exposure
3. Administer high-flow O_2 via non-rebreather or positive-pressure ventilations.

ABSORBED e.g., organophosphates, DEET

This can be a HAZMAT scene—be especially aware of pesticides. **SLUDGEM** (mnemonic for nerve agent poisoning: salivation, lacrimation, urination, defecation, gastrointestinal upset, emesis, miosis)

1. Ensure scene safety.
2. Remove the poison.
3. Remove any contaminated clothing.
4. Immediately decontaminate the patient with soap and water.

INJECTED e.g., reptile/insect envenomations (see Bites & Stings), drug overdose

1. Scrub and clean any obvious wounds.
2. Lightly wrap the wound site proximally with an elastic bandage.
3. Immobilize the extremity.
4. Monitor for signs of anaphylaxis and be prepared to treat it.

Group Preventative Medicine

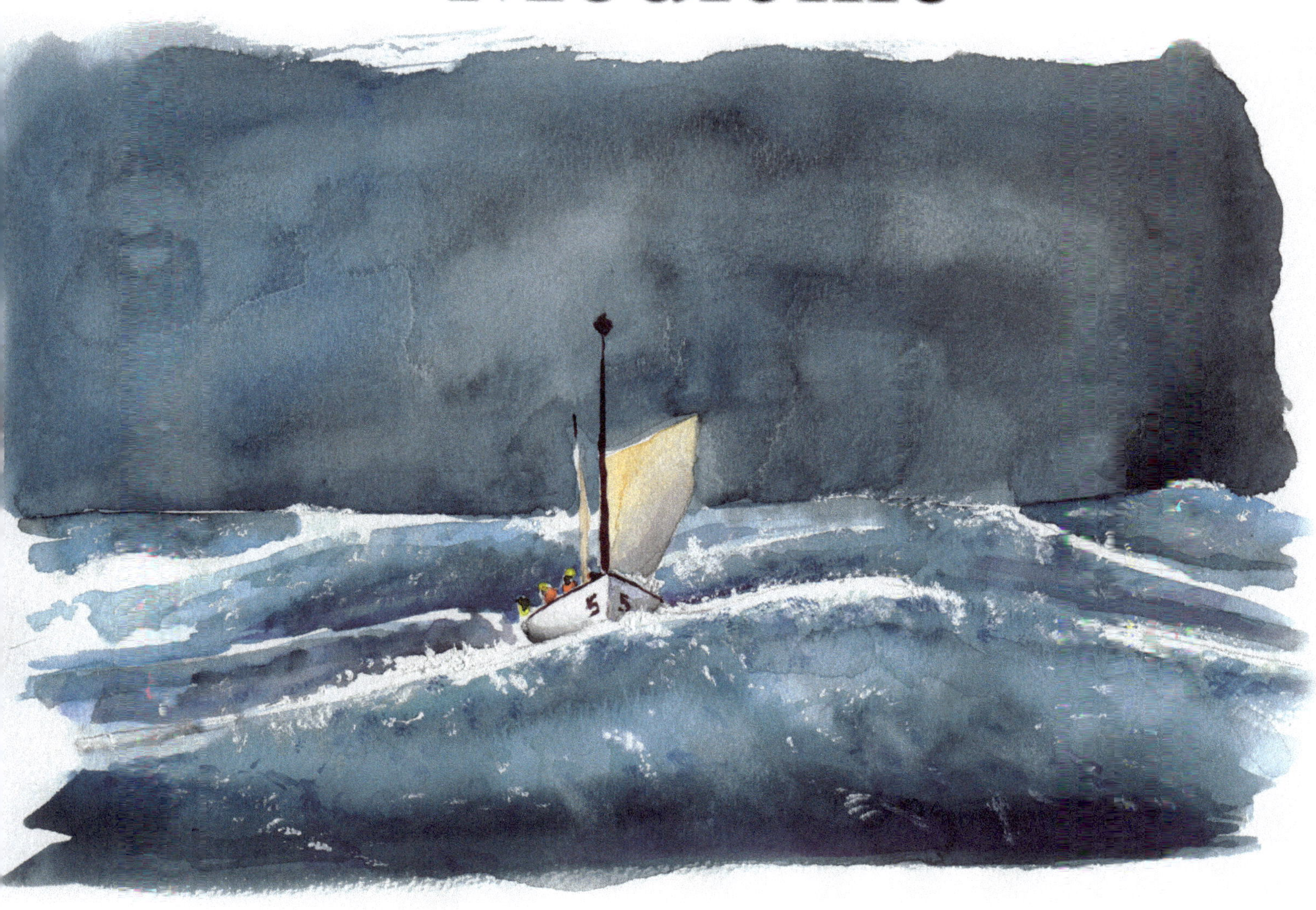

WATER PURIFICATION

WATERBORNE DISEASES ARE SOME OF THE MOST COMMON DISEASES known to man. They are spread primarily via the oral-fecal route when a pathogen in human or animal waste contaminates the drinking water supply. The disease-causing pathogen is transmitted to people when they drink the water, consume food that was washed in the contaminated water or handled by dirty hands that prepared the food, or by washing their own hands in the contaminated water.

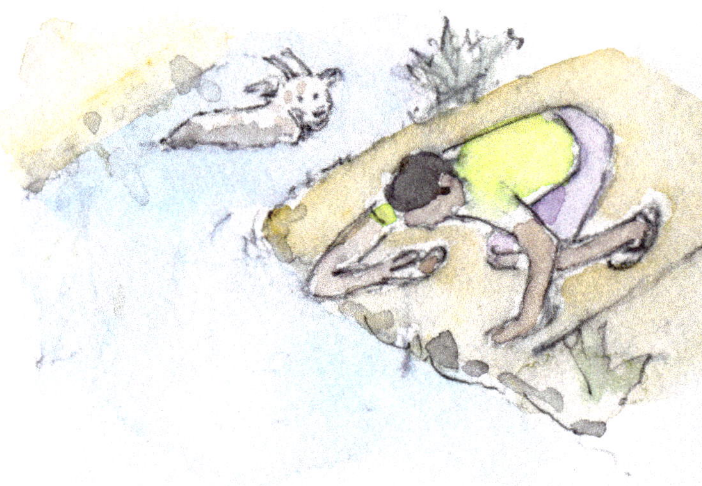

Most waterborne illnesses affect the gastrointestinal tract and present as an upset stomach, gas, bloating, abdominal cramping, fever, chills, and most importantly, diarrhea.

PRECAUTIONS

- Only consume potable water.
- Sterilize your water.
- Properly wash vegetables.
- In developing countries:
  - ☑ Avoid ice cubes—freezing won't kill all the little nasties. And no, alcohol (as in a mixed drink) will not kill the organisms in a melting ice cube.
  - ☑ Make sure that bottle water still has the factory seal—it is not uncommon for bottled water bottles to be refilled with tainted local tap water.
  - ☑ Canned drinks are always safe—they have been pasteurized.
- Wash your hands frequently—carry hand sanitizer and use it frequently.
- Swimming
  - ☑ Swimming in contaminated water is dangerous, and there is almost no way to protect yourself from bacteria and viruses.
  - ☑ If in doubt, don't take the plunge—err on the dry side.

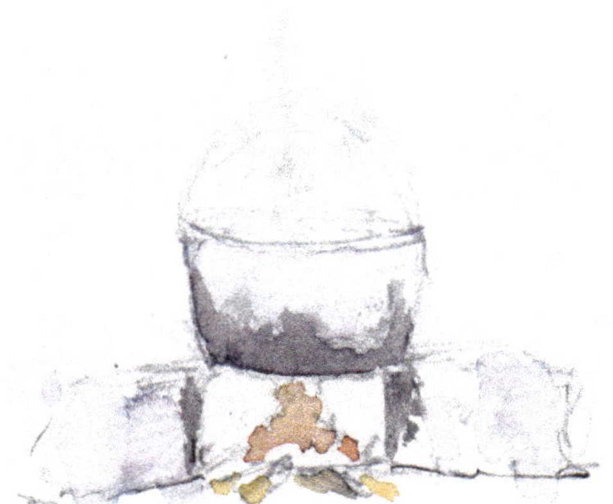

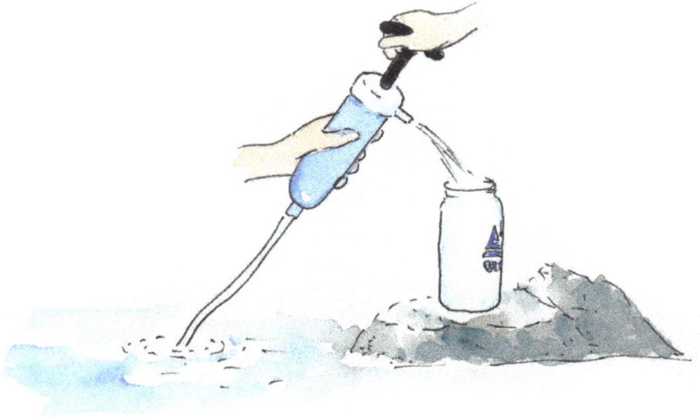

METHOD	CONSIDERATIONS	ADVANTAGES	DISADVANTAGES
BOILING	■ Rolling boil kills all disease-causing pathogens. ■ Below 8,000 feet, bringing water to a rolling boil is sufficient. ■ Above 8,000 feet, boil water for several minutes.	■ It is absolutely reliable. ■ You can see it working. ■ No precision is needed—when the water has boiled for the appropriate amount of time (see above), it's sterile.	■ It requires fuel/fire or a stove. ■ It takes time and effort. ■ You end up with hot water.
CHEMICALS (iodine and chlorine)	■ Iodine or chlorine, when added to water in appropriate quantities, are very effective disinfectants. ■ Effectiveness requires proper contact time—the chemical has to be in the water long enough to work (30 minutes minimum, 60 minutes for dirty, very cold, or very acidic water). ■ Reducing the amount of debris in the water before adding chemicals makes the chemicals more effective. ■ Dosages vary depending on chemical and water volume. ■ The cap and threads must be treated, too!	■ Both are readily available, cheap, lightweight, and safe. ■ Chlorine bleach is available just about everywhere in the world. ■ Easy to use—just add to your water and wait. ■ Small amounts are needed (as tablets, crystals, or drops).	■ Iodine should not be used by people with thyroid disease or if they are allergic to it. ■ You must wait 30 – 60 minutes. ■ The chemicals can make the treated water taste unpleasant: drink-mix crystals can help; also, dissolving a vitamin C tablet will neutralize the bad taste—flavor the water after the sterilization time is over.
FILTRATION	■ Filtration is very effective; bacteria and protozoa are easily strained out (they are relatively big) ■ Filtration alone is not effective against viruses—they are too small. ■ Multi-stage filters will also kill viruses : 1st stage filters sediment, 2nd stage kills bacteria and protozoa, 3rd stage uses iodine to kill viruses, 4th stage (optional) uses activated charcoal to remove aftertaste.	■ Convenient and easy to use: simply pump or use a gravity feed. ■ Speed: you don't have to wait—pump and you're done. ■ No unpleasant aftertaste.	■ Can be heavy and expensive. ■ Unless multi-stage, will not filter out viruses—chemical treatment may be required after filtration. ■ Undetected defects (e.g., a cracked filter) can compromise effectiveness without your knowledge. ■ Filters can become plugged. ■ Maintenance (both at home and in the field) required. ■ Not suitable for large groups. ■ With multistage filters, it can be hard to tell when the chemical has run out.
UV LIGHT	■ Uses UVS (ultraviolet-C, short wave, or germicidal) light to kill everything. ■ Water must be clear: turbid water will not be treated effectively so must be filtered first.	■ Easy to use and effective. ■ Fast: typically less than two minutes for a liter of water.	■ Although its effectiveness against bacteria and protozoa (e.g., giardia) is high, some resistant viruses require much higher dosages (10 – 30 times). ■ Requires batteries. ■ Relatively expensive. ■ Not suitable for groups.
ELECTROLYSIS	■ Uses electricity to convert salt and water into a powerful disinfectant.	■ Destroys viruses , bacteria, and giardia in 30 minutes, cryptosporidium (protozoa) in 4 hours. ■ Compact, rugged, submersible. ■ Safety indicator shows when water is safe. ■ No health risks or unpleasant aftertaste.	■ Requires batteries. ■ Relatively expensive.

COMMON EXPEDITION PROBLEMS

From a survey of outdoor programs

ALLERGIES
- Remove the problem, or remove the patient from the problem.
- Use specific allergy medications if patient has them.
- Know how to identify and treat anaphylaxis.

BLISTERS
- Prevent first with correct sock/boot combination.
- It's best if blisters can heal by themselves, but they are difficult to hike on.
- To prevent surface skin from tearing, draining is recommended.
- Make a small pinhole at the base.
- Cover the area with a moleskin doughnut, lubricating the layer inside the hole; cover entire area with moleskin, tape, etc.
- Use tincture of benzoin to help adhere the bandage to the skin; it's very sticky and it toughens skin.

BURNS
- Remove the source; cool for 15 – 20 minutes.
- You may need to remove charred clothing or other burnt material from wound.
- Cover 1st and 2nd degree burns with moist, sterile dressing.
- Cover 3rd degree burns with a dry, sterile dressing.
- Keep the patient hydrated.
- Monitor for shock, dehydration, and infection.

COLDS/COUGH
- Probably related to allergies or adjusting to different environment.
- Treat with allergy medication and rest.
- Keep hydrated.

CONTACT DERMATITIS
- Poison ivy/oak/sumac skin allergies.
- Wash area with cool water and soft, mild soap.
- Sores are not contagious once the oil has been washed from the area.
- Severe reactions may need additional drugs.
- May need to evacuate.

DEHYDRATION
- Prevent.
- Rehydrate.
- Drink a lot.
- Drink often.

DIARRHEA
- The body is trying to flush out whatever the cause of the problem—help it.
- Keep the patient well-hydrated.
- Watch for nausea, fever, vomiting, etc.
- Patient can be given rice water or an over-the-counter medication such as Pepto-Bismol® or Imodium.
- Electrolytes will be lost and must be replaced (ORS, etc.).

FROSTBITE
- Prevention is best.
- Skin-to-skin rewarming for 1st and 2nd degree frostbite.
- Leave third degree frostbite frozen.
- Do not field rewarm.
- Insulate to prevent further freezing.
- Evacuate.

HEADACHE
- Probably associated with dehydration.
- Try rehydration before drugs.
- Follow local protocols.

INSECT BITES
- Protect with clothing and insecticides/repellents.
- Use topical itch cream on bites.
- Know how to recognize and treat anaphylaxis.

HEAT EXHAUSTION
- Prevention is easy.
- Don't overexert yourself, especially in hot/humid weather.
- Rest before you get overheated.
- Eat and drink enough (both quantity and frequency).
- Supplement plain water with beverages such as Gatorade, which help replenish electrolytes.
- Mild cases are relatively common.
- Can progress to heat stroke (which is life-threatening— please refer to the heat stroke section).

MINOR FRACTURES

- Splint and evacuate.

MINOR HYPOTHERMIA

- Remove the patient from environment.
- Get wet stuff off and put dry stuff on.
- Stoke the fire with warm, sweet liquids.
- Encourage light exercise if the patient feels up to it and the weather allows.
- Apply heat packs to the core and specific chilled areas.

MINOR MUSCULOSKELETAL INJURIES: STRAINS AND SPRAINS

- RICE
- Remove boot if it's an ankle sprain.
- Apply cold for 20 – 30 minutes.
- Rewarm to normal body temperature.
- Test it—have the patient try to use it.
- Splint it if necessary.

MINOR SOFT TISSUE INJURIES

- Stop the bleeding.
- Prevent infection.
- Promote healing.

OBJECTS IN THE EYE

- Flush the eye thoroughly with clean water.
- Check for eye injuries.
- If a bandage is necessary, bandage both eyes to avoid sympathetic movement in the uninjured eye.
- Leave a pinhole in the uninjured eye so the patient can walk on their own.
- Do not remove objects impaled in the eye.
- Immobilize the object with a doughnut bandage.
- Evacuate.

RASHES: ATHLETE'S FOOT, JOCK ITCH

- Wash the area.
- Keep the area clean and dry.
- Use powder if available.

SMALL IMPALED OBJECTS

- Remove them.
- Wash area thoroughly with soap and water.
- Monitor for infection.

SUNBURN

- Prevention is best.
- Wear clothing that protects the arms, legs, neck, and head.
- Limit sun exposure, especially in the middle of the day.
- Use sunscreen with a minimum SPF of 15 (50 is overkill).

URINARY TRACT INFECTIONS

- More prevalent in women.
- Potentially severe if the infection travels to the kidney.
- Painful, burning, frequent urination.
- There may be blood in urine.
- Keep well-hydrated.
- Drink cranberry juice to offset pH in bladder.
- Evacuate the patient, as antibiotics will most likely be required.

VAGINITIS

- Itchy, painful inflammation with possible discharge.
- Caused by bacteria, yeast or parasite.

ACRONYMS

(S)AMPLE	Signs/Symptoms, Allergies, Medications, Past Pertinent History, Last Oral Intake, Events
a&O	Alert and Oriented
a&O x 1	Alert and Oriented times one (person)
a&O x 2	Alert and Oriented times two (person, place)
a&O x 3	Alert and Oriented times three (person, place, time)
a&O x 4	Alert and Oriented times four (person, place, time, events)
AAA	Abdominal Aortic Aneurysm
ABCDE	Airway, Breathing, Circulation, Disability, Environment/Exposure
ADL	Activities of Daily Living
AED	Automated External Defibrillator
AEIOU TIPS	Acidosis (or alcohol), Epilepsy, Infection, Overdose, Uremia, Trauma, Insulin, Psychosis, Stroke
AEMT	Advanced Emergency Medical Technician
AGE	Arterial Gas Embolism
AHA	American Heart Association
ALOC	Altered Level of Consciousness
ALS	Advanced Life Support
AMI	Acute Myocardial Infarction
AMS	Acute Mountain Sickness
APGAR	Appearance, Pulse, Grimace, Activity, Respiration
ART	Attitude, Resources, Techniques
ASAP	As Soon As Possible
ASTM	American Society for the Testing of Materials
AV	Atrioventricular Node
AVPU	Alert, Verbal, Pain, Unresponsive
BEAM	Body, Elevation, And Movement
BID	Twice a Day
BLS	Basic Life Support
BP	Blood Pressure
BSA	Body Surface Area
BSI	Body Substance Isolation
BUFF	Big, Ugly, Fat, Fluffy
BVM	Bag Valve Mask
C/C	Chief Complaint
CDC	Centers for Disease Control and Prevention
CHF	Congestive Heart Failure
CISD	Critical Incident Stress Debriefing
CNS	Central Nervous System
C/O	Complaining Of
COPD	Chronic Obstructive Pulmonary Disease
CP	Command Post
CPR	Cardiopulmonary Resuscitation
CSF	Cerebral Spinal Fluid
CSM	Circulation, Sensation, and Motion
CVA	Cerebrovascular Accident
CVD	Cardiovascular Disease
CVS	Cardiovascular System
DEET	Diethyltoluamide
DNR	Do Not Resuscitate
DO	Doctor of Osteopathy
DOA	Dead On Arrival
DOT	Department of Transportation
DRT	Dead Right There
DT	Diphtheria & Tetanus Booster
DTs	Delirium Tremens
ECG	Electrocardiogram
ED	Emergency Department
EGTA	Esophageal Gastric Tube Airway
EKG	Electro-cardiogram (also ECG)
EMR	Emergency Medical Responder (the street term for FR)
EMS	Emergency Medical Services
EMT	Emergency Medical Technician
EOA	Esophageal Obturator Airway
ER	Emergency Room
ETA	Estimated Time of Arrival
ET	Endotracheal Tube
ETOH	Alcohol
FAST	Face, arms/legs, speech, time
FBLP	Full Bore Linear Panic
FBAO	Foreign Body Airway Obstruction
FEMA	Federal Emergency Management Agency
FOAM	Free of Any Movement
FR	First Responder (see EMR)
FUS	Fat Ugly Splint
Fx	Fracture
GI	Gastrointestinal
H7	Hypothermia, Hyperthermia, Hypoglycemia, Hyperglycemia, Hypoxia, Hypovolemia, Head Injury
HAC	High-Altitude Cachexia (extreme weight loss)
HACE	High-Altitude Cerebral Edema
HAFE	High-Altitude Flatulent Expulsion
HAPE	High-Altitude Pulmonary Edema
HARH	High-Altitude Retinal Hemorrhage
HAV	Hepatitis A Virus
HAZMAT	Hazardous Materials
HBV	Hepatitis B Virus
HIV	Human Immunodeficiency Virus
HMO	Health Maintenance Organization
HPI	History of Present Illness
HR	Heart Rate
HTN	Hypertension
Hx	History
IC	Incident Commander
ICP	Intracranial Pressure
ICS	Incident Command System
ICU	Intensive Care Unit
IM	Immediate Treatment
IV	Intravenous
JVD	Jugular Vein Distention
KED	Kendrick Extrication Device
KTD	Kendrick Traction Device
LAF	Look, Ask, Feel
LLQ	Left Lower Quadrant
LOC	Level of Consciousness
LPM	Liters per Minute
LT RX	Long-Term Treatment
LUQ	Left Upper Quadrant
MAST	Medical Anti-shock Trousers
MCI	Mass (Multiple) Casualty Incident
MD	Medical Doctor
MDI	Metered Dose Inhaler
MI	Myocardial Infarction
mmHg	Millimeters of Mercury
MMI	Marine Medicine Institute
MMR	Measles, Mumps, and Rubella
MOI	Mechanism of Injury
MVA	Motor Vehicle Accident
NAEMT	National Association of Emergency Medical Technicians
NOI	Nature of Illness
NPA	Nasopharyngeal Airway
NRB	Non-rebreather (oxygen mask)
NREMT	National Registry of Emergency Medical Technicians
NSAID	Non-steroidal Anti-inflammatory Drugs (e.g., ibuprofen)
N/V	Nausea and/or Vomiting
OBGYN	Obstetrics and Gynecology
OPA	Oropharyngeal Airway
OPV	Oral Polio Vaccine
OPQRST	(re: pain) Onset, Palliates/Provokes, Quality, Radiates, Severity, Time
OR	Operating Room
OSS	Oregon Spine Splint
OTC	Over-the-Counter
PAS	Patient Assessment System
PASG	Pneumatic Anti-shock Garment
PCR	Patient Care Report
PERRL	Pupils Equal, Round, Reactive to Light
PNS	Peripheral Nervous System
PO	By Mouth (for administering medications)
PR	By Rectum (for administering medications)
POC	Position of Comfort

POF	Position of Function
PT	Patent
QD	One a Day
QID	Four Times a Day
RBC	Red Blood Cell
RICE	Rest, Ice, Compression, Elevation
RLQ	Right Lower Quadrant
RMSF	Rocky Mountain Spotted Fever
ROM	Range of Motion
RR	Respiratory Rate
RRQ	Rate, Rhythm, Quality
RUQ	Right Upper Quadrant
Rx	Prescription (Treatment)
S/S	Signs and Symptoms
SA Node	Sinoatrial Node
SAR	Search and Rescue
SCTM	Skin, Color, Temperature, Moisure
SHARP	Swollen, Hot, Achy, Red, Pus (signs of infection)
SOAP	Subjective, Objective, Assessment Plan
SOB	Shortness of Breath
SOLO	Stonehearth Open Learning Opportunities
STI	Soft Tissue Injury
TBO	"The Big One" (Heart Attack)
TBSA	Total Body Surface Area (pertaining to burns)
TIA	Transient Ischemic Attack
TID	Three Times a Day
TIL	Traction-In-Line
Tx	Traction
UTI	Urinary Tract Infection
VF	(V-Fib) Ventricular Fibrillation
VS	Vital Signs
VT	(V-Tach) Ventricular Tachycardia
WBC	White Blood Cell
WEMT	Wilderness Emergency Medical Technician
WFR	Wilderness First Responder
WHO	World Health Organization
WMS	Wilderness Medical Society

Prefixes (with examples)

a/an—without; absence of (asystole)

brady—slow (bradycardia)

cardio—having to do with the heart (cardiovascular)

cerebro—having to do with the brain (cerebrospinal)

contra—opposed to (contraindicated)

cyan—blue (cyanosis)

dys—difficult (dyspnea)

epi—above, upon (epidermis)

gastro—having to do with the stomach (gastroenteritis)

glyco—sugar (glycogen)

hepato—having to do with the liver (hepatitis)

hemi—half (hemiplegia)

hemo or **hema**—having to do with the blood (hemoglobin)

hyper—too much (hypertension)

hypo—too little (hypothermia)

intra—inside (intracranial)

myo—muscle (myocardium)

neo—new (neonate)

peri—around (periosteum)

pneumo—air (pneumothorax)

pulmo—lungs (pulmonary)

poly—many, much (polyuria: too much urine)

retro—behind (retroperitoneal)

sub—below, under (subdural)

tachy—rapid (tachycardia)

vaso—having to do with the vessels (vasogenic)

Suffixes (with examples)

algia—pain, painful condition (neuralgia)

ectomy—to remove surgically (appendectomy)

emia—blood (hypoglycemia)

esthesia—sensation (paresthesia)

genic—originating from (neurogenic)

gram—record (electrocardiogram)

ia—state or condition (pneumonia)

ion—process (extraction)

itis—inflammation (arthritis)

ology—science of (osteology)

opia—vision (myopia)

(o) stomy—to make an opening (tracheostomy)

(o) tomy—cutting into (lobotomy)

pathy—disease of (osteopathy)

plegia—paralysis (hemiplegia)

paresis—weakness (hemiparesis)

pnea—breathe, breathing (dyspnea)

GLOSSARY

Abolition — Elimination or stopping of

Abscess — Localized collection of pus

Abrasion — An area of the epidermis and dermis that is scraped

Accessory muscles — Secondary muscles used to assist breathing during respiratory distress—many accessory muscles are located in the neck

Acidosis — An abnormal increase of hydrogen ion concentration in the body that causes the blood pH to fall below normal levels, as in diabetic ketoacidosis

Acute — Characterized by rapid onset, severe symptoms, and a short course

Adrenaline — A hormone released by the body in response to stress—it has many effects on the body including increased heart rate, respiratory rate, and blood pressure (Synonym epinephrine)

Agonal — Very painful—associated with the pain of dying

Alkalosis — Excess of alkali or reductions of acid in the body; common causes include hyperventilation, excessive vomiting/diarrhea

Allergen — A substance that produces a hypersensitive reaction in the body; there are many different kinds of allergens (pollen, various foods, etc.), and the reactions they cause range from insignificant to life-threatening; related terms anaphylaxis, histamine

Alveoli — Extremely small air sacs in the lungs where gas exchange occurs

Ambient — Surrounding—in the context of wilderness emergencies it typically refers to the pure temperature of the environment without taking into account other factors, such as wind

Amniotic sac — (aka "bag of waters") sac of fluid containing the developing fetus

Anaerobic — Living without oxygen—relating to microorganisms that can live and grow without the presence of oxygen

Ana-kit — A kit consisting of epinephrine and antihistamines used to treat someone in anaphylactic shock (aka, "bee-sting kit")

Anaphylaxis — An exaggerated, life-threatening allergic reaction that causes bronchoconstriction and vasodilation

Aneurysm — A ballooned-out area of a blood vessel caused by the weakening of the vessel wall

Angina — A condition marked by intense, suffocating pain; one who suffers angina pectoris usually has severe substernal pain that can radiate to the jaw, arms and abdomen

Anoxia — A deficiency of oxygen

Anterior — Toward the front; on the belly side

Antibody — A specific, protective protein made in response to an antigen; antibodies fight antigens

Antigen — A foreign protein or substance that stimulates the formation of antibodies

Antivenom — An antitoxin specific to an animal or insect venom

Aphasia — Difficulty in speaking and/or understanding speech caused by an injury or disease that affects the speech centers in the brain

Apnea — An absence of breathing

Arrhythmia — Abnormality in the rhythm of the heart

Arteriole — A small artery

Artery — A muscular, thick-walled blood vessel that carries blood away from the heart

Asphyxia — Suffocation

Aspiration — The accidental inhalation of fluid and/or particles into the lungs

Asystole — Absent ventricular contractions resulting in a loss of a detectable balance

Ataxia — Lack of coordination—the inability to coordinate muscles correctly

Atherosclerosis — The thickening and hardening of arteries

Atria — The upper chambers of the heart—the right atrium receives blood from the body; the left atrium receives blood from the lungs

Atrophy — The deterioration or decrease in size of tissue due to lack of use

Aura — A peculiar sensation or warning of an impending attack (e.g., seizure)

Auscultate — To listen through a stethoscope

Avulsion — A soft tissue injury that leaves a flap of skin partially attached to the body

Axillary — Region of the body commonly called the armpit

Bandage — Any material used to hold a dressing in place

Baroreceptor — A sensing mechanism located in the aortic arch and carotid sinus that detects changes in blood pressure

Barotrauma — Physical damage to body tissues caused by a difference in pressure between an air space inside or beside the body and the surrounding fluid—scuba divers sometimes suffer barotrauma as a result of the combination of extreme water pressure and insufficient time spent decompressing

Bifurcate — To divide into two branches

Bleb — Blister

Bounding — Leaping—often used to describe a patient who has an abnormally strong, throbbing pulse

Brachial — Pertaining to the arm—A brachial pulse can be taken between the biceps and triceps muscles of the upper arm

Bradycardia — Slow heart rate, less than 60 beats per minute

Bronchi — The two tubes that the trachea splits into at its lower end

Bronchospasm — A sudden constriction of the bronchial tubes due to involuntary plain muscle in their walls

Bronchus — One of the main branches of the lungs

Cardiac — Pertaining to the heart

Carotid — Either of two main arteries, one on either side of the neck, that supply blood to the head

Cartilage — Tough, relatively elastic tissue that works like bone to support the body; among other places, cartilage is found in the nose, ears, and joints

Cephalic — Pertaining to the head

Cerebral — Pertaining to the brain

Cervical — Pertaining to the neck, as in the cervical vertebrae

Cervix — The neck, or lower part, of the uterus; also, any neck-like structure

Cheyne-Stokes breathing — An abnormal breathing pattern characterized by a series of quick breaths followed by no breaths at all

Chronic — Long, drawn out—used to describe a disease that is not acute, e.g., chronic bronchitis

Coccyx — Pertaining to the lowest part of the spine—the coccyx vertebrae

Colostomy — Establishment of an artificial cutaneous opening into the colon

Compensatory — Stabilizing; serving as a substitute or counterbalance; used to describe the first stage of shock in which the body tries to compensate

Compliance — The act of following another's will; in medical terms, it describes the stiffness of the lungs; as compliance decreases, the lungs become more difficult to artificially ventilate

Concussion — An injury to an organ, especially the brain, caused by violent jarring and followed by a temporary or prolonged loss of function

Conduction — The transfer of heat through one object to another—A person lying directly on cold ground loses heat via conduction

Congenital — Any condition that exists or was acquired before birth

Contraindication — A situation that prohibits the use of a drug or treatment

Contusion — A bruise—an injury that causes hemorrhaging in or beneath the skin without breaking the skin

Convection — The transfer of heat in gas or liquid caused by the circulation of currents; a person standing in the wind loses heat via convection

Coronary — Pertaining to the blood vessels that supply blood to the heart itself

Costal — Pertaining to the ribs

Crackles — Fine or coarse bubbling sounds produced by fluids in the lower airway

Cranial — Pertaining to the skull

Cravat — A piece of material used for bandaging and/or making slings

Crepitus — Grating and crunching of fractured bone ends—crepitus can be felt and heard

Crowning — The stage during childbirth when the presenting part of the baby can be seen at the opening of the vagina

Cyanosis — Bluish coloration of the skin due to lack of oxygen and excess carbon dioxide in the blood

Cardiothoracic — Pertaining to the heart and chest cavity

Carina — Where the trachea splits into the two main branches

Cosmesis — Appearance and shape

Dead space — That portion of inhaled air that does not reach the alveoli and so is not involved in gas exchange

Death, biological — Irreversible brain damage

Death, clinical — The moment that the heart stops

Debridement — Excision of devitalized tissue and foreign matter from a wound

Decompensatory — Characterized by the inability of the heart to maintain adequate blood circulation—describes the second stage of shock in which all body functions fail rapidly

Defibrillate	Use of electric shock to stop ventricular fibrillation
Dementia	General mental deterioration due to organic or psychologic factors
Dependent lividity	A bruising or darkened discoloration on the bottom side of the body, caused by blood leaking from the vasculature after death
Dermis	The inner or middle layer of skin that contains hair follicle roots, sweat glands, nerves, and blood vessels
Diagnosis	Identification of a disease or condition
Diaphoretic (sweating)	Often used to describe patients who are pale, cool and clammy
Diastole	The period of ventricular relaxation when the ventricles rest and refill with blood
Differential diagnosis	A systematic method used to identify unknowns, typically through a process of elimination—used by medical professionals to help make a diagnosis
Dilate	To get wider or larger, to expand
Diplopia	Double vision, seeing two objects when only one is present
Distal	Farther from the heart as a point of reference—the ankle is distal to the knee
Dorsal	Toward the back, posterior
Dressing	Sterile material that is placed directly on a wound
Dyspnea	Difficulty breathing, shortness of breath
Ecchymosis	Discoloration or bluing of the skin
Eclampsia	A condition that occurs during pregnancy and is characterized by high blood pressure and seizures—also called toxemia
Ectopic	Located away from normal position as in an ectopic pregnancy where the embryo develops in a space other than the uterus
Edema	Swelling
Embolism	A solid, liquid, or gaseous mass that circulates in the blood and can potentially block blood vessels
Endotracheal	Within or through the trachea
Epidermis	The outermost layer of skin
Epinephrine	See adrenaline
EpiPen	An auto-injectable means of delivering epinephrine, used to treat someone in anaphylactic shock
Epistaxis	A nosebleed
Evaporation	The changing of a liquid into a gas—sweating works as a cooling mechanism because of the heat transfer that occurs as the moisture on the skin evaporates
Evisceration	An injury that causes organs in the abdomen to protrude from the body
Exacerbate	To make worse, to aggravate
Extension	To stretch out, the act of bringing the distal portion of a joint in continuity with the long axis of the proximal portion—opposite of flexion
Febrile	Characterized by fever
Femoral	Pertaining to the femur or the thigh—the femoral artery delivers blood to the leg
Fibrillation	Disorganized movements of the heart muscle resulting in ineffectual contractions of the heart chambers
Flaccid	Soft, limp
Flail	To wave or swing vigorously as in a flail chest that moves erratically because it is unstable
Flexion	The act of flexing or bending; bending of a joint so as to approximate the parts it connects—opposite of extension
Gastric	Pertaining to the stomach
Glucose	Simple sugar used by the cell for energy
Halogenation	Using one of the chlorine group of elements (iodine or chlorine, specifically) to disinfect water
Hematoma	Swelling filled with blood
Hematopoiesis	The formation of blood
Hyperbaric	A condition of increased pressure
Hemiparesis	Weakness on one side of the body
Hemiplegia	Paralysis of one half of the body
Hemoglobin	A protein that carries oxygen in the blood
Hemorrhage	Bleeding, especially severe bleeding
Hemothorax	Bleeding into the pleural cavity of the lungs
Hernia	Protrusion of any organ into a space where it does not belong
Histamine	A protein released by the body in response to an antigen—histamine can cause inflammation, vasodilation, and bronchoconstriction
Hitch	A fastening loop or knot, often which can be released by pulling against the strain that holds it
Homeostasis	A tendency to constancy and stability in the body, equilibrium
Hydration	The taking in of water

SOLO Wilderness First Responder

Hydrophobia — Literally, a fear of water, one of the signs/symptoms of rabies (rabies is sometimes referred to as hydrophobia)

Hyperglycemia — Abnormally high concentration of sugar in the blood

Hypoglycemia — Abnormally low concentration of sugar in the blood

Hypokalemia — Abnormally low concentrations of potassium in the blood

Hyponatremia — Abnormally low concentration of sodium in the blood

Hypoperfusion — Lack of supply of oxygenated blood to cells (shock)

Hypotension — Low blood pressure systolic <110, diastolic <70

Hypothalamus — A region of the brain that regulates many fundamental body functions, including temperature

Hypovolemia — Abnormally decreased amount of blood and fluids in the body

Hypoxic — Used to describe someone who has a deficiency of oxygen at the cellular level—someone who is hypoxic may be restless, short of breath, confused, and/or lethargic

Ileostomy — Establishment of a passage through which the ileum discharges directly to the outside of the body

Incontinence — The inability to control the elimination of urine or feces

Indications — The circumstances under which a drug or treatment is suited for use

Inebriated — Intoxication, especially from alcohol

Infarction — Death of tissue caused by cutting off the blood supply to that tissue

Inhale — An apparatus for administering pharmacologically active agents by inhalation

Irrigation — The washing out of a cavity or wound with fluid

Insulin — A hormone that helps the body utilize sugar

Integument — Skin

Intravenous — Within or into a vein

Intubation — The placement of a tube into the trachea or esophagus

Ischemia — Lack of oxygen in a tissue as a result of lack of blood-flow to that tissue

Jugular — Pertaining to the throat or neck as in the jugular veins that carry blood away from the head

Ketoacidosis — A condition in which the body metabolizes fat and produces too many ketones and acids in the blood causing thirst, urination, nausea, vomiting, and sometimes coma

Kussmaul's breathing — Deep, heavy breathing that attempts to blow off body wastes—Kussmaul's breathing is characteristic of a diabetic in ketoacidosis

Labored — Requiring a lot of effort, strained

Laceration — A cut or tear in the skin—lacerations vary in dimension and severity depending upon their location and whether they have gone through any major blood vessels

Laryngospasm — Convulsive involuntary muscular contraction of the larynx, usually accompanied by spasmodic closure of the glottis

Larynx — Voice box, a structure made of cartilage and muscles that is located between the pharynx and the trachea

Lateral — Of or towards the side, away from the midline of the body

Lethargic — Extreme sleepiness combined with apathy and sluggish behavior

Ligament — Fibrous tissue that connects bones to other bones

Lumbar — Pertaining to the lower back as in the lumbar vertebrae

Lymph — Colorless fluid that circulates in the lymphatic system and helps remove bacteria and certain proteins from cells

Lysis — Disintegration of membranes of cells or bacteria

Mania — An emotional disorder characterized by euphoria, increased psychomotor activity, rapid speech, flight of ideas, decreased need for sleep, distractibility, grandiosity, and poor judgment—usually occurs in bipolar disorder

Meconium — Fetal intestinal content that stain the amniotic fluid green or black

Medial — Toward the midline of the body

Mediastinum — The space between the lungs

Meninges — Highly vascular membranes that separate the brain from the skull

Metabolism — The sum of the chemical changes occurring in tissue

Midline — Imaginary line running vertically from the nose through the belly button thus splitting the body in half

Myocardial — Pertaining to the muscular of the heart (myo = muscle)

Narcosis — Unconscious state caused by narcotics or other toxic substances in the body

Necrosis — Death of tissue, usually caused by lack of blood supply

Nematocyst — A stinging cell of coelenterates consisting of a poison sac and a coiled barbed stinger capable of being ejected and penetrating the skin of an animal on contact—of considerable consequence in large jellyfish and Portuguese man-of-war, whose large numbers of these stinging cells can cause great pain and even death

Neurogenic — Originating in or pertaining to the nervous system

Obligate — Characterized by the ability to survive only in a particular set of environmental conditions

Occlusion — Obstruction, blockage—a blood clot can cause the occlusion of a vessel

Palliate — To make less severe or intense, to mitigate, to relieve

Pallor — Extreme or unnatural paleness

Palpate — To examine or explore by touching

Palpitate — To move with a tremulous motion, to tremble, shake, or quiver

Paradoxical — Contradictory, when used to describe respirations, paradoxical refers to the collapse of the chest upon inhalation (as opposed to the expected chest rise)

Paresis — Slight paralysis or weakness

Paresthesia — A numbness or pins-and-needles sensation that indicates some disturbance in nerve function

Parietal — Pertaining to a wall

Patent — Not blocked, open; expanded

Pathogen — An agent that causes a disease

Pedal — Pertaining to the foot

Perfusion — The flow of blood through tissue such that the tissue has an adequate supply of oxygen and nutrients

Pericardium — The thin sac surrounding the heart

Peripheral — Pertaining to an outside boundary or outer edge—the peripheral nervous system consists of all the nerves that extend from the brain and spinal cord

Pertinent — Relevant, having logical, precise relevance to the matter at hand

Pharynx — The portion of the airway between the nasal cavity and the larynx—The pharynx includes the nasopharynx, oropharynx and laryngopharynx

Pituitary — A gland located in the brain and responsible for regulating all other glands

Pleura — Membranes that line the outer surface of the lungs, the inner surface of the chest wall, and the thoracic surface of the diaphragm

Pneumothorax — Air trapped in the pleural space that can cause the underlying lung to collapse

Polydipsia — Excessive thirst that is relatively chronic

Polyphagia — Excessive eating

Polyuria — Excessive excretion of urine

Posterior — On the back or dorsal side

Postictal — Pertaining to the period after the convulsive state of a seizure

Priapism — Sustained erection of the penis, sometimes associated with spinal cord injury

Primigravida — A woman in her first pregnancy

Prognosis — Probable outlook for recovery

Prone — Lying flat with the face downward

Prophylactic — Preventative—e.g., taking one aspirin a day as a prophylactic measure

Proteinuria — The presence of urinary protein

Proximal — Closer to the heart as a point of reference—the knee is proximal to the ankle

Psychogenic — Arising from the mind, as opposed to the body

Pulmonary — Pertaining to the lungs

Purulence — The condition of containing or forming pus

Radial — Pertaining to the wrist—a radial pulse can be taken at the wrist

Radiation — Emission of energy in rays or waves—a campfire radiates heat

Rales — Fine breath sounds that represent the opening of collapsed alveoli—the sound can be simulated by rubbing hair between the fingers

Renal — Pertaining to the kidneys

Rigor — A shaking chill

Rigor mortis — The stiffening of the body after death

Sacrum — Pertaining to the lower spine as in the sacral vertebrae

Sepsis — Infection, contamination

Septum — A dividing wall that usually separates two cavities

Shock — Inadequate tissue perfusion caused by a number of conditions including but not limited to heart failure, nerve failure, and loss of blood volume

Sign — An indication of injury or illness that the examiner observes

Sling — A securing device that runs around the arm and the back of the neck such that it immobilizes the arm

Splint — A device that supplies stabilization and immobilization to an unstable body part

Sprain — An injury in which a ligament is stretched or torn

Sputum	Expectorated (coughed-up) matter, especially mucous associated with lung diseases
Strain	The over-stretching of a muscle or the injury of a muscle, often from overuse
Stridor	A harsh, high-pitched sound associated with severe upper airway obstruction
Subcutaneous	Underneath the skin
Sublingual	Beneath the tongue
Superficial	On the surface
Supine	Lying flat with the face upwards
Swathe	Something tied around the body to enhance the immobilization of a part
Symptom	An indication of illness or injury that is not observable and must be related by the patient
Syncope	A brief lapse in consciousness
Systemic	Throughout the entire body
Systole	Period during which the ventricles contract and are active
Tachycardia	Rapid heart rate, over 100 beats per minute
Tachypnea	Increased rate of respirations
Tendon	A tough band of fibrous connective tissue that attaches to muscle to bone
Thoracic	Pertaining to the thorax, as in the thoracic vertebrae
Thready	Weak and shallow, as in a thready pulse
Thrombolysis	The process of dissolving blood clots
Tidal volume	The volume of one breath
Tonic-clonic	Tonic—state of continuous muscular contraction; Clonic—series of intermittent muscular contraction and relaxation
Tracheal shift	Movement of the trachea away from midline
Traction	The act of drawing or pulling, a pulling or dragging force exerted on a limb in a distal direction
Urticaria	Hives
Vasoconstriction	The narrowing of blood vessels
Vasodilation	The widening of blood vessels
Vector	A carrier, often an invertebrate animal (tick, mite, mosquito, fly, etc.) capable of transmitting an infectious agent among vertebrates, transmitting a pathogen from a reservoir to a host
Vein	A blood vessel that carries blood toward the heart
Ventral	Toward the front, anterior
Ventricle	A thick-walled lower chamber of the heart that receives blood from the atrium and pumps it out to the lungs and body
Vertigo	A sensation of irregular or whirling motion, either of oneself or of external objects, imprecisely used as a general term to describe dizziness
Visceral	Pertaining to the organs of the chest or abdomen

Frank Hubbell worked as a ski patrol director, rescue squad captain, and on the mountain rescue service before graduating from medical school. He is the past president of the American Alpine Club medical committee and past vice president of the European UIAA (International Union of Alpine Associations) Medical Commission.

Dr. Hubbell currently serves as the medical director for NH Region V EMS Council and is a 28-year representative on the NH EMS Medical Control Board and NH EMS Coordinating Board. He is a founding partner of the Saco River Medical Group in Conway and Glen, New Hampshire, and is the Director of the Conway Walk-In-Care and Spine Center.

Dr Hubbell along with his wife, Lee Frizzell, founded Stonehearth Open Learning Opportunities (SOLO) in 1976. The school teaches wilderness and emergency medicine and the home campus is in Conway New Hampshire. This book is one of many Dr. Hubbell has written for use in SOLO courses.

www.ingramcontent.com/pod-product-compliance
Lightning Source LLC
Chambersburg PA
CBHW041415100425
24807CB00001B/2